BY THE EDITORS OF *CONSUMER GUIDE*®

WOMEN'S
HOME REMEDIES
HEALTH GUIDE

BOBBIE HASSELBRING
BRIANNA L. POLITZER

CONSULTANTS:

MICHELLE HARRISON, M.D.
JOHN H. RENNER, M.D.,
CONSUMER HEALTH
INFORMATION RESEARCH INSTITUTE

PUBLICATIONS INTERNATIONAL, LTD.

CONSULTANTS

Dr. Michelle Harrison is internationally known in the area of women's health. She is a family physician and psychiatrist who has written *Self-Help for Premenstrual Syndrome* and numerous articles in the popular and academic press. Dr. Harrison was founder and President of a New York chapter of the American Medical Women's Association and has served as vice president of one of its branches.

Dr. John H. Renner is the president and medical director of the Consumer Health Information Research Institute (CHIRI), a nonprofit organization dedicated to providing reliable and accurate patient health education for preventive care, wellness, and self-help. Dr. Renner also serves as a member of the Board of Directors of the National Council Against Health Fraud and as Clinical Professor of Family Practice at the University of Missouri.

WRITERS

Bobbie Hasselbring is the former editor of *Medical Self-Care Magazine* and has authored five books on health and psychology, including portions of *The Home Remedies Handbook*. She currently writes a column for the *Oregonian* and has become a nationally recognized health writer. The American Heart Association awarded her its 1991 Award for Media Excellence.

Brianna L. Politzer is a freelance writer specializing in health, medicine, and nutrition. She has worked as a newspaper reporter and an editor and has contributed to many health publications, including *Medical Tribune News Service, American Health, AIDS-Patient Care,* and *The Home Remedies Handbook*.

OTHER CONTRIBUTING WRITERS

Sue Berkman, Linda J. Brown, Jenny Hart Danowski, Susan G. Hauser, Susan Nielsen, and Diana Reese.

ILLUSTRATIONS
Lane Gregory

COVER PHOTO
Chas Studio, Atlanta Georgia

Copyright ® 1994 Publications International, Ltd. All rights reserved. This book may not be reproduced or quoted in whole or in part by mimeograph or any other printed or electronic means, or for presentation on radio, television, videotape, or film without written permission from:

Louis Weber, C.E.O.
Publications International, Ltd.
7373 North Cicero Avenue
Lincolnwood, Illinois 60646

Permission is never granted for commercial purposes.

Manufactured in U.S.A.

8 7 6 5 4 3 2 1

ISBN 0-7853-0185-2

●Contents

●Contents

FROM ACNE TO MENSTRUAL CRAMPS TO yeast infections, *Women's Home Remedies Health Guide* addresses the common health problems that women often face.

Each chapter starts out with basic information about a health problem, its causes and symptoms, and what it means to you as a woman. Tips for home treatment and, wherever possible, strategies for prevention follow.

The remedies described in this book are all simple, safe, commonsense steps you can take to care for yourself. The idea behind all the remedies and prevention strategies is to help you get healthy and stay healthy, as well as to save you some of the time and money you spend on seeking and receiving medical care for common health problems.

That said, however, keep in mind that your doctor should be your principal health-care provider. Some problems cannot be treated without the help of a physician. For others, you should see a physician if your symptoms persist beyond a certain period of time. So, as you read, remember these points:

• Pay attention to the warnings given with some of the treatments. If you are advised to consult your doctor about a certain remedy, pick up the phone and give her a call. If you have certain medical conditions, such as high blood pressure, avoid remedies that are not recommended for you. Pregnant and breast-feeding women need to be especially careful and should not take any medications, even those available over the counter, without first checking with a doctor.

• Be very cautious when deciding whether you have the health problem profiled in this book. Self-diagnosis is often unreliable. If you have never had this particular problem before or if, for any reason, you are not sure you have it now, check with your doctor before trying any home-care remedies.

• Don't try every treatment suggestion simultaneously. Read the entire profile on your condition and decide which remedies seem the most appropriate for you. If one remedy does not work, consider trying another one. Use your common sense in applying the information in this book.

• Remember that your doctor is your health-care partner. Throughout this book, you will frequently be advised to consult your physician. This is because your primary-care physician knows you best and will know if any other conditions you may have are likely to impair the effectiveness of a remedy or treatment. In addition, your doctor should be made aware of any persistent or chronic health problems you may be having. You and your doctor share the responsibility of keeping you well. Keeping her informed of what's going on is part of your end of the deal.

Above all, keep in mind that when it comes to staying well, no book can replace living a healthful lifestyle and using your common sense. *Women's Home Remedies Health Guide* provides you with the information you need to help you cope with individual health problems and make good decisions about your health in general. But exercising, eating a healthful diet, getting regular checkups, and being well informed about health matters are crucial steps only you can take to ensure that you stay as well as you can.

●Acne

How to Battle

Unsightly

Blemishes

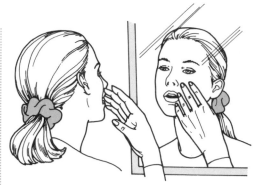

If you've turned to this page, you probably weren't one of those clear-skinned girls who survived high school without ever having to stare at a single pimple in the mirror. Then again, most of us weren't. Acne is one of the curses of adolescence that we're only too happy to say goodbye to. Unfortunately, this unattractive skin condition follows some of us long into adulthood and middle age.

Acne is so common that more than 80 percent of the population suffers from it at least once or twice in a lifetime. Because the male hormone testosterone plays a role in its development, boys are more likely than girls to have severe acne during adolescence. In contrast, women are much more likely than men to have acne in their 20s, 30s, and 40s. Women are also more likely to visit a dermatologist for treatment.

Acne can occur anywhere on the body but appears most frequently on the face, neck, back, chest, and shoulders. In severe cases, there may be pus-filled sacs that break open and discharge fluid. If untreated, severe acne can leave permanent scarring.

Symptoms

Most of us think of pimples when we think of acne. We don't bother dividing up the different annoying spots we see on our face. But dermatologists have broken pimples down into the following categories:

Comedones: Ducts that are plugged up with oil, dead skin cells, and bacteria.

Whiteheads: Closed comedones with skin covering the top. These appear as tiny, white bumps.

Blackheads: Open comedones, or comedones that do not have skin covering them. These appear black, not because they contain dirt, as many people believe, but because the material inside the duct has been exposed to oxygen.

Papules: Ruptured comedones in which there is inflammation and secondary infection. These look like small, hard, red bumps.

Pustules: Ruptured comedones in which there is inflammation and secondary infection. However, in contrast to the papule, the pustule has more pus near the surface, giving it a yellowish center.

Nodules: Sometimes called cysts, these ruptured comedones are generally larger, deeper, and more painful than pustules and are more likely to result in scarring. Nodules characterize the most severe form of acne.

If you're over 40 and have suddenly developed severe acne, you may be suffering from acne rosacea, which is a different disease from acne vulgaris, the medical name for garden-variety acne.

How can you tell the difference? Acne rosacea is characterized by redness, inflammation (swelling), and dilated blood vessels. Further clues: You don't have any blackheads, the acne is located mainly on the central part of your face (your nose and cheeks), and you have a lot of pustules (pus-containing pimples). You're more likely to suffer from this type of acne if you're light-skinned.

Unfortunately, there's not much you can do on your own for acne rosacea, although you should be especially careful to avoid the sun, since sun exposure can worsen the condition. Acne rosacea can, however, be treated by a dermatologist.

CAUSES

The first thing to know is that those annoying pimples aren't your fault. You couldn't have prevented them from popping up, even if you had washed your face a thousand times a day. In fact, the tendency to develop acne is hereditary.

Experts differ in their opinions on what causes acne, but they generally agree that it often results from the hormonal changes that accompany puberty. At this time, increasing amounts of certain hormones—particularly the male hormone testosterone—stimulate the skin's oil glands. Most of the excess oil leaves the skin through the hair follicles. Sometimes, however, the follicles become clogged with oil, bacteria, and dead skin cells, causing the lumps that are the first sign of acne.

Although the changes accompanying adolescence are the most notorious cause of acne, many factors in an adult's life can bring on breakouts, as well. In women, hormonal changes resulting from pregnancy, menstruation, and the use of birth control pills can all cause fluctuations in acne. In some women, low-dose oral contraceptives improve acne; in others, they make it worse. If you have acne along with menstrual irregularities, you may want to see a physician to determine whether abnormal hormone levels are to blame.

Dermatologists agree that high levels of stress can affect hormone levels, as well. While a tough week probably won't cause acne in a woman who has never suffered from it, it can worsen a mild case.

Other common causes of acne include wearing heavy, oily makeup; occupational exposure to grease, such as standing over a deep-fat fryer as a fry cook or working as a mechanic; and taking certain drugs (such as Dilantin, which is used in the treatment of epilepsy).

The role of diet in the development of acne is unclear. Experts do know that diet alone does not cause or cure the skin condition. However, some cases of acne appear to improve after eliminating certain foods, particularly chocolate and other fatty foods.

AT-HOME TREATMENT

No matter what's causing your acne, there are several steps you can take to help clear up your skin and get it blemish-free.

Don't mess with it. In other words, don't pick, press, rub, or otherwise manipulate those pimples. If you do, you will risk spreading the bacteria and increasing the chances for scarring. The oil plug at the top of a whitehead is like a balloon. You can pop it, but below the surface, the sebum, bacteria,

WARNING!

Avoid most prescription and over-the-counter acne treatments when:
- **You are pregnant.**
- **You are breast-feeding.**
- **You are allergic to any of the ingredients contained in the preparation.**
- **You have a special medical condition requiring that you avoid certain drugs.**

If any of these conditions applies to you, consult your doctor for the safest and most appropriate way to handle your acne.

and skin cells may leak into the surrounding tissue, causing even worse inflammation.

Try benzoyl peroxide. A number of over-the-counter products contain benzoyl peroxide, which helps break up the plug of dead skin cells, bacteria, and oil in pores and cuts down on the bacteria as well. Start with the lowest concentration of benzoyl peroxide and work your way up, especially if you have sensitive skin, because the higher the concentration, the more irritating it may be. Use it once or twice a day. If your skin does become dry and sore, applying a mild, oil-free moisturizer may help.

Browse the supermarket shelves. Other over-the-counter acne products contain sulfur or resorcinol, which help unplug oil glands by irritating the skin. These may be helpful, although most dermatologists believe that benzoyl peroxide is the most effective over-the-counter ingredient for acne.

Hit it before it has a chance. While it is useful to apply benzoyl peroxide and other acne medications to existing pimples, it is more effective to cover the whole acne-prone area with the treatment. That may include your entire face (avoiding the lips and eyes), back, and chest.

Treat your face with tender loving care. Many people with acne think it's a good idea for them to use hot water, a washcloth, and a highly drying soap to wash their acne away. However, those stubborn pimples aren't likely to let you off the hook that easily. Although bacteria does play a role in acne's development, a lack of cleanliness is not a cause of breakouts. Washing removes oils from the surface of the skin, not from within the plugged ducts. And, since adults can certainly suffer from both acne and dry skin, a too-aggressive quest for cleanliness may very well leave you with skin that is far more irritated than it was when you began your scrubbing regimen.

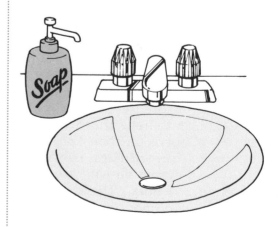

Use tried-and-true washing techniques. Replace your harsh soap with a mild, doctor-recommended cleansing bar, such as Dove Unscented, Tone, Basis, or Neutrogena. Rub lightly with your fingertips and warm water. Do not use a washcloth. If your skin is oily, use a soap with benzoyl peroxide for its drying properties. No more than once or twice a day should be sufficient.

Say "no thanks" to exfoliation. The word exfoliation refers to removing the top layer of dead skin cells. Some dermatologists recommend using a rough washcloth or specially designed product to do just that. However, your skin is already irritated if you have acne. Don't use brushes, rough sponges, cleansers with granules or walnut hulls, or any other product of that nature on delicate facial skin. For the back and chest areas where the skin is less sensitive, you can try one of the commercially available acne scrub pads, along with a soap that contains benzoyl peroxide.

Pass on the oily products for hair and skin. That includes oily pomades on your hair, heavy oil-based moisturizers, and even oily cleansers. Many women believe that by using cold cream on their face they will avoid wrinkles. (Dry skin doesn't bring on wrinkles—sun exposure does.) These types of cleansers may just aggravate acne. Look for oil-free makeup.

If you're not sure—and some labels can be misleading—set the bottle of makeup on the counter. If it separates into water and powder, it's water-based. If it doesn't, it contains oil. Dermatologists also recommend choosing powder blushes and loose powders over oil-containing alternatives. Lipstick and eye makeup that contain oil are not risky, since the areas to which these products are applied are not oily.

Avoid salon facials. Doctors warn that most people who give salon facials aren't trained to

16 STEPS TO CLEARER SKIN

- Don't pick, prod, or rub your pimples.
- Experiment with products containing benzoyl peroxide.
- Try over-the-counter products containing sulfur or resorcinol.
- Don't just apply products to existing pimples; cover all acne-prone areas.
- Don't try to dry skin out by washing with harsh soaps and hot water.
- Use gentle cleansing products.
- Don't irritate facial skin further by scrubbing with a washcloth, brush, sponge, or exfoliating cream.
- Avoid oily hair treatments, facial moisturizers, and cleansers.
- Use only oil-free makeup, powder blushes, and loose powders.
- Don't go to the salon for a facial.
- Avoid touching your face.
- Absorb excess oil with commercially available powdered papers.
- Don't try to dry out your skin by exposing it to the sun.
- Avoid salt, food supplements, and vitamins that contain high levels of iodine.
- Keep your hair clean.
- Try hairstyles that keep your locks out of contact with your face.

treat acne-prone skin properly. They may end up doing more harm than good. Some dermatologists will do medical facials during patient visits. These are the only types you should have.

Take up a new pensive look. Don't rest your chin in your hands or otherwise touch your face. People who do a lot of telephone work often get chin-line acne from the constant contact with their hands and the phone. The contact can also cause trauma to acne, just like picking the pimples does. Tight sweatbands and chin straps from sports equipment can have the same effect.

Get rid of the oil. Some cosmetic companies make a paper product that can be pressed onto the skin to soak up oil that often forms on acne-prone skin. These products are easy to use and may reduce shine. Unfortunately, this won't help the acne go away, but it may help you feel a bit better.

Use sunscreen. At one time, sun exposure was believed to help acne. However, too much sun can lead to skin cancer and premature aging, creating risks that outweigh the benefits. Dermatologists suggest protecting skin with a sunscreen that has a sun protection factor (SPF) of 15 or higher. Look for one that's oil-free or noncomedogenic. Unfortunately, many waterproof products are too likely to clog oil glands to use on the face, so you'll have to be diligent about reapplying the sunscreen often.

Don't overdo iodine. This piece of advice is still somewhat controversial, but some doctors believe that high levels of iodine, found in some multiple vitamins, food supplements like kelp, and iodized salt, may encourage acne.

Shampoo regularly. Oily hair, particularly if it touches the face, can sometimes bring on or aggravate breakouts. Wash your hair frequently enough to keep the oil to a minimum.

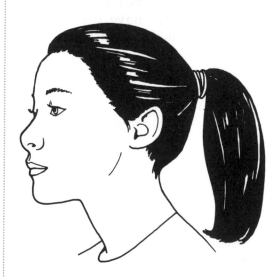

Tie your hair back. Minimize your hair's contact with your face by tying it into a ponytail or a braid. A headband that doesn't touch the face may also be helpful.

AT THE DOCTOR'S

With today's drugs, there's no reason for anyone to put up with serious or persistent acne. While acne doesn't pose a threat to physical health, it can affect your self-esteem and your confidence, prompting you to withdraw from social and romantic situations. These psychological effects are especially apparent in teenagers who suffer from the skin condition.

The good news is, you're never too young or too old to seek medical treatment for acne. When should you see a dermatologist for your condition? Most dermatologists answer that by saying, "When it bothers you." Severity is in the eye of the beholder in this case.

It's probably time to see a dermatologist if you have used benzoyl peroxide products for six to eight weeks and still have problems, if you have pustules larger than a match head, if you have nodules the size of the end of your little finger, or if you have any scarring from your acne. However, it's much better to see a dermatologist before any scarring occurs.

Today's arsenal of treatments includes combinations of topical and oral antibiotics and a class of medications called retinoids. It's the latter that have revolutionized acne treatment. Tretinoin (Retin-A) is applied to the skin, while isotretinoin (Accutane) is taken orally. Pregnant women should not take isotretinoin; it has been shown to cause miscarriage and birth defects. Isotretinoin is considered a last-ditch treatment, but it's especially effective for cystic acne. One course of this treatment generally is enough.

While these treatments can be very effective, all have their own class of side effects. The topical medications, such as Retin-A and erythromycin gel, can dry or irritate

WHEN TO SEE A DERMATOLOGIST

It's time to seek medical treatment when:
- **Your acne is severe enough to cause you bother or embarrassment.**
- **You have used benzoyl peroxide products for six to eight weeks and still have problems.**
- **You have pustules (pimples containing pus) larger than a match head.**
- **You have nodules (painful cysts characterizing the most severe kind of acne) the size of the end of your little finger.**
- **Your acne has caused scarring.**

skin. Oral antibiotics are notorious for causing yeast infections and stomach upset. Accutane can cause skin to dry out and sport a deep red tone for the duration of treatment. Your doctor will be able to advise you on the course of treatment that is most appropriate for you.

Some dermatologists also use special treatments, such as medical facials or ultraviolet lamps. Others may recommend that you use certain skin products. Be wary, however, of any dermatologist who insists that you purchase special skin cleansers from his or her office. Most reputable doctors will not sell their own products and if they do, won't insist that you buy them.

Sources: Vincent A. DeLeo, M.D., Assistant Professor of Dermatology, Columbia-Presbyterian Medical Center, New York, New York. **Alan D. Klein, M.D.,** Spokesperson, American Academy of Dermatology; Teaching Staff, Ventura County Medical Center, Ventura, California. **Albert M. Kligman, M.D., Ph.D.,** Emeritus Professor of Dermatology, University of Pennsylvania School of Medicine, Philadelphia, Pennsylvania. **Alan N. Moshell, M.D.,** Director, Skin Disease Program, National Institute of Arthritis and Musculoskeletal and Skin Diseases, National Institutes of Health, Bethesda, Maryland.

○ALLERGIES

How to

Fend Off

an Attack

MAYBE IT WAS YOUR FRIEND'S CAT that got your goat. But, then again, maybe it's just that spring has sprung and an acacia tree is in full bloom right outside your window. Whatever the culprit, you've been sneezing for hours and tears are running down your cheeks from your itchy eyes. You're in the midst of a full-scale allergy attack.

Millions of people all over the world suffer from allergies. For people with common hay fever and allergies, symptoms may range from a continuous, annoying postnasal drip to a full-scale, coughing-sneezing-itchy-eyed allergy attack. For other allergy sufferers, such as those with allergic asthma or an allergy to bee stings, an allergy attack can actually be fatal.

There are four categories of allergens (substances that cause allergic reactions): inhalants, contactants, ingestants, and injectants. Inhalant allergens are those that are breathed in, including such items as dust, molds, pollen, feathers, and animal dander. Contactant allergens are those that touch the skin, including substances such as poison ivy, poison oak, cosmetics, detergents, fabrics, and dyes. Ingestant allergens are those that are swallowed, such as foods and medications. Some common ingestant allergens include milk, eggs, shellfish, fish, peanuts, chocolate, strawberries, tomatoes, and citrus fruits. Injectant allergens are substances that penetrate the skin, such as insect venom and injected drugs.

SYMPTOMS

Common allergy symptoms can include watery eyes, a runny nose, itching or inflamed skin, hives, and a swollen mouth or throat. Some allergic reactions may be accompanied by headaches, sinus stuffiness, a reduced sense of taste or smell, or breathing difficulties.

An extremely severe allergic reaction, called anaphylactic shock, is characterized by sudden breathing difficulties (caused by swelling of the throat and larynx and narrowing of the bronchial tubes in the lungs), itching skin, hives, and the collapse of the blood vessels. Other symptoms include vomiting, diarrhea, cramps, low blood pressure, and unconsciousness. If left untreated, this type of allergic reaction may be fatal. If you think that you or someone near you may be having an anaphylactic reaction, call for help immediately.

How can you tell whether you have an allergy? Only an allergist can give you a medical diagnosis, but your symptoms will usually be a pretty good indication. There is one exception, however: Many people believe that if they have an adverse reaction to a food, such as congestion after eating dairy products or a headache after eating sugar, they have an allergy to that food. Often, they are incorrect. Allergists stress that there is a big difference between having a food sensitivity and having a food allergy. The distinction is important, since a real food allergy can be fatal and a food sensitivity cannot be.

If you are truly allergic to a food, the reaction will be almost immediate, occurring from within a few minutes to two hours after you eat it. The most common symptoms are hives, diffuse swelling around the eyes and mouth, and abdominal cramps. A less common reaction is anaphylactic shock with difficulty breathing. In severe cases, extremely low blood pressure, dizziness, or loss of consciousness may result. In these instances, call for emergency medical assistance.

CAUSES

No one knows why allergies develop in response to seemingly benign substances, such as milk or dust. However, doctors do know that an allergy can appear, disappear, or reappear at any time and at any age. They also know that the tendency to be allergic to certain substances runs in families.

The immune system's job is to build up antibodies to protect the body against foreign substances. However, in the case of an allergy, these antibodies overreact against the substance, producing chemicals called histamines. These histamines are what cause the symptoms associated with the allergy attack.

Although an allergic reaction may develop the first time a person is exposed to an allergen, it usually takes time for the body to develop such a sensitivity.

AT-HOME TREATMENT

In many cases, it is difficult to differentiate between allergy symptoms and the symptoms of other disorders and illnesses, such as a cold, a deformity of the nose, or a food intolerance. For this reason, many doctors suggest that allergies be properly diagnosed by a board-certified allergist (a medical doctor who treats allergies) to avoid the self-administration of inappropriate medications or other remedies. Also, many allergy sufferers can benefit from today's wide range of available treatments, such as new prescription antihistamines that don't cause drowsiness, nasal corticosteroids, and allergy injections that can provide immunity to a specific allergen. If you don't go to the doctor, you may be missing out on a treatment that could be of great help to you.

It's probably time to see an allergist if your allergies are causing you to cough, wheeze, or have trouble breathing. These symptoms may be caused by allergic asthma, which must be supervised by a doctor. Allergic asthma is often treated with inhalers and other drugs. Self-treatment may be dangerous.

However, many mild allergies, such as seasonal hay fever or an allergy to cats, can be treated with a combination of properly used, over-the-counter antihistamines and a wide range of strategies to reduce or eliminate your exposure to particularly annoying allergens.

The following tips are designed to help reduce the discomfort caused by the most common allergies. They may be used in combination with an allergist's treatment or, if your allergies are mild, by themselves.

Put the cat out. Sometimes, the best way to reduce allergy discomfort is to avoid exposure to the allergen as much as possible. For example, if you are allergic to cats, avoid visiting the homes of friends who own them. If you must be around a cat, make the visit as short as possible and avoid touching the animal or sitting in the cat's favorite chair.

Rinse it away. If your eyes are itchy and irritated and you have no access to allergy medicine, rinsing your eyes with cool, clean water may help to soothe them somewhat. Be sure to use only clean water from the tap. Although it is not as effective as an antihistamine, this remedy certainly can't do any damage and may give you some relief until you can get your medicine.

---

23 ALLERGY-TREATMENT TIPS

- Reduce or eliminate your exposure to substances that cause you problems.
- Flush itchy, irritated eyes with cool water.
- Try holding a warm, wet washcloth on your forehead to relieve painful sinus congestion.
- Use saline solution to soothe a dry nose and to remove irritants that become lodged in nasal passages.
- Wash your hair to remove traces of pollen that collected while you were outside.
- Take a hot shower to wash off pollen residues.
- Wear sunglasses or goggles when you are outside to shield your eyes from airborne allergens.
- Keep windows and doors shut during allergy season.
- Wear a surgical mask when exercising outdoors.
- Don't allow smoking in your home.
- Reduce your time outside during pollen season.
- Use a filter on the exhaust port of your canister vacuum.
- Invest in an industrial-strength vacuuming system.
- Avoid feather dusters; dust only with a damp cloth.
- Have someone else mow the lawn.
- Dehumidify your house with an air conditioner or dehumidifier.
- Don't burn household or construction refuse.
- Avoid wood smoke.
- Don't "choke down" a wood stove.
- Bathe your pet every other week.
- Double-rinse your laundry.
- When planning a vacation or business trip, call ahead to find a hotel that will be easy on your allergies: second floor or higher, no pets allowed.
- Bring your own vinyl- or plastic-encased pillow with you on trips.

Try a warm soak. If sinus passages feel congested and painful, a washcloth soaked in warm water may make things flow a little more easily. Place the washcloth over the nose and upper-cheek area and relax for a few minutes.

Flush it out. Irrigating the nose with saline solution may help soothe upper-respiratory allergies by removing irritants that become lodged in the nose, causing inflammation. The solution may also remove some of the inflammatory cells themselves.

Leave no trace. If you've spent long hours outdoors during the pollen season, wash your hair after you come inside to remove traces of pollen. The sticky stuff tends to collect on the hair, making it more likely to fall into your eyes.

Slip into the shower. If you wake up in the middle of the night with a coughing, sneezing allergy attack, a hot shower may wash off any pollen residues that have collected on your body throughout the day. The warm water will also relax you and may even help you go back to sleep.

Shield your eyes. On a windy day in pollen season, a pair of sunglasses may help shield your eyes from airborne allergens. For extra protection, try a pair of sunglasses with side shields or even a pair of goggles.

Stay inside. Some allergists believe that air pollution may cause or augment allergies. They recommend being outside as little as possible on smoggy days or wearing a surgical mask, especially while exercising outside. The mask won't remove everything, but it will help.

Put up a smoke screen. Since tobacco smoke is a notorious irritant that can cause or aggravate respiratory allergies, try banning smoking from your home or confining it to the garage or porch.

Close the windows. The majority of us, unless we work outdoors, spend most of our time inside. During pollen season, this can be a terrific advantage for hayfever sufferers. Keep pollen out by keeping doors and windows closed. Remember: For hayfever sufferers during pollen season, there is really no such thing as fresh air. Air purifiers may help eliminate indoor pollen, but they also tend to stir up dust.

Invest in a vacuum filter. If your vacuum cleaner allows small particles of dust to be blown back into the air as you vacuum, you're recycling the allergy factors right back into your home. A filter placed on the exhaust port of your canister vacuum may help. (Uprights don't usually have an exhaust port). If dust really bothers you and you've got the money, you can invest in an industrial-strength vacuuming system. Some allergists recommend a brand called Nilfisk, which has an excellent filtering system and which retails for about

$500. To find out where you can purchase filters or special vacuums, talk to your allergist or write to the Asthma and Allergy Foundation of America, Department CG, 1125 15th Street NW, Suite 502, Washington, D.C. 20005.

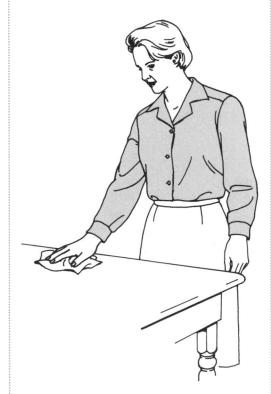

Contain the dust. Dusting at least once a week is important. However, if it is done improperly, dusting may actually aggravate respiratory allergies. For example, feather dusters tend to spread dust around, rather than containing it, and dusting sprays may give off odors that can worsen allergies. The best dusting tool is a damp cloth.

Delegate the dusting. If dusting aggravates your allergies, don't do it. Instead, ask a spouse or family member to do the dirty work or hire a housekeeper, if possible. Then stay out of the house for a few hours while it is being dusted.

Dry out. Dust mites (microscopic insects that are usually the allergy culprits in dust) grow very well in humid areas. To keep the moisture level down, you can invest in a dehumidifier or use the air conditioner, which works equally well. A dehumidifier can also help prevent mold, another allergen, from growing. When cooking or showering, use the exhaust fan—another way to help keep humidity down.

Throw out the trash. Although it is common to burn household and construction refuse, this may not be such a wise idea for allergy sufferers. Wood that is treated with heavy metals or other chemical-laden materials can bring on an allergy attack. It's best to take this refuse down to the local dump. If you must burn it, your best bet is to stay away from the fireplace when it's in use.

Don't light a fire. Many people with respiratory allergies find that wood smoke poses a particular problem. With wood stoves, the biggest problem is "choking down" the stove, or decreasing the amount of oxygen in order to cool down the fire. Choking down throws irritating toxins into the air and can aggravate allergies.

Pay a local high-school kid to mow your lawn. During pollen season, a grass-allergic person is

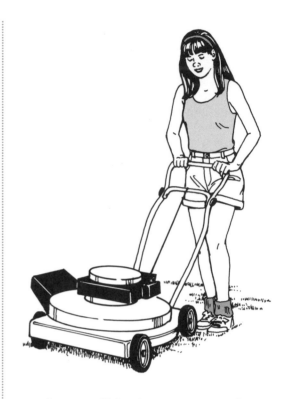

better off letting someone else mow the lawn. Find out when the pollination season in your area is, and delegate the mowing during that time.

Hose down the cat. A little-known trick for cat or dog owners who are allergic to fur: Bathe your pet frequently. There is strong evidence that simply bathing animals in warm water substantially reduces the amount of allergens on their fur. Animals secrete substances from their sweat glands and their saliva. When these substances dry, they flake off and are easily breathed in, causing allergies to act up. However, these chemicals are water soluble and are easily rinsed off.

If you're a cat owner and can't imagine bathing your furry friend for fear of being scratched, take heart: One out of ten cats actually enjoys being bathed. If they are exposed to baths as kittens, chances are higher that bath time will be a harmonious experience. A twice-monthly bath in warm water, with no soap, should be sufficient. In addition to bathing your pet, try to wash your hands soon after you've had direct contact with your furry friend. Also be sure to avoid rubbing your eyes after touching the cat.

Rinse it twice. Chemicals in detergents and other laundry products can cause skin irritation in many people. Because of this, it's important to make sure that the final rinse cycle on your machine thoroughly rinses the detergent from your clothes. To be sure, run clothes through an additional rinse cycle and skip the dryer sheets.

Anticipate your needs. When planning a vacation or business trip, call ahead to find a room that will be easier on your allergies. Ask for a room that's not on the lower level, because such a room may have been flooded in the past and may still be a haven for mold growth. Shop around for a hotel or motel that doesn't allow pets, so you won't be subject to the leftover dander of the last traveler's dog or cat. If possible, bring your own vinyl- or plastic-encased pillow.

AT THE DOCTOR'S

If you've got severe or persistent allergies that don't seem to respond to home treatment (or if you suffer from wheezing and coughing), you should consider seeing an allergist for treatment. If you know what's causing the problem, you're halfway to feeling better. If you haven't uncovered the culprit, your doctor will be able to help identify the offender by using a skin-scratch test (in which small amounts of suspected allergens are applied to tiny scratches in the skin) or by injecting you just under the skin with suspected allergens.

Once the allergy has been identified, your practitioner will map out a course of treatment. Three types of medicines are commonly prescribed for allergies: antihistamines, which combat the effects of the histamines that the overly sensitive immune system is producing; corticosteroids, which reduce inflammation and swelling; and bronchodilators, which ease breathing by opening bronchial tubes.

Your doctor may also prescribe immunotherapy, or "desensitization," which consists of injections of an allergen in gradually increasing quantities. This allows the body to build up a tolerance to the offending substance. It works best in controlling allergies to pollen, insect venoms, and house dust.

PREVENTION

One great way to prevent an allergy attack is to use an over-the-counter antihistamine (be sure to consult your doctor about taking any medication, however, if you're pregnant, breast-feeding, or have any special medical conditions). Although many people misuse these drugs, believing them to be an on-the-spot fix for whenever they feel itchy-eyed or prone to attacks of sneezing, antihistamines actually work best when they are used before the attack occurs.

If you suffer from hay fever, you'll get the maximum benefit from antihistamines if you start taking them a week or two before the allergy season begins. (When it begins depends on where you live.) People with pet allergies who know they will be exposed to someone else's cat or dog should also begin taking antihistamines ten to fourteen days in advance.

Many allergists recommend an over-the-counter antihistamine that contains chlorpheniramine maleate, one of the oldest, safest allergy drugs. It can take care of symptoms such as sneezing; itchy, runny nose; and itchy eyes. (If you also have nasal stuffiness, you can try a combination product that contains chlorpheniramine and pseudo-ephedrine, a nasal decongestant.) Start with about one-fourth of the dose that the package recommends, then slowly build up to 24 milligrams per day (12 milligrams in the morning and 12 milligrams in the evening), providing you can maintain that dosage without drowsiness. Since drowsiness tends to go away in a week or two, try starting with evening doses, then adding a morning dose as you begin to tolerate the medication. (Be sure to avoid operating a motor vehicle or heavy machinery if the medication makes you drowsy.)

If you have an allergy to dust, antihistamines may not be enough. In this case, your prevention strategy can be made more effective by scrupulously ridding your home of dust mites, microscopic insects that live in dusty, humid environments. The feces and corpses of mites are thought to be the irritating components in dust. Allergists believe that since we spend most of our time at home in the bedroom, that's the most important place to allergy-proof. The following tips will help you do just that:

Get rid of the breeding grounds. Invest in airtight plastic or vinyl cases or special covers that are impermeable to allergens for your pillows and mattresses (except for waterbeds). Pillows and mattresses contain fibrous material that is an ideal environment for dust-mite growth. These cases are usually available at your local department store or through mail-order companies. You can also contact the Asthma and Allergy Foundation of America for more information on where to purchase cases and covers.

11 PREVENTION STRATEGIES

- Begin to take antihistamines 10 to 14 days before you will be exposed to an allergen, if possible.
- Buy plastic or vinyl pillowcases and mattress covers.
- Avoid down and feather pillows and comforters.
- Wash sheets and bedding in hot water every seven to ten days.
- Have someone else dust once a week.
- Replace overstuffed furniture with wood, vinyl, and leather.
- Get rid of carpeting; opt for wood floors instead.
- Invest in washable curtains.
- Have the blinds vacuumed weekly.
- Try to store miscellaneous items outside the bedroom or wrap them tightly in plastic garbage bags.
- Have the air conditioner and heating ducts cleaned monthly.

Clean them out. Down, kapok, and feather comforters and pillows are not for people with allergies. The feathers have a tendency to leak and can wreak havoc on your respiratory tract. Comforters and sheets should be washed every seven to ten days in water as hot as they can tolerate. Wash your mattress pads and synthetic blankets every two weeks.

Once a week, be meticulous. Putting off cleaning for longer than a week may allow an excessive amount of dust to collect. However, since cleaning raises dust, it's best not to clean more than once a week. If necessary, you can spot dust with a damp cloth more often.

Change the decor. Overstuffed furniture is another breeding ground for dust mites. If possible, replace overstuffed items with wood, vinyl, and leather. Since carpeting makes an excellent dust-mite lair, opt instead for bare floors or look into getting a product for killing dust mites in carpets.

Wash the curtains. If possible, invest in curtains that can be washed, since their fabric is often a place where dust mites hide.

Use your vacuum on the blinds. The slats of venetian blinds are notorious dust collectors. If you can't replace your venetian blinds with washable curtains, at least run the vacuum lightly over them or dust them well during your thorough weekly cleaning.

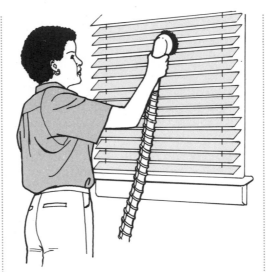

Use the attic for storage space. Stored items tend to collect dust and have no place in an allergy-proof bedroom. If the bedroom is the only storage space you have, wrap items tightly in plastic garbage bags.

Don't neglect the air conditioner and the heating ducts. Every month or so, clean out the vents on your heating and air-conditioning units, or have someone clean them for you. These ducts are breeding grounds for mold, dust mites, and bacteria. If you let such nasties collect, they'll be blown into the room each time you turn on the appliance.

Sources: **Clifton T. Furukawa, M.D.,** Past Chairman, Professional Education Council, American Academy of Allergy and Immunology; Clinical Professor of Pediatrics, University of Washington School of Medicine, Seattle, Washington. **Anthony Montanaro, M.D.,** Associate Professor of Medicine, Division of Allergy and Immunology, Oregon Health Sciences University, Portland, Oregon. **Edward J. O'Connell, M.D.,** Past President, American College of Allergy and Immunology; Professor of Pediatrics, Allergy/Immunology, Mayo Clinic, Rochester, Minnesota. **Abba I. Terr, M.D.,** Clinical Professor of Medicine, Director, Allergy Clinic, Stanford University Medical Center, Stanford, California.

●ARTHRITIS

How to Relieve

the Pain and

Stiffness

ARTHRITIS HURTS WHEN YOU NEED IT least, when you most want to feel your best; in the morning, when you're buttoning your shirt; when you thought you were going to enjoy a relaxing bike ride with your family. Sometimes it makes you feel like you're getting old. Other times, it just makes you angry with its uncanny timing and inconvenience.

You're not alone. An estimated 37 million Americans are caught in the grip of some form of arthritis or rheumatic disease. And few of us will make it to a ripe old age without joining the fold.

There are more than 100 different forms of arthritis and rheumatic disease, according to the Arthritis Foundation of Atlanta. Some of the more widely known are osteoarthritis, rheumatoid arthritis, gout, and lupus. Osteoarthritis is marked by a breakdown and loss of cartilage, the tough tissue that separates and cushions the bones in a joint. As cartilage is worn away and the bones begin to rub against each other, the joint becomes aggravated. In osteoarthritis, this breakdown of cartilage is accompanied by inflammation, hardening of the bone beneath the cartilage, and bone spurs (growths) around the joints. At least a mild manifestation of this disease is almost a certain eventuality of the aging process.

Rheumatoid arthritis, on the other hand, is not an inevitable aspect of the aging process. With this disease, the synovial membrane, or lining, of a joint becomes inflamed, causing pain, swelling, heat, and redness.

With gout, needle-shaped uric acid crystals collect in the joints, due to a fault in the body's ability to metabolize, or process, purines. Purines are naturally occurring chemicals found in certain foods, such as liver, kidney, and anchovies. The disease primarily targets overweight, fairly inactive men over the age of 35.

Lupus, on the other hand, affects many more women than men. It is a condition in which the body's own immune system attacks healthy cells.

SYMPTOMS

If you've got arthritis, you probably know it from the swelling, pain, stiffness, and redness in your joints. For many arthritis sufferers, the pain is greatest in the morning and subsides as the day progresses. Damp weather and emotional stress may make the symptoms worse.

With rheumatoid arthritis, symptoms may be accompanied by more generalized feelings of fatigue and fever. There may be periods where the symptoms disappear completely, only to return with greater severity.

Lupus may cause fatigue, fever, severe joint pain, and mouth sores. (See the lupus profile.)

CAUSES

Researchers are still not clear on what predisposes some people to develop arthritis. One theory is that arthritis sufferers may have defective collagen, a protein that helps form the body's cartilage. Experts do know that arthritis is not an inherited disease. Nonetheless, people who have a family history of arthritis are more likely to develop the disease.

Being overweight, which puts excess strain on the joints, is a factor in the disease's development. Constant sports- or job-related joint abuse also plays a role. However, a sedentary lifestyle may aggravate an existing problem.

AT-HOME TREATMENT

Frustrated by the chronic pain of arthritis, some sufferers pursue an endless succession of promises for 100 percent relief—whether from an unproven drug, a new diet, or another questionable treatment. Unfortunately, at this time, arthritis has no cure. So, before you jump at the next hot-sounding testimonial, proceed with caution. Get all the facts. Consult your physician or other health-care provider before following any new course of treatment. And remember, if something sounds too good to be true, it probably is.

There are a variety of steps you can take that will leave you more active and in control of your pain. Here are some tips to help relieve discomfort and get you back into the swing of things.

Use heat, cold, or both. There are no hard and fast rules when it comes to deciding which—heat, cold, or a combination of the two—will give you the best results. The bottom line is to use whichever feels the best over time.

Heat relieves pain by relaxing muscles and joints and decreasing stiffness. It is excellent for osteoarthritis, which causes minimal inflammation. When applied before exercise, heat may also loosen up the muscles and help them perform better.

A hot compress is a good way to apply heat to small areas. However, compresses tend to cool down quickly. An electric blanket or heating pad can provide sustained dry heat to larger areas. A warm shower, bath, or whirlpool can keep the wet heat coming.

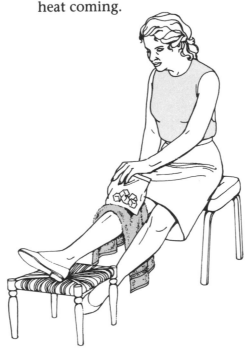

In some instances, however, heat may aggravate a joint that is already "hot" from inflammation, as sometimes occurs with rheumatoid arthritis. In these cases, a cold pack may be the answer. There are many ways to make a cold pack, such as filling a plastic bag with crushed ice, or using a package of frozen peas or blue ice. Wrap the cold pack in a towel and apply it to only one or two joints at a time, so you don't get a chill. Cold packs are ordinarily used to reduce pain in specific joints, not over large areas. They should not be applied without a doctor's approval where vasculitis (inflammation of the blood vessels) or Raynaud's phenomenon (a condition characterized by spasms of the arteries in the fingers and toes) exist.

You may find that alternating heat and cold gives you the most relief. For the best results, the Arthritis Foundation recommends the contrast bath: Soak your hands and/or feet in warm water (no more than 110 degrees Fahrenheit) for about three minutes, then soak them in cold water (about 65 degrees Fahrenheit) for about a minute. Repeat this process three times, then finish with a warm-water soak.

Let your hands do some swimming. Doing hand exercises in a sink full of warm water may help ease discomfort.

Don't try to cream it away. Over-the-counter creams may give temporary relief by heating up the joints. However, you should not rely exclusively on these creams. They should just be a part of a comprehensive treatment program for your arthritis.

Tie it up. Try tying a wool scarf around the elbow or knee joint when it aches. Be careful not to wrap it too tightly, however; you don't want to hamper your circulation.

Glove your hands. The tightness caused by stretchy gloves may reduce the swelling that often accompanies arthritis. The warmth created by covered hands may also make the joints feel better. Wearing thermal underwear may provide the covered joints with the same warming effect.

Go electric. The same battery-operated mitts used by hunters to keep their hands toasty on cold mornings in the woods can also keep your hands warm and pain-free. Try wearing them at night while you sleep.

Sleep on a water bed. According to the National Water Bed Retailers' Association in Chicago, many water-bed owners claimed in a study that their rheumatoid arthritis was helped by a water bed. This may be because the slight motions made by the water can help reduce morning stiffness. The heat of the water under you as you sleep may also help relieve joint pain.

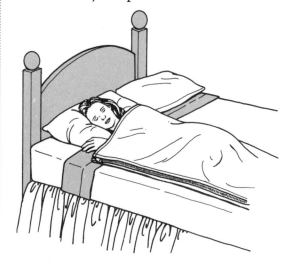

Camp out in your bedroom. If a water bed is out of the question, you might consider camping gear. The cocoon-like effect of a sleeping bag traps heat, which can help relieve morning aches and pains, some doctors believe. You don't have to leave home to use one: Try it on top of your bed. If your spouse suffers from arthritis, too (or even if he doesn't), you can always invest in a double bag.

Sleep in downy comfort. One doctor from Norway tells the story of staying in a bed-and-breakfast while he was on a business trip to New York. The doctor, who was suffering from arthritis pain, slept peacefully each night in the B&B's bed and awoke each morning pain-free. The bed was outfitted with a goose-down comforter and pillow. The doctor felt that the bedding's warmth and minute motion brought on the relief. For those who are allergic to down, an electric blanket may be a good alternative.

Lose the spare tire. Being overweight puts more stress on the joints. A weight gain of only 10 pounds can mean an equivalent stress increase of 40 pounds on the knees. So if you carry excess pounds, losing weight can help improve joint function. It may even slow the progress of osteoarthritis.

Stay active. Maintain movement in your joints as best you can. This can help keep your joints functioning better for a longer amount of time and, at the same time, brighten your outlook on life. Even small movements mean a lot. If all you can tolerate is a little housecleaning or gardening, or a stroll around the block, that's enough for the time being.

Exercise, when it feels better. When the inflammation has calmed down, that's the time to build up the amount of exercise that you do.

Range-of-motion exercises can be done by almost any arthritis sufferer. They help maintain good movement by putting the joints through their full range of motion. Isometrics, in which you create resistance by tightening a muscle without moving the joint, can help to strengthen muscles. Weight-bearing exercises, such as walking, also build muscle strength. While strengthening exercises can be beneficial to you, they should only be done under the supervision and care of a therapist or physician, especially if you also suffer from cardiovascular disease. Stretching, which helps make the muscles more flexible, is often recommended as the first step in any regular program of exercise.

Warming up before beginning any exercise makes the joints more flexible. Massage your muscles and/or apply hot or cold compresses or both—whichever you prefer. You may find that a warm shower is the quickest way to warm up.

The following range-of-motion exercises are recommended by the Arthritis Foundation. For best results, carry out the exercises in a smooth, steady, slow-paced

23

13 WAYS TO EASE DISCOMFORT

- Apply hot or cold compresses (whichever feels best) to stiff joints.
- Do hand exercises in a sink full of warm water.
- Don't overuse over-the-counter "heat" creams.
- Tie a wool scarf around a stiff, painful joint.
- Wear stretchy gloves.
- Invest in a pair of electric gloves.
- Try a water bed.
- Sleep in a sleeping bag on top of your bed.
- Use down comforters and pillows or an electric blanket if you're allergic to feathers.
- Try to lose any excess body weight.
- Maintain an active lifestyle.
- Start a program of gentle exercise.
- Try water aerobics or do stretches in a heated jacuzzi.

manner; don't bounce, jerk, or strain. Don't hold your breath; breathe as naturally as possible. Do each exercise five to ten times, if possible. If any exercise causes chest pain, other pain, or shortness of breath—stop. When your joints are inflamed, it's best to skip the exercises and rest. If you have any questions, contact your therapist or physician. And remember: It may be some time before you feel the benefits of regular exercise, so be patient with yourself.

1) Shoulders: Lie on your back and raise one arm over your head, keeping your elbow straight. Keep your arm close to your ear. Return your arm slowly to your side. Repeat with the other arm.

2) Knees and hips: Lie on your back with one knee bent and the other as straight as possible. Bend the knee of the straight leg and bring it toward the chest. Extend that same leg into the air and then lower the straightened leg to the floor. Repeat with the other leg.

3) Hips: Lie on your back with your legs straight and about six inches apart. Point your toes upward. Slide one leg out to the side and return, keeping your toes pointing upward. Repeat with other leg.

4) Knees: Sit in a chair that is high enough so that you can swing your legs. Keep your thigh on the chair and straighten out your knee. Hold a few seconds. Then bend your knee back as far as possible to return to the starting position. Repeat with the other knee.

5) Ankles: Sit on a chair and lift your toes off the floor as high as possible while keeping your heels on the floor. Then return your toes to the floor and lift your heels as high as possible. Repeat.

6) Fingers: Open your hand with your fingers straight. Bend all of the finger joints, except the knuckles. Touch the top of the palm with the tips of your fingers. Open and repeat.

7) Thumbs: Open your hand with your fingers straight. Reach your thumb across your palm until it touches the base of the little finger. Stretch your thumb out again and repeat.

Take care to pace yourself. Here's a useful recipe to assess whether you've overdone your exercise routine: See how you feel a few hours after you exercise and then again after twenty-four hours. If your pain has increased considerably, then it's time to cut back on the frequency and the amount of exercise. Of course, if the activity brought relief, you've found a worthwhile exercise. Tailor your routine to include the exercises that give you the most relief and the most enjoyment.

Go jump in a pool. If you find that even simple movements give you discomfort, a heated pool or whirlpool may be the perfect environment for exercise (unless you also have high blood pressure, in which case you should avoid whirlpools and hot tubs). Try a few of your simpler exercises while in the water. The buoyancy will help reduce the strain on your joints. The warm water will also help loosen joints and maintain motion and strength. Even a warm bath may allow you some increased movement. In a pinch, a hot shower may do: Running the stream of water down your back, for instance, may help relieve back pain long enough to do some simple stretches.

COPING STRATEGIES

In addition to easing discomfort, you can learn to live well with arthritis by protecting your joints. What's more, with a little planning and reorganizing, you can learn to do daily tasks more efficiently, so that you'll have more energy to spend on activities you enjoy. Here are some tips from the Arthritis Foundation that may help.

Arrange your day. Prepare a realistic, written schedule of what you would like to accomplish each day. That way, you can carry out your most demanding tasks and activities when you think you'll have the most energy and enthusiasm.

Loosen up. As a general rule, you want to avoid activities that involve a tight grip or that put too much pressure on your fingers. Use the palms of both hands to lift and hold cups, plates, pots, and pans, rather than gripping them with your fingers or with only one hand. Place your hand flat against a sponge or rag instead of squeezing it with your fingers. Avoid holding a package or pocketbook by clasping the handle with your fingers. Instead, grasp your goods in the crook of your arm—the way a football player holds the ball while running across the field—and you won't be hit by as much discomfort.

Change position often. Keeping joints locked in the same position for any length of time will only add to your pain and stiffness. Relax and stretch your joints as often as possible.

Unhand it. Whenever possible, use your arm instead of your hand to carry out an activity. For example, push open a heavy door with the side of your arm rather than with your hand and outstretched arm.

Get off your feet. Sitting down to complete a task will keep your energy level up much longer than if you stand.

Buy new knobs. Replace round doorknobs with the kind that have long, thin handles. They require a looser, less stressful grip to operate, so you'll put less strain on your joints.

Pad your tools. For a more comfortable grip, tape a layer or two of thin foam rubber, or a foam rubber hair curler, around the handles of household tools such as brooms, mops, and rakes. Replacing heavier eating and cooking utensils with lighter-weight ones may also minimize hand pain.

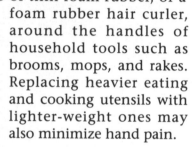

Get on the wagon. Heavy loads of groceries and laundry will be easier to tote if you use a wagon or cart that glides along on wheels.

Automate your life. Automatic appliances can do much of the work for you. Electric can openers and knives, for example, are easier to operate than manual versions. An electric toothbrush has a wider handle and is easier to grip than a regular toothbrush.

Rearrange your priorities. Arranging your possessions so that they are within easy reach can help minimize the amount of reaching you do. Adjust the shelves and racks in any storage area so that you don't have to strain to get the items you need. Buy clothes with pockets to hold things you use often,

like a pair of reading glasses. Use an apron with pockets to carry cleaning supplies with you as you do chores.

Grab a gripper. For those items you can't store nearby, buy a long-handled gripper, a long stick of the kind used in grocery shops to grab items from top shelves. Make household chores easier with a long-handled feather duster or scrub brush. Extract your clothes from the dryer with an extended-reach tool.

Forgo the buttons and laces. Buying clothing and shoes with Velcro self-fastening tape closures can save you frustration.

Learn a new way to walk. When climbing stairs, lead with your stronger leg when you are going up and your weaker leg when you are coming down.

Don't bend over. When reaching for or lifting something that's low or on the ground, bend your knees and keep your back straight as you lift.

Go loopy. Tying loops around refrigerator- and oven-door handles can make a tight grip unnecessary. Have loops sewn on your socks, too, then use a long-handled hook to help you pull them up.

Buy a shower seat. A specially made stool can give you a steady place to shower and can ease your way in and out of the bathtub.

Don't kneel while you garden. Sitting, rather than stooping, over your flower beds or vegetable garden may help reduce the stress on your back and legs.

Don't be proud. Don't be afraid to ask your family members or friends for assistance when you need it. As the saying goes, many hands make light work. By sharing the load, you'll have more time and energy for the people and activities you enjoy.

Lay out the newspaper while you read. Likewise, lay a book flat or use a book stand to give your hands a break as you read.

Set goals you can meet. Instead of making long to-do lists, try setting a more forgiving pace. Plan on tackling only one major cleaning chore per day, whether it is doing the laundry or cleaning the kitchen. Spread out the work and you'll be spreading out the strain.

Call the Arthritis Foundation. The Arthritis Foundation can keep you up-to-date on products made especially for arthritis sufferers. Call the Arthritis Foundation Information Line at 800-283-7800, Monday through Friday, 9:00 A.M. to 7:00 P.M., Eastern time, to talk to a skilled operator who can answer your questions about arthritis.

Sources: **Earl J. Brewer, Jr., M.D.,** Former Head, Rheumatology Division, Texas Children's Hospital, Houston, Texas; Former Clinical Professor, Former Head, Rheumatology Division, Department of Pediatrics, Baylor College of Medicine. **John Staige Davis IV, M.D.,** Margaret Trolinger Professor of Medicine, University of Virginia School of Medicine, Charlottesville, Virginia. **Arthur I. Grayzel, M.D.,** Senior Vice-President for Medical Affairs, Arthritis Foundation. **Janna Jacobs, P.T., C.H.T.,** President, Section on Hand Rehabilitation, American Physical Therapy Association (APTA). **John R. Ward, M.D.,** Professor of Medicine, University of Utah School of Medicine, Salt Lake City, Utah.

22 STRATEGIES TO HELP YOU COPE

- Schedule your most important tasks for when you have the most energy.
- Try not to grip objects too tightly.
- Avoid activities that put too much pressure on your fingers.
- Don't stay in one position too long.
- Relax and stretch your joints whenever you can.
- Use your arms, rather than your hands, to hold and carry things.
- Conserve energy by sitting down to complete a task.
- Buy long, thin door handles to replace harder-to-turn round knobs.
- Tape foam rubber around broom, mop, and tool handles for a more comfortable grip.
- Invest in lightweight eating and cooking utensils.
- Replace manual can openers and other appliances with electric ones.
- Arrange your home so that your possessions are within easy reach.
- Choose clothing and shoes that have Velcro self-fastening tape closures instead of buttons and laces.
- Climb stairs by leading with your stronger leg going up and your weaker leg coming down.
- Bend from your knees, instead of from your waist.
- Try tying loops around refrigerator- and oven-door handles.
- Tote heavy loads in a wagon or shopping cart.
- Invest in stools for the shower and for the garden.
- Ask for help when you need it.
- Don't hold on to newspapers and books while you read; lay them down instead.
- Set realistic goals.
- Make friends with the Arthritis Foundation.

●BACK PAIN

How to Ease

the Ache

IT WAS EARLY MORNING. YOU WERE walking toward the coffeemaker when you heard a knock at the door. You turned around, a bit too quickly perhaps. That's when the searing pain shot up your back, making you yell out in pain. Now, hours later, you're flat on your back, wishing either for a miracle or for a quick demise.

Take heart—you're not alone. Back pain is one of the most common physical ailments, affecting a full 80 percent of all Americans at some point in their lives.

CAUSES

Back pain can arise as a result of a variety of different physical causes. Strains are the most common reason for the pain. Strains occur when overworked or underexercised back muscles are pushed beyond their normal capacity. The muscles may contract or go into spasm, bunching together in a tight, hardened mass. Meanwhile, the body sends out a sharp pain signal as nearby muscles tighten in an effort to protect strained muscles and prevent further damage. A strain can be caused by participation in a sport, a sudden jerking motion (such as a car braking), or a reflex action, such as a sneeze.

Overweight is a major cause of backache, because it increases the stress on back muscles. Similarly, pregnancy can produce back pain because of the weight or position of the fetus. For some women, menstruation is also associated with dull back discomfort.

Many people experience back pain as they age and their joint tissues deteriorate or shift. Osteoporosis is another cause of back pain, when brittle vertebrae begin to disintegrate. Other causes include sitting at a desk for long periods of time, psychological tension, stress, and anxiety over everyday problems. In addition, back pain can result from diseases of the kidneys, heart, lungs, intestinal tract, or reproductive organs.

Backache occasionally stems from a physical malformation. In these cases, the pain is often due to the effect of the malformation on the surrounding tissues. For example, having one leg that is much shorter than the other or having a curvature of the spine may force muscles out of alignment, making pain a likely result.

AT-HOME TREATMENT

Unfortunately, your doctor may not be able to do much to help, beyond prescribing some pain medication or muscle relaxants and advising you to rest. (If the doctor finds a major injury or a disk problem, he or she may be able to prescribe other treatments.) On the bright side, you can usually be on your feet again in just a few days if you follow some simple steps to take care of yourself.

The following remedies are appropriate for anyone who is suffering from back pain as a result of tight, aching muscles or a strain. However, if you are experiencing pain, weakness, or numbness in the legs or a loss of bowel or bladder control, see a doctor without delay.

Take a load off. Bed rest may be the best way to relieve the strain on the muscles. The optimal way to lie is flat on your back with two pillows underneath your knees. Don't lie facedown, since this position forces you to twist your head to breathe and may cause neck pain. Try to get up and start moving around after about three days, since longer periods of bed rest may weaken the muscles and make them more prone to strain.

Cool it down. To help keep inflammation and discomfort to a minimum, apply an ice pack to the painful area within 24 hours of the injury. Ice decreases the nerves' ability to relay the pain signals that are making you suffer. To create an ice pack, fill a plastic bag with ice cubes or use a bag of frozen peas. Wrap the bag in a thin towel and place it on the injured area for 20 minutes. Wait for 30 minutes, then put the ice pack back on for another 20 minutes. Do not put the ice pack directly on your skin.

Soak it. If it's been more than 24 hours since you injured your back, ice will not help reduce pain or inflammation. At this stage of the game, heat may help by relaxing and loosening up the muscle spasms. A 20-minute soak in the bathtub may be enough to get you back on your feet again. Pregnant women, however, should not sit in a hot tub or hot bath for too long, since raising the body temperature over 100 degrees Fahrenheit for long periods may cause birth defects or miscarriage. People with high blood pressure should also avoid such hot spots.

Buy a new bed. Sleeping on a soft, sagging mattress may contribute to the development of back pain or worsen an existing problem. If you can't afford a new mattress, you might try putting a three-quarter-inch-thick piece of plywood between the mattress and box spring. No matter how you solve the mattress problem, however, try to sleep on your back with two pillows underneath your knees or on your side with one pillow between your knees.

Massage it away. Ask your spouse, friend, or roommate to give you a back rub. You might also find a local massage therapist who makes house calls. Check the yellow pages for listings or ask friends for a referral.

Slow down. Many cases of back pain are the result of muscles made tight by stress and emotional tension. You may want to consider practicing relaxation and deep-breathing exercises, such as closing your eyes, breathing deeply, and counting backward from 100.

Take a painkiller. An over-the-counter analgesic, such as aspirin, acetaminophen, or ibuprofen, may help relieve your pain. However, be aware that not all medications—not even nonprescription ones—are for everyone. Pregnant women, for example, should not take

8 WAYS TO EASE DISCOMFORT

- Take some time out to rest your back. Lie flat on your back with two pillows under your knees.
- As soon as the pain starts, apply an ice pack to the injured area to reduce pain and inflammation (20 minutes at a time should be sufficient).
- After the first 24 hours of pain, take a hot bath to relax muscle spasms.
- Buy a firmer mattress or place plywood between your mattress and box spring.
- Get a massage.
- Learn to relax.
- Take an over-the-counter analgesic, such as aspirin, acetaminophen, or ibuprofen—with your doctor's approval.
- See a doctor if the pain persists, or if other symptoms, such as loss of bladder or bowel control or radiating pain, develop.

any medication without first checking with their doctor. People with ulcers should stay away from analgesics containing aspirin. Ask your physician to recommend the best medication for you.

Call the doctor. If back pain persists for more than two weeks, if it continues to get worse, or if you have any numbness, tingling, or burning in your legs, it's time to visit a physician, who will check for underlying disorders that may be responsible for the pain.

PREVENTION

Many of the activities you engage in each day—sitting, lifting, bending, carrying—can put a strain on your back. By learning new ways of going about these activities, you can help prevent back pain and ensure the health of your back for years to come. The tips that follow can help.

Try creative cushioning. If you have to stay seated for extended periods in an unsupportive chair and don't have a cushion, try rolling up a towel or an article of clothing so that it has about the same circumference as your forearm. Slide the rolled-up cloth between your lower back and the chair. If necessary, you can simply slide your forearm between your lower back and the back of the chair to ease the strain on your back. Even with the best support, however, sitting is still stressful for your back, so try to make small adjustments in the curvature of your lower back every few minutes or so.

Practice back-friendly lifting. The large muscles of your legs and buttocks are stronger and better equipped to bear heavy weights than your back muscles are. So, instead of bending from the waist when you lift, practice squatting while keeping your back straight and erect—as if you were balancing a book on your head. Then, straighten your legs to come up again. Keep your weight balanced over an erect spine. Hold heavy objects close to your body when you pick them up and carry them. This way, the weight is carried by the erect spine, and your muscles are not required to do as much work. If you have to reach something on a high shelf, try getting underneath the object and resting it on your head.

Pay attention. The primary cause of back injury is careless activity, according to experts. If you are prone to back pain, try moving more consciously. Avoid bending, twisting, and lifting. Avoid being caught off-guard. If you can, ask others to do strenuous tasks, such as yard work or carrying around heavy suitcases.

Lose the spare tire. Extra weight puts extra strain on back muscles. The equation is simple: The less you have to carry, the less load you have. Also, when you gain weight in your abdomen, you may become sway-backed, which can accentuate back pain. Sensible, gradual weight loss may help ease the stress on your muscles.

Go swimming. Orthopedic surgeons have long believed that swimming is the best aerobic exercise for a bad back. Doing laps in the pool can help tone and tighten the muscles of the back and abdomen. Walking is second best. You can also try the back-saving exercises that follow.

Sit supported. The seats of most cars and trucks were not designed with back support in mind. Airplane seats are particularly bad for you since they curve away from the back. Seats should support the small of your back. If yours doesn't, invest in a small cushion that can be fitted to provide the missing support. The most desirable sitting position is not one in which your back is straight up and down. It's better to be leaning back at an

angle of about 110 degrees. If you sit for long hours, you should periodically get up and walk around.

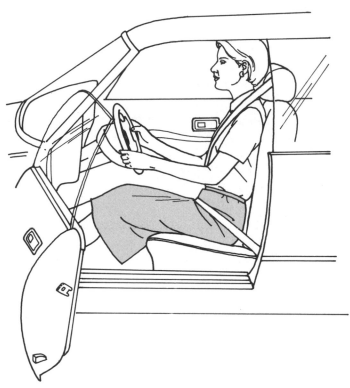

Exercise your back. Back exercises can be used to ease the pain of an already troubled back, but they are best used to prevent the injury from recurring. For maximum results, do the following exercises daily. Don't discontinue them, even after the pain gets better, since strength and flexibility can only be maintained through consistent exercise. Stretches may be done twice a day. Although these exercises are safe and effective for most back pain caused by muscle strain or spasm, people with disk or other structural problems should not engage in any type

31

8 TIPS FOR KEEPING YOUR BACK PAIN-FREE

- Buy a cushion to use in the car or on an unsupportive seat.
- When you have to sit for long periods of time, periodically stand up and stretch.
- Lift by squatting, then straightening your legs, not by bending over from the waist.
- Carry objects by holding them close to your body.
- Move consciously; don't be careless in your activity.
- Maintain ideal body weight.
- Start a program of lap swimming.
- Do back exercises every day.

of exercise, except under the supervision of a doctor.

1) *Single Knee-to-Chest.* Lie on your back with your knees bent and your feet on the floor. Grasp the back of one thigh with both hands; gently and slowly pull toward your chest until you feel mild tension—not to the point of pain. Hold to the count of ten, without bouncing, then release. Repeat four to five times with the same leg, then switch sides. This exercise stretches muscles in the hips, buttocks, and lower back—all muscles that become shortened and tight after a long day of sitting or standing. It is a good warm-up to the other exercises.

2) *Double Knee-to-Chest.* Lie on your back with your knees bent and your feet on the floor. This time, grasp both thighs and gently and slowly pull them as close to your chest as you can. Again—pull only to the point of slight tension, and don't bounce. Hold to the count of ten, then release. Repeat four or five times before doing the next exercise.

3) *Lumbar Rotation.* Lie on your back with your hips and knees bent,

your feet flat on the floor, and your heels touching your buttocks. Keeping your knees together and your shoulders on the floor, slowly allow your knees to rotate to the right, until you reach a point of mild tension. Hold for a count of 10, then return to the starting position. Repeat four to five times on the right side, then switch to the left.

4) *Partial Sit-Up.* Lie on your back with your knees bent, your feet flat on the floor, and your hands gently supporting your head. Slowly curl up just to the point where your shoulders come off the floor. Avoid bending your neck. Hold for a few counts, then roll slowly back down. Exhale as you rise, inhale as you lower. Repeat 10 to 15 times. This exercise strengthens the abdominal muscles; strong abdominal muscles help you maintain good posture and reduce the possibility of back injury.

5) *Active Back Extension.* Lie down with your chest on the floor. You can put a pillow under your stomach (not under your hips) if that feels comfortable. Put your arms at your sides, with your hands next to your buttocks. Slowly extend your head and neck and raise your upper body off the floor. Hold for five to ten counts. Slowly lower yourself back to the starting position. Remember to breathe as you do the exercise. Repeat five to ten times.

6) *Posture Enhancer.* Stand with the back of your head, your shoulders and shoulder blades, and your buttocks held firmly against a wall. Your heels should be about six inches away from the wall. Do not allow your lower back to curve excessively. Start with the backs of your hands against the wall at thigh level.

Slowly slide the backs of your hands up the wall, without allowing your elbows, head, buttocks, or shoulder blades to lose contact with the wall. (The movement is similar to making angels in the snow.) Stop at the point where your arms are so high that the above-mentioned body parts cannot stay against the wall. Repeat five times.

7) *Office Exercises*. If you spend many hours a day hunched over paperwork at a desk, chances are your lumbar, or lower, spine is being stretched and pulled in the wrong direction. (The lower spine's natural curve is slightly inward, toward the abdomen. Hunching forward causes the lower spine to be curved outward, toward the chair.) Poor sitting posture puts stress on the ligaments and other tissues. To give your lower back a break, periodically get up to a standing position, with your feet shoulder-width apart and your hands on your hips. Slowly lean back to a point of mild tension and hold for a count of ten. Repeat four to five times.

You should also practice getting out of your chair properly with your feet shoulder-width apart, your head up, your eyes focused straight ahead, and your buttocks stuck out. Use the strength of your arms, legs, and buttocks—instead of your back—to help you rise.

Sources: **Henry J. Bienert, Jr., M.D.**, Orthopedic Surgeon, Tulane University School of Medicine, New Orleans, Louisiana. **Daniel S.J. Choy, M.D.**, Assistant Clinical Professor of Medicine, Columbia University College of Physicians and Surgeons; Director, Laser Laboratory, St. Luke's-Roosevelt Hospital Center, New York, New York. **Billy Glisan, M.S.**, Director, Injury Prevention Program, Texas Back Institute, Dallas, Texas. **Jerold Lancourt, M.D.**, Orthopedic Surgeon, North Dallas Orthopedics & Rehabilitation, P.A., Dallas, Texas. **Willibald Nagler, M.D.**, Anne and Jerome Fisher Physiatrist-in-Chief, Chairman of the Department of Rehabilitation Medicine, The New York Hospital-Cornell Medical Center, New York, New York.

●BAD BREATH

How to Make a

Better First

Impression

THERE'S A REASON FOR ALL OF THOSE mouthwash and breath-mint commercials we see on television. Some of us—indeed, many of us—believe we have a problem with bad breath. After all, we live in a society that is obsessed with first impressions—visual and otherwise. We don't want to risk offending someone simply by opening our mouths. Halitosis, more commonly called bad breath, has plagued us for centuries. There is evidence that the ancient Greeks rinsed with white wine, aniseed, and myrrh to get rid of any traces of bad breath. The Italians mixed up a mouthwash of sage, cinnamon, juniper seeds, root of cypress, and rosemary leaves to freshen their mouths, according to the Academy of General Dentistry.

Today, Americans spend more than a half-billion dollars a year for mouthwashes that often contain little more than alcohol and flavoring. But still, we worry. Indeed, *New York Times* health columnist Jane E. Brody has written that she receives more questions about bad breath than about any other common medical problem.

Maybe one explanation for our preoccupation with our breath is the fact that we don't really know when it smells less-than-fresh. Sure, you can try breathing into a handkerchief or running floss between your teeth, but the bottom line is that it's pretty difficult to smell your own breath. (And who wants to find out the unfortunate news by being told by a spouse, colleague, or prospective love interest?)

CAUSES

The route to better-smelling breath depends on what's causing the odor. In 80 to 90 percent of cases, bad breath has to do with something in the mouth. Plaque, the nearly invisible film of bacteria that's constantly forming in your mouth, is a common halitosis culprit. Cavities and gum disease are other principal offenders. While tooth decay by itself doesn't smell bad, you can bet food trapped in the spaces between your teeth does.

Occasionally, bad breath can be attributed to something in the lungs or the gastrointestinal tract. The strong odors of foods such as garlic, onions, and alcohol are carried through the bloodstream and exhaled by the lungs. Another big loser when it comes to turning your breath sour—and harming your health—is tobacco. Some health problems, such as sinus infections or diabetes (which may give the breath a chemical smell), can also cause bad breath.

AT-HOME TREATMENT

Uncovering the culprit will bring you one step closer to kissing your halitosis goodbye. Here's what you can do to keep your breath fresh:

Clean up your act. Meticulous oral hygiene is the basic tenet in the fight for fresh breath. That means a thorough brushing twice a day. It also means flossing regularly. Food and bacteria trapped between teeth and at the gum line can only be removed with floss. If it's left to linger, it's guaranteed to ruin a first kiss.

To avoid having bacteria constantly reintroduced into your

mouth, replace your tooth-brush frequently. You can also wash your toothbrush in the diswasher to kill bacteria.

Don't leave your tongue out of this. Bacteria left on your tongue can also contribute to less-than-fresh breath, so be sure to brush your tongue after you've polished your pearly whites.

Don't dry out. A dry mouth is another cause of smelly breath. Saliva's natural antibacterial action cleans your mouth and washes away food particles. In fact, the reduced saliva flow we experience at night is to blame for morning breath. Chewing sugarless gum or sucking on sugarless candy can step up your saliva production during the day.

Wash it away. If you just can't get around to brushing between meals, at least rinse your mouth with plain water. Swishing the water around in your mouth may help to remove some of the food parti-cles left after a meal.

Try a natural breath freshener. That green sprig of parsley that came with your meal can do more than just decorate your plate. While munching on parsley or spearmint won't cure bad breath, the scent of the herb itself can temporarily help cover up offending oral odor.

Eat breath-healthy foods. Foods that help fight plaque may also help fight mouth odor. Opt for celery, carrots, peanuts, or a bit of low-fat cheese if you want something to snack on.

---

7 STEPS TO FRESHER BREATH

- Brush your teeth twice a day and floss regularly.
- Use your toothbrush on your tongue after you've finished brushing your teeth.
- Keep your mouth moist with sugarless gum or candy.
- Rinse your mouth out with plain water if you can't get around to brushing between meals.
- Chew on parsley or spearmint after eating.
- Eat plenty of hard, crunchy vegetables to clean teeth when you're hungry for a snack.
- Use mouthwashes that contain fluoride or plaque-fighting ingredients.

Use mouthwash, in a pinch. Mouthwashes do cover odors, dentists agree. However, their effects are short-lived: any-where from 20 minutes to two hours. These products don't prevent bad breath, either. While they may be able to kill bacteria that contribute to bad breath, a new batch of bacteria crops up fairly quickly. If you do decide to use a mouthwash, it's best to choose a product that contains cavity-fighting fluoride or one that is accepted by the American Dental Association for removing plaque.

Sources: **Erwin Barrington, D.D.S.,** Professor of Periodontics, University of Illinois at Chicago, Chicago, Illinois. **Sebastian G. Ciancio, D.D.S.,** Past President, American Academy of Periodontology; Professor and Chairman, Department of Periodontology, Clinical Professor of Pharmacology, Director, Center for Clinical Dental Studies, School of Dental Medicine, State University of New York at Buffalo, Buffalo, New York. **Linda Niessen, D.M.D., M.P.H.,** Associate Professor and Chair, Geriatric Oral Medicine, Department of Community Health and Preventive Dentistry, Baylor College of Dentistry, Dallas, Texas. **Virginia L. Woodward, R.D.H.,** Past President, American Dental Hygienists' Association; Private Practice Clinician, Louisville, Kentucky.

●Bladder Infection

Get Rid of the

Bathroom

Blues

YOU WOKE UP HAVING TO GO—AND GO and go. You're afraid to get more than a few feet from an available bathroom. You feel like you have to go now, but when you do, not much happens and it burns like fire.

If this sounds like what you're experiencing, it's likely you have a bladder infection, also called cystitis, urinary tract infection, or UTI. This condition is usually caused by a bacterial invasion of the bladder and urinary tract. Normally urine in the bladder is sterile, but if it becomes contaminated with bacteria, you can wind up with a painful bladder infection. Some women have cystitis without bacteria present. The bladder is inflamed, or irritated and painful, but no organisms are found.

WARNING!

Untreated bladder infections can spread into the kidneys and cause a serious kidney infection (acute pyelonephritis). Kidney infections cannot be treated at home. They must be treated with antibiotics and often require hospitalization. Call your doctor if you develop these symptoms:
- Mid-back pain on one or both sides
- Groin pain
- Fever
- Chills
- Nausea and vomiting
- Difficult and painful urination

SYMPTOMS

The bacteria in contaminated urine can cause pain or burning during urination, a frequent urge to urinate, and/or blood in the urine. In some cases, bladder infection symptoms can also include fever and back and groin pain. However, a high fever, chills, and one-sided back pain usually indicate that the infection has gone to the kidneys, which demands the immediate attention of a doctor.

CAUSES

Men, women, and children can all get bladder infections. But the odds seem especially high for women. For one thing, the female urethra, the tube leading from the bladder to the outside of the body, is only about one-and-a-half inches long—a short distance for bacteria to travel. (In contrast, a man's urethra is about eight inches long.) Also, in women, the anus and outside openings of the urethra and vagina are so close together that it's easy for bacteria to travel from one to the other.

Sexual intercourse can also cause women to suffer bladder infections more frequently. Because many women contract their first UTIs right after marriage, the term "honeymoon cystitis" has sometimes been used for this condition.

Doctors don't agree about how intercourse may contribute to women's bladder infections. Some believe sexual intercourse helps transport bacteria from the anal area and vagina into the bladder. Others think intercourse may irritate the bladder tissues and make them more "receptive" to infection or inflammation.

Intercourse is not the only factor in bladder infections. They can occur in women of any age, whether or not they are having intercourse. Bladder infections are not unusual in little girls.

Pregnant women often suffer from frequent bladder infections. The changing hormones of pregnancy and the pressure exerted by the enlarged uterus on the bladder and the ureters, the two tubes that carry urine from the kidneys to the bladder, make moms-to-be perfect candidates for UTI.

Bladder infections are usually caused by the normally harmless intestinal bacteria, *Escherichia coli (E. coli)*, needed for digestion. *E. coli* and other bacteria become incorporated into the stool. If the bacteria travels into the bladder, an infection can result. In 10 to 15 percent of cases, bladder infections are caused by another organism, such as *Chlamydia trachomatis*.

AT-HOME TREATMENT

Bladder inflammation can sometimes be treated at home with the self-care tips that follow. However, if your symptoms are severe and persist for more than 24 hours, if they don't respond to home remedies, if you have a fever, or if you suspect your symptoms may be due to a sexually transmitted disease or other infection, see your doctor.

Bottoms up. At the first sign of bladder discomfort, begin drinking water and don't stop. During the first 24 hours, drink at least one eight-ounce glass of water every hour. The water will wash out some of the bacteria and dilute the urine, thus making it less hospitable for bacteria. Be careful about increasing your fluids if you suffer from urinary leakage, however; it can make both your infection and your incontinence worse.

Try baking soda. Some women experience greater relief if they add a teaspoon of baking soda (sodium bicarbonate or bicar-

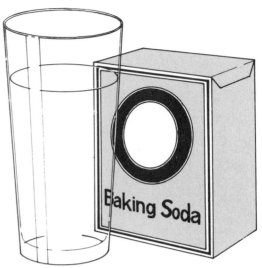

bonate of soda) to each glass of water. The soda counteracts the acidity of the urine. (Don't use baking soda if you're on a salt- or sodium-restricted diet, and don't use it for extended periods of time.)

Warm it up. Take hot baths or use a hot water bottle or heating pad for lower abdominal pain. The heat will relieve symptoms. (Pregnant women should not sit in a hot bath or hot tub for too long, since raising the body temperature above 100 degrees Fahrenheit for long periods may cause birth defects or miscarriage.)

Sitz it. Sitting in a warm sitz bath can ease the discomfort. Fill the bathtub with three or four inches of water and soak.

Take a load off. A bladder infection can make you feel lousy. Take the opportunity to rest in bed and conserve your energy.

Lay off the caffeine. The caffeine in tea, coffee, and cola stimulates the kidneys and makes the bladder fill up faster during a time when it's painful to urinate. If caffeine seems to make your bladder pain worse, lay off until the problem clears up.

Ease the pain. Bladder infections can be painful. Acetaminophen, ibuprofen, or aspirin, especially if taken before bedtime, can ease your discomfort.

5 Tips for Taking Care of it at Home

- Drink eight ounces of water every hour.
- Add baking soda to your drinking water.
- Use hot pads or hot baths.
- Take a sitz bath.
- Rest in bed.

At the Doctor's

Not all bladder discomfort can be self-treated. You should see your doctor if you have unusual pain or vaginal discharge or if you have any of the following:

- Your bladder symptoms don't respond to home remedies within 24 hours.
- You have symptoms and fever that increase after 24 hours of home treatment.
- You are diabetic.
- You have a personal history of kidney problems.
- You develop shaking spells or have vomited within the last 12 hours.
- You have blood in your urine.
- You have had an abdominal or back injury within the last two weeks prior to the onset of your symptoms (may indicate kidney injury).
- You have high blood pressure.
- You have or suspect you may have a sexually transmitted disease.

Your doctor will likely want to do a urine analysis and urine culture. He or she will ask you to get a "midstream catch" urine sample, which will then be examined for bacteria and large numbers of white blood cells. In a few cases, the doctor may want to take the urine specimen with a catheter to ensure an uncontaminated sample.

In difficult or chronic cases of bladder infection, the physician may want to take special X rays to find out if something is blocking the bladder or urethra during urination. Sometimes a lighted, flexible tube (cystoscope) is used to examine the bladder.

Oral antibiotics are usually effective against bladder infections. Recurrent bladder infections may require larger doses or longer-term medication (four to six weeks). It's important that you take the entire course of the drug, even after symptoms have stopped. If you're susceptible to yeast infections after taking antibiotics, eat live-culture *(Lactobacillus acidophilus)* yogurt to help replenish helpful bacteria, and if necessary, use an over-the-counter yeast medication such as miconazole (Monistat) or clotrimazole (Gyne-Lotrimin).

Black women should not take sulfa antibiotics, which are frequently used to treat UTIs, until they've been tested for G6PD deficiency. About 10 percent of blacks have this hereditary deficiency and should not take sulfa drugs.

If you use the preventive tips outlined in this chapter and you still have chronic or persistent bladder infections, talk with your doctor about possible physical causes. You may have an anatomic defect, such as a narrowed urethra. Or kidney stones may be present, which can be removed. If no anatomic problems are discovered, talk with your doctor about using low-dose antibiotics as a preventive measure. If your infections follow intercourse, talk to your doctor about using antibiotics as preventative therapy.

PREVENTION

The best news about bladder infections is that with a few simple lifestyle changes, you may be able to avoid getting one in the first place.

Let go. Studies have confirmed that women are notorious for not going to the bathroom when they first feel the urge. You know how it is: The boss wants the report by this afternoon, your phone hasn't stopped ringing, and you're already late for your first appointment. You don't have time to go to the bathroom.

Holding urine allows it to concentrate in the bladder and creates a perfect place for bacteria to grow. Over time, not going when you feel the urge can cause chronic infections and leakage (incontinence) problems. The bladder, which is a hollow muscle, distends and stretches when it's filled with urine. If you repeatedly stretch it, it won't empty completely and can become a breeding ground for bacteria. Repeated stretching can also damage the muscles that allow you to shut off the urine stream completely and may leave you facing the prospect of wearing adult diapers to control leakage.

When you feel the urge, go. Even if you don't feel the urge, go anyway. Make sure you urinate every two or three hours.

Go for the H$_2$O. Drinking plenty of water is generally good for your health, but when it comes to preventing bladder infections, it's essential. Water dilutes the urine, which gives the bacteria less nourishment. Drink eight to ten 8-ounce glasses of water every day.

Keep it clean. Wash your vaginal and anal areas frequently with a mild soap. Avoid perfumed, deodorant soaps that can irritate tender skin. Ask your partner to wash thoroughly before sex, too.

Wipe from front to back. Wiping away from the urethra can dramatically reduce the incidence of bladder infections.

Bring on the cranberry. Research shows that drinking cranberry juice, an old-time bladder infection remedy, actually works best preventively. It acidifies the urine, making it less friendly to bacterial growth, and it appears to interfere with the bacteria's ability to attach to the wall of the bladder. Try to drink two to four glasses of cranberry juice daily. You might try alternating cranberry juice with baking soda diluted in water every two to three days, making the urine more and then less acidic. This may kill bacteria.

Stay loose. Restrictive, tight-fitting clothing like leotards tends to trap heat and promote bacterial growth. Opt instead for comfortable, loose-fitting clothing that allows air circulation.

Go with cotton. Wear cotton underwear, which is less irritating and "breathes."

Reconsider your birth control. If you use a diaphragm and are bothered by frequent bladder infections, check with your doctor about switching to a smaller size or to another brand of diaphragm or trying another form of birth control.

---

9 WAYS TO PREVENT BLADDER INFECTION

- Drink plenty of water.
- Keep your vaginal and anal areas clean.
- Wipe from front to back.
- Wear loose-fitting clothing.
- Choose cotton underwear.
- Check into alternative birth control.
- Empty your bladder after intercourse.
- Avoid intercourse during menstruation.
- Change tampons/napkins frequently.

Empty your bladder after intercourse. Right after intercourse, empty your bladder and wipe off the moisture from front to back. This can help wash out any bacteria that might have entered the urethra.

Be a creative lover. For some women, intercourse, particularly during menstruation, may precipitate bladder infections. During the friction of sex, blood can enter the urethra, allowing bacteria to multiply rapidly. For other women, intercourse appears to trauma-

tize the urethra and disrupt its lining, making it more susceptible to infection.

There are plenty of ways to pleasure one another besides sexual intercourse. If it causes bladder problems, avoid intercourse during menstruation and explore other lovemaking options.

Change tampons/napkins. Blood makes an excellent growth medium for bacteria. Therefore, during your menstrual period, change your tampons and/or napkins frequently.

Track your infections. Keep a bladder-infection diary, noting the patterns that precede an attack. Some women find their bladder infections are related to stress, intercourse, menstruation, or other factors. Discover what brings on your bladder infections.

Avoid caffeine and alcohol. Alcohol is a bladder irritant and caffeine is a bladder stimulant. If you are prone to bladder infections, you're better off avoiding both these beverages, or at least keeping your consumption to a minimum.

Sources: **Amanda Clark, M.D.,** Assistant Professor, Department of Obstetrics and Gynecology, Oregon Health Sciences University, Portland, Oregon. **Sadja Greenwood, M.D.,** Assistant Clinical Professor, Department of Obstetrics, Gynecology, and Reproductive Sciences, University of California at San Francisco, San Francisco, California. **Theodore Lehman, M.D.,** Associate Clinical Professor of Surgery (Urology), Oregon Health Sciences University; Director, The Oregon Impotence Center, Portland, Oregon. **Anne Simons, M.D.,** Coauthor, *Before You Call the Doctor;* Family Practitioner, San Francisco Department of Public Health; Family Practitioner and Assistant Clinical Professor, Family and Community Medicine, University of California San Francisco Medical Center, San Francisco, California.

How could something so tiny be such a pain in the foot? But you just couldn't resist a bargain. After all, they were Italian leather, and they were half-price. This morning they felt a little tight when you put them on, but you figured they would stretch out as the day went on. How can you break in your new shoes if you don't wear them? Now it's midafternoon and you're wondering how your poor feet are going to get you through the rest of the day. Your beautiful new shoes have given you a couple of painful blisters. Now you're cursing the designer as you limp down the hallway to your next meeting.

CAUSES

Blisters are tender spots that fill up with fluid released by tiny blood vessels in an area where delicate skin tissues have been burned, pinched, or just irritated. Virtually everyone has experienced friction blisters, the kind caused by hot, sweaty, or ill-fitting shoes. If you have one now, read on to find out how to take care of it. Then go on reading to learn how you can help protect your precious feet in the future.

AT-HOME TREATMENT

The following tips will protect your blister and set it firmly on the road to healing:

Give it some space. Instead of simply placing an adhesive bandage directly on the blister's surface, "tent" the bandage by bringing in its sides so the padding in the middle of the bandage raises up a bit. This will not only protect the blister but allow air to circulate, which will aid in healing.

Medicate it. A special type of bandage, available in pharmacies, contains a gel and antiseptic to cushion and "clean" the blister. These may work better than run-of-the-mill bandages. Ask your pharmacist about them.

Let the air in. Some physicians believe that a blister should not be covered at all, to allow for maximum aeration. If you don't have shoes that leave the blistered area uncovered, try slipping your shoe off while you sit at your desk at work.

Take steps to prevent infection. Regardless of whether your blister is covered or not, you should apply an antibacterial/antibiotic ointment to it several times a day. Doctors generally recommend Bacitracin or Polysporin. These varieties may be less likely than other over-the-counter ointments to cause an allergic reaction or irritation.

Cushion the blow. If a bandage just isn't enough to stop the pain, you may want to cover the tender area with a pad, which provides more of a cushion. A good choice is to use circular pads of foam adhesive, which can be found in the foot-care aisle of drug and beauty-aids stores. Pharmacies also carry sheets of padding that you can cut to size for a more exact fit. Cut the padding in the shape of a doughnut, and place it on the skin surrounding the blister so that the blister fits in the

11 WAYS TO TREAT A BLISTER

- Tent a bandage by bringing in its sides so the padding in the middle of the bandage raises up a bit.
- Try medicated bandages made specifically for blisters.
- Expose the blister to air.
- Apply antibacterial/antibiotic ointment to the blister several times a day.
- Apply foam to the blister.
- Elevate the blistered area.
- Use a sewing needle sterilized in alcohol to drain blisters that cause extreme pressure.
- Do not remove the skin from the top of a popped blister.
- Soak tough-skinned areas in Burow's solution before draining blisters that have developed there.
- Watch for signs of infection.
- Use patience in waiting for the blister to heal.

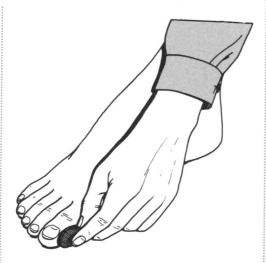

hole of the doughnut. Then gently cover the blister with an antibacterial ointment and a bandage.

Put your feet up. Elevating a blistered area may temporarily relieve the pressure.

Pop it. Many doctors believe that a blister should never be drained, because of the risk of infection presented when the skin is broken. However, most experts do concede that a blister causing extreme pressure may benefit from being drained. Blisters that may be especially likely to cause pressure are those located on the fingers or toes or under a nail.

If you decide to pop your blister, use a sewing needle that has been sterilized with rubbing alcohol. Never use a needle that has been sterilized over a flame, since the soot on the tip of the needle can tattoo, or dirty, the blister's surface. Next, wipe the skin with alcohol and prick the blister once or twice near its edge. Slowly and gently press out the fluid.

Avoid overexposure. Once you have popped the blister and drained the fluid, do not remove the deflated top layer of skin. This skin protects the blister from infection and helps new cells move in to heal the site. Also, since the outer skin protects the tender area underneath from friction and injury, removing it will probably make the blister hurt even more.

Soften it up. To drain a blister on a tough-skinned area, such as on the sole of the foot, it's best to start by soaking the blister in Burow's solution, which is available from pharmacies in packets or tablets (follow the directions on the package). Soaking the blister for 15 minutes, three to four times a day, will soften it and make draining easier. A day or two of this should be sufficient.

Keep an eye on it. Be watchful for signs of infection in an intact or drained blister. If you notice any redness, red streaks, or pus, contact your physician.

Wait it out. As the old adage goes, time heals all wounds. You can expect the blister's fluid to be reabsorbed by the body in about a week to ten days. With any luck, the pain will go away in less time than that.

PREVENTION

Once your blister feels better, it's wise to adopt strategies to keep it from recurring. The following tips will help you to do just that.

Skip the morning shoe shopping. Since one of the principal causes of friction blisters is a shoe that is too tight or that doesn't fit properly, take steps to ensure that you buy shoes with plenty of breathing room. Since your feet may swell by as much as half a shoe size over the course of a day, shop for shoes late in the day.

Come prepared. Make sure that the shoes you are buying will have room for the socks you plan to wear with them. Bring a pair with you when you shop.

Go one step further. Your feet will spread out more when you walk on cement or tiled floors than when you walk on carpeted floors. If the shoe store you shop in is carpeted, you may be prevented from accurately gauging a shoe's fit. Here's a veteran shoe-buyer's tip: Ask the salesperson if you can take a few steps behind the counter or in the back room, if either area is uncarpeted.

Choose leather. Unlike nonporous vinyl and plastic materials, leather has microscopic pores that allow air to circulate, keeping the foot drier. The clusters of perforated holes found on many styles of sports footwear promote the same effect. A dry foot is less likely to develop blisters. Another advantage of leather: It stretches and softens with time.

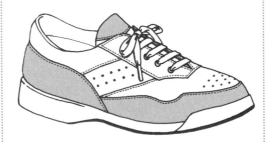

Don't risk it, first time out. Ideally, a shoe should feel comfortable when you try it on. Often, however, new shoes have stiff areas that take time to soften up. Resist the temptation to take off for work in a brand-new pair. Instead, break them in gradually. One way to do this is to wear the new shoes for limited amounts of time, switching to your old pair of shoes in between.

Take the heat off. The heat of midday, especially in the summer, can cause feet to perspire more, making them more prone to developing blisters.

Keep it dry. One cardinal rule in blister prevention is: Never wear wet shoes. The moisture can cause more "dragging" between the foot and the shoe, resulting in a friction blister. If you jog twice a day, for instance, you may want to buy a second pair of running shoes for your second run.

Anticipate and protect danger zones. If you have a chronic hot spot—a place where blisters often develop—apply petroleum jelly to the area before putting on your sock. Foam or felt pads, without the jelly, can also absorb the friction and protect problem areas. For best results, make sure the padding covers the entire danger zone, since the irritation may occur in a larger area than you anticipate.

Invest in padded socks. There are a number of socks on the mar-

ket that sport extra padding in certain spots, such as the toe, the heel, or the arch. Choose socks that provide cushioning in the areas where you often develop blisters.

Choose socks that let your feet breathe. Natural fibers, such as cotton and wool, tend to keep the feet dry by absorbing moisture. However, recent research suggests that acrylic fibers may, through a wicking action, actually move moisture away from the foot, keeping it drier and making it less prone to blistering. Your best bet is to try them both and see which type of fiber keeps your feet drier and more comfortable.

Size your socks. Make sure that you buy a sock that fits your foot well to reduce the chances of it bunching up inside the shoe and causing a blister. Also, cotton and wool socks can stretch out with wear, making them looser and more likely to slip inside the shoe. If this is a recurrent problem for you, switch to acrylic socks.

Take a powder. Foot powders may aid in keeping the foot dry and preventing painful blisters.

Sources: **Wilma Bergfeld, M.D., F.A.C.P.,** Head, Clinical Research, Department of Dermatology, Cleveland Clinic Foundation, Cleveland, Ohio. **Glenn B. Gastwirth, D.P.M.,** Deputy Executive Director, American Podiatric Medical Association, Bethesda, Maryland. **Jerome Z. Litt, M.D.,** Author, *Your Skin: From Acne to Zits;* Assistant Clinical Professor of Dermatology, Case Western Reserve School of Medicine, Cleveland, Ohio. **Nelson Lee Novick, M.D.,** Author, *Super Skin: A Leading Dermatologist's Guide to the Latest Breakthroughs in Skin Care;* Associate Clinical Professor of Dermatology, Mount Sinai School of Medicine, New York, New York.

12 WAYS TO KEEP BLISTERS AT BAY

- Shop for shoes in the afternoon.
- Bring the appropriate socks or hosiery with you when you shop for shoes.
- When buying shoes, try them out on a hard, uncarpeted floor.
- Buy only leather shoes and sport shoes that have tiny holes for ventilation.
- Break in shoes gradually.
- Don't exercise in the afternoon.
- Don't wear wet shoes.
- Apply foam or petroleum jelly to areas where blisters chronically develop.
- Buy padded sport socks.
- Buy socks that absorb or wick moisture away from your feet.
- Make sure socks fit well.
- Try using foot powder to help keep feet dry and blister free.

How to Keep

Undesirable

Scent at Bay

BODY ODOR IS NOT EXACTLY A TOPIC OF polite conversation, but it doesn't have to be. If you've got it, you know it. You're also probably eager to get rid of it.

In some cultures and countries, intense body odor is considered to be a desirable characteristic, signifying sexual attractiveness and potency. But let's face it, here in the U.S.A. a pungent aroma emanating from your armpits is not going to make you the life of the party. So powerful is our cultural distaste for body odor that every day, some 95 percent of all Americans over the age of 12 reach for one product or another that will enable them to feel safe in the company of others.

CAUSES

Body odor begins with sweat. The body has two types of sweat glands, both of which produce sweat that is made up largely of water. The eccrine glands, which are located on almost every part of the body, produce sweat that cools the body. The apocrine glands, which are located in the armpits, around the nipples, and in the groin, produce sweat whose function is unclear. However, one characteristic of the apocrine glands' sweat does not need any scientific probing to be brought to light—its smell. This is the sweat that makes you smell, well—overly fragrant. The reason for its pungency is that apocrine sweat contains a substantial amount of oil, which provides food for bacteria. It's this bacterial feeding frenzy that causes unwelcome odor.

AT-HOME TREATMENT

The following tips are sure to have you smelling like roses in no time:

Become a clean machine. The strength of the odor a person produces depends on how much sweat that person's glands secrete, combined with the number of bacteria present on the skin. In fact, people with strong underarm odors carry two to three times more underarm bacteria than do those who have a less-intense aroma.

You can control the odor by washing the area frequently. Washing eliminates the sweat that forms near the apocrine glands and reduces the number of bacteria waiting to feed on it. The underarm and groin areas are prime candidates for a frequent once-over with soap (a deodorant soap is your best bet) and water. Once a day is the bare-bones minimum; feel free to wash more often, if necessary.

Tame your laundry. The smell of sweat that seeps into your clothing may come back to haunt you (and others) at inopportune moments. Bacteria-containing sweat can also harm your clothing if it is left to dry into the fibers. Good advice is to wash your clothing after each wearing.

Deodorize. A good deodorant may be sufficient to counteract a minor case of body odor. The Food and Drug Administration (FDA) considers deodorants to be

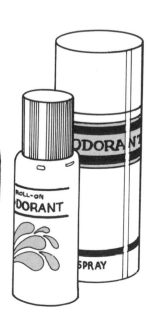

5 DEODORIZING TIPS

- Wash problem areas frequently—at least once a day.
- Wash your clothing after each wearing.
- Try a deodorant. If that doesn't seem to eliminate the problem, buy some antiperspirant.
- If antiperspirants and deodorants irritate your skin, try using an antibacterial soap, antibiotic ointment, baking soda, or talcum powder.
- Eliminate sweat- and odor-producing foods from your diet.

cosmetics, not drugs, unlike antiperspirants. Deodorants work in two ways: They contain a substance to kill some of the bacteria that feed on your sweat, and they mask the unpleasant odor with a scent of their own.

Go one step further. If your deodorant just doesn't cut it, an antiperspirant is the next logical weapon in your war against smell. Antiperspirants seek to control the odor by controlling the amount you sweat. Experts say that an antiperspirant can reduce the amount you perspire by as much as 50 percent.

The FDA classifies antiperspirants as over-the-counter drugs, because they are designed to alter a natural body function, namely, the amount of eccrine sweat we produce. (Actually, apocrine sweat is what contains the oil upon which bacteria feed, but neither an antiperspirant nor a deodorant can decrease apocrine sweat production.) By reducing eccrine sweat production, antiperspirants reduce the moisture that is vital to the breeding of bacteria. Antiperspirants usually also have an antibacterial agent, for additional protection. (For more tips on choosing an antiperspirant and staying dry, see Excessive Perspiration.)

Try washing with antibacterial soap. Antiperspirants and deodorants may cause skin irritation. If you have a sensitivity to them, try using an antibacterial soap, such as chlorhexidine (Hibiclens), or an over-the-counter antibiotic ointment. Talcum powder and baking soda are also effective wetness and odor fighters that won't irritate the skin.

Avoid sweat- and odor-producing foods. Your diet can affect your body odor in two ways. Some spicy foods, such as hot peppers, can cause you to perspire more, adding to the existing problem. Other pungent foods, such as garlic, can actually be carried by your sweat, complicating matters with extra, unwanted aromas. If you're concerned about body odor and don't mind making a few sacrifices, consume only minimum amounts of onions, garlic, hot spices, and beer, and avoid excessive doses of vitamins.

Sources: **Allan L. Lorincz, M.D.,** Professor of Dermatology, University of Chicago Medical Center, Chicago, Illinois. **Donald Rudikoff, M.D.,** Assistant Clinical Professor of Dermatology, Mount Sinai School of Medicine, New York, New York. **Alan Shalita, M.D.,** Chairman, Department of Dermatology, State University of New York Health Science Center at Brooklyn, Brooklyn, New York.

•BREAST DISCOMFORT

Soothing

Strategies to

Ease the Pain

BREASTS REPRESENT MANY THINGS TO women: feminine identity, sensual pleasure, maternal bonding with breast-feeding babies. But there are times when our breasts can become sources of discomfort, pain, worry, and anxiety.

If you suffer from breast pain and discomfort, you're not alone. Most women experience breast soreness, tenderness, or pain at some time. Breast discomfort is a normal part of being a woman. The best news is that breast discomfort is rarely a sign of breast cancer and many home care remedies are available to provide relief.

CAUSES

The breasts are highly sensitive mammary glands that can respond with swelling, tenderness, soreness, or pain to a woman's normal hormonal changes, especially changes in estrogen levels. Most women experience these kinds of breast changes in association with menstruation, pregnancy, and menopause. In addition, some women suffer from a fibrocystic breast condition, or "lumpy breasts," that can be a source of discomfort.

Menstruation. Each month, a woman's body undergoes major shifts in the reproductive hormones, estrogen and progesterone, as the body prepares for a possible pregnancy. These changes in hormones can cause the breasts to become engorged, swollen, and tender. For most women, these breast changes occur premenstrually, days before the onset of menstrual blood.

Pregnancy. During pregnancy, the hormonal shifts that begin before menstruation continue and the mammary glands develop in antici-

pation of milk production. While many moms-to-be fantasize about the miracle of breast-feeding their newborns, often the reality of lactating breasts can be uncomfortable. Sometimes mother's milk comes in too early or too heavily and causes a painful condition called engorgement. Some breast-feeding mothers develop sore, cracked, and bleeding nipples. (Rest assured, these problems are temporary.) Milk ducts can become backed up, leading to a painful breast infection that's called mastitis.

Menopause. Many women believe breast discomfort ends with fertility and that with menopause, they will no longer have to worry about

---

WARNING!

While some causes of breast discomfort can be effectively treated at home, see your doctor if you have any of the following symptoms:
• A lump or firmness
• Soreness in only one breast (nonlactating breasts)
• Any nipple discharge in a nonlactating woman
• Any nonhealing redness or sore on the breasts
• A change in your breast self-exam
• Nipple discharge on one side (Lactating breasts may secrete white/yellow discharge for up to a year after nursing is discontinued.)

---

painful, swollen, tender, premenstrual breasts.

Normally, estrogen levels drop off dramatically at menopause. But today, many women opt for hormone therapy to reduce menopausal symptoms such as hot flashes and to reduce their risk of developing the bone-thinning disease osteoporosis. Since each woman's body is unique, it often takes some time for physicians to determine just the right combination and dosage of hormones for each woman. It is during this transition period that many menopausal women experience breast discomfort.

Fibrocystic Breast Condition. A source of breast discomfort for many women is a common condition called fibrocystic breast disease, known more commonly as "lumpy breasts." Fibrocystic breasts are really just a normal variation in breast tissue. All women's breasts are somewhat lumpy. If you feel your own breast tissue, the tissue around structures like the mammary glands should feel granular, like a sack filled with small pebbles. In some women, many of these "pebbles" are larger. In fact, it's estimated that more than half of all women have some degree of breast lumpiness, and at least one-third of women suffer from fibrocystic breasts. Many of these women experience intense breast swelling, tenderness, and lumpiness a week or two before their menstrual periods. In some women, these noncancerous (benign) lumps are temporary and may appear and then disappear for no apparent reason. Others develop lumps that stay with them throughout their childbearing years.

No one knows exactly what causes fibrocystic breasts, although some researchers believe that the condition may be inherited. For reasons not yet understood, fibrocystic breasts are more common in women who have never breast-fed a child.

Most women with fibrocystic breasts need not fear an increased risk of breast cancer. Only one subcategory of fibrocystic breast condition, duct hyperplasia, is associated with increased risk of cancer.

Fibrocystic breast lumps can, however, make it more difficult to detect new, possibly dangerous growths. Women with fibrocystic breasts have one or more of these three types:

Fibrosis. With fibrosis, the connective tissue that supports the milk glands thickens and becomes quite fibrous. This condition may or may not be painful. Sometimes it is accompanied by cysts.

Cysts. The breast's milk ducts become blocked by an overgrowth of the surrounding tissue and can't drain properly. The blocked ducts swell into tender, fluid-filled cysts that can be tiny or quite large.

Duct Hyperplasia. This is the only type of fibrocystic breast condition that may increase the risk of breast cancer. The lining of the ducts that carry milk to the nipples becomes overgrown. To diagnose this condition, it's necessary to have a biopsy.

AT-HOME TREATMENT

None of us can escape the normal hormonal fluctuations that cause our breasts to undergo sometimes painful changes. We can, however, use self-care strategies to make ourselves more comfortable.

Start with BSE. One of the most important reasons for doing regular breast self-exams (BSE) is to become familiar with what your breasts ordinarily feel like, what your degree of lumpiness is, and how it may change during your menstrual cycle. If you do this month after month, year after year, your fingers will become familiar with your breast tissue, and you are more likely to notice any changes.

While breast cancer rarely causes pain, tenderness, or soreness, if you suddenly develop these symptoms, a breast self-exam is a good place to start to ensure you haven't developed any suspicious lumps. Remember that 90 percent of women's breast lumps are found by the woman or her lover, not by her physician. The best time to examine your breasts is during the week following your menstrual period. A monthly BSE is recommended, but a self-exam is warranted any time you notice changes in your breasts. If you don't know how to do a breast self-exam or if you're unsure whether you're doing it properly, talk with your doctor.

1. Conduct a visual exam. Stand with your arms at your sides and look at your breasts. Are there any noticeable bulges, wrinkles, or dimpling? Bring your arms over your head and then bend at the waist and look for the same changes. Squeeze each nipple gently. Is there any discharge?

2. Conduct a manual exam. Lie with a pillow under one shoulder to flatten and elevate the breast. Using the opposite hand, flatten the fingers, and starting at the armpit, use small, circular patterns to examine the entire breast to the center of the chest. Then examine the opposite breast.

If you discover any changes, report them to your doctor without delay. Remember that most breast lumps are benign (noncancerous). For lumps that are cancerous, early detection and treatment are important.

14 WAYS TO EASE PAINFUL BREASTS

- **Do a monthly breast self-exam.**
- **Have a pregnancy test if your period is late.**
- **Wear a comfortable, supportive bra.**
- **Eliminate caffeine.**
- **Cut down on salt.**
- **Apply hot and cold packs.**
- **Stay within healthful weight range.**
- **Exercise regularly.**
- **Try vitamin/mineral supplementation for premenstrual or birth-control-induced soreness.**
- **Cut dietary fat.**
- **Quit cigarette smoking.**
- **Try aspirin, ibuprofen, or acetaminophen for pain.**
- **Use natural rather than prescription diuretics.**
- **Check your cosmetics.**

Test for pregnancy. If you experience breast changes such as tenderness and swelling and there's any possibility you might be pregnant, get tested as soon as possible. If you are pregnant, it's important that you begin proper prenatal care immediately.

Nix the caffeine. Research is mixed on whether or not eliminating caffeine helps lumpy, fibrocystic breasts. One study conducted by the National Institutes of Health found no relationship between caffeine consumption and breast lumps. On the other hand, some women have found that cutting out caffeinated coffees, teas, colas, and chocolate has a positive effect on fibrocystic breasts. If you suffer from lumpy breasts, try eliminating caffeine and see if your breast discomfort decreases.

Slow down on salt. Some women have problems with fluid retention premenstrually. If your breasts become swollen, try cutting down on salt to minimize fluid retention.

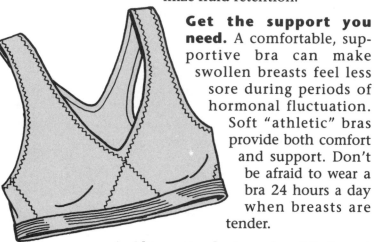

Get the support you need. A comfortable, supportive bra can make swollen breasts feel less sore during periods of hormonal fluctuation. Soft "athletic" bras provide both comfort and support. Don't be afraid to wear a bra 24 hours a day when breasts are tender.

Alternate hot and cold. Breast pain can be minimized in some women by alternating warm heating pads with ice packs. Apply the heat for 30 minutes, then ice for 10 minutes. Repeat as often as needed.

Keep off the excess weight. In women, body fat is the producer and storehouse of estrogen. Being excessively overweight can predispose you to fibrocystic breasts.

Exercise regularly. Aerobic exercise helps release endorphins, the body's natural pain relievers.

Try vitamin and mineral supplements. If your breast discomfort arises premenstrually or is caused by taking birth control pills, consider looking into the "PMS formula" vitamin and mineral supplements offered by vitamin companies. While research is still scanty on supplements and PMS breast dis-comfort, some women say they've been helped by vitamin B$_6$, magnesium, B-complex, vitamin C, and vitamin E. Keep in mind that vitamin B$_6$ can be toxic if taken in doses that are too high. Before taking any B$_6$ supplements, consult your doctor about the correct dosage for you, and take it in conjunction with other B vitamins.

Don't experiment with vitamin or mineral supplements if you're pregnant or breast-feeding. You should be sure to talk with your physician before taking any supplement or medication, even over-the-counter drugs.

Forego the "water pills." Some women take "water pills," diuretics, to reduce fluid retention. While diuretics can help flush excess fluids from the body and reduce breast swelling, over time they can also deplete your stores of potassium, unbalance your electrolyte system, and interfere with glucose production. Instead, try eating a diet high in natural diuretics such as parsley, cucumbers, cabbage, and teas like nettle, juniper, dandelion, and sarsaparilla. (Pregnant women should discuss any herbal tea with their physician before using.)

Kick the nicotine habit. If you smoke cigarettes, quit. Some researchers believe that nicotine stimulates fibrous tissue growth and the buildup of cyst-causing estrogen.

Try OTC pain relievers. Aspirin, ibuprofen, or acetaminophen can ease the pain of premenstrual breasts. If your problem is fibrocystic disease, try ibuprofen for pain relief. Pregnant or breast-feeding mothers should always talk with their doctor before taking any medications, including over-the-counter drugs.

Go low-fat. A high-fat diet, especially one high in saturated fats such as those found in meat, butter, lard, and coconut and palm oils, promotes the secretion of hormones that stimulate breast tissue growth. Eat a lower fat diet that contains plenty of whole grains, legumes, rice, and fresh fruits and vegetables. This diet will also promote your general health.

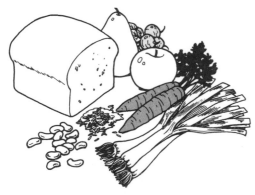

Watch those cosmetics. Some herbal cosmetics and remedies, such as those made with ginseng, can have steroidal effects similar to estrogen. If you're using such a product, try stopping for a time. Then, if you find that your breast condition improves, consider switching to another type of cosmetic.

BREAST CARE FOR NURSING MOTHERS

Toughen up. During the final weeks of your pregnancy, you can "toughen" your nipples and get them ready for breast-feeding by massaging them between the thumb and forefinger or by rubbing them with a bath towel. Exposing nipples to the air tends to toughen them, too.

Once you begin nursing, keep your nursing bra flaps open or go braless, if it's comfortable, especially after feeding. If you immediately put on your bra and nursing pads after nursing, you'll probably have some leakage and the pad will hold the moisture against the nipple, which softens it. Opt for disposable paper or washable liners instead of plastic ones that can cause irritation or even nipple infection.

Check the baby connection. Often, breast-feeding mothers experience nipple soreness because the baby is "latched on" at the very end of the nipple and the baby's gums mash tender tissues. The key is to get the baby to close down on the areola (the darkened area around the nipple) rather than on the nipple itself. Get the baby's mouth open wide, lift your breast from underneath, and pull the baby in close as quickly as possible. If you bring her toward the breast too slowly, she will clamp down as soon as her lips touch the nipple. If you feel general tenderness or a sharp pain when the baby latches on, she's latched on incorrectly and you'll need to reposition her in order to nurse without pain.

Take tea. Another way to toughen and condition breasts for nursing is to apply black-tea bags to the nipples. Dip the tea bags in boiling water, let them cool, and apply them directly to the nipples. The tannin in the tea toughens the nipple tissue.

Once you've started nursing, warm black-tea bags placed on the nipples can soothe sore nipples. Soak the tea bags in hot water for a few minutes, squeeze them out, and apply.

Prop up. The baby tugging on the nipple during breast-feeding causes irritation. To minimize the downward tugging on the breast, lift the baby up by placing her on a pillow on your lap during breast-feeding.

Start slowly. While the first few times you breast-feed your child can be very exciting, it can also be hard on your breasts. Expect discomfort in the first few days. You can try limiting each nursing time to five minutes, but you may then have to nurse very often.

Let 'em nurse. Once your milk comes in, which can occur any time from two to five days after you give birth, let your baby nurse at will for as long as he or she wants. Most babies go through a marathon nursing period at this time. It's fine to let the baby nurse constantly for a few days.

One of the advantages of letting the baby nurse at will during initial engorgement is that the baby siphons off the excess milk. Most mothers' breasts produce enough milk for twins before readjusting the amount for just one baby. If you only allow the baby to nurse every three to four hours, the milk will come in and painfully engorge the breasts for the first 36 to 48 hours.

Nix the pump. If your breasts do become engorged, don't use a manual breast pump. The body can't tell the difference between a breast pump and a baby. If you pump out the excess milk, the body will simply produce more milk.

Of course, you may need to use a breast pump if you have to go on a trip away from your nursing baby and plan to continue nursing regularly when you return, or if your baby becomes ill and loses her appetite. In those cases, the pump will help keep your normal milk supply flowing.

Try warm water. To help reduce the pressure from the breasts, stand under a warm shower and let the water hit your breasts. Or stand over a sink filled with warm water and splash the water onto them.

Skip the soap. Keep your lactating breasts clean with warm water, but forego soap. All soaps are drying and can promote nipple cracking.

Strap on an "ice chest." If painful engorgement is a problem, try filling your bra with ice between feedings. For a more comfortable ice pack, try a bag of frozen peas, which will mold to the shape of the breasts.

Warm up before feeding. Having a baby latch onto an empty nipple can be quite painful. To stimulate the milk flow for nursing, 15 minutes before feeding, take a hot shower or soak a bath towel in hot water, wring it out, and place it across your breasts with a plastic bag on top to keep it warm.

Switch breasts. If you've developed a sore nipple on one side, start feeding on the sore side first, but switch to the other breast after about five minutes, burping the baby in between. Keep switching until the baby is finished eating. This will ensure the baby drains both breasts evenly, rather than leaving one full and one drained.

Ice 'em. For temporary sore-nipple relief, apply ice to the nipples.

Try OTC pain relievers. If you develop a low-grade fever (100.2 to 100.6 degrees Fahrenheit), take acetaminophen to lower it. If you feel achy, ibuprofen can relieve the aches and discomfort. But remember, always check with your doctor before taking any over-the-counter medication while you are nursing. If your fever is persistent, call the doctor.

Strap 'em up. Not every mother can or wants to breast-feed her baby. Non-nursing mothers must wait until their breast milk dries up for engorgement to subside. For temporary relief, wear a tight bra or wrap a towel

---

13 SOOTHING STEPS FOR LACTATING BREASTS

- Toughen nipples.
- Ensure baby is "latched on" properly.
- Start nursing slowly.
- During initial engorgement, breast-feed frequently.
- Don't pump milk from breasts.
- Stand in a hot shower.
- Avoid using soap on nipples.
- Wear a bra full of ice.
- Massage nipples with ice.
- Warm your breasts before nursing.
- Alternate breasts often during feedings.
- Try over-the-counter pain relievers.
- Use pressure/ice/aspirin to reduce milk supply.

---

or Ace bandage around your breasts. The pressure decreases the milk supply because it collapses the milk glands so they can't hold as much milk.

Applying ice packs and taking aspirin can also reduce the engorgement and swelling. Apply the ice pack for 20 minutes; remove it for ten before reapplying it.

Sources: Amanda Clark, M.D., Assistant Professor of Obstetrics and Gynecology, Oregon Health Sciences University, Portland, Oregon. **Raven Fox, R.N., I.B.C.L.C.,** Registered Nurse and Lactation Consultant, Evergreen Hospital and Medical Center, Kirkland, Washington. **Phyllis Frey, A.R.N.P.,** Nurse Practitioner, Bellevue, Washington. **Sadja Greenwood, M.D.,** Assistant Clinical Professor, Department of Obstetrics, Gynecology, and Reproductive Services, University of California at San Francisco, San Francisco, California. **Deborah Purcell, M.D.,** Past Chair, Department of Pediatrics, St. Vincent Hospital and Medical Center, Portland, Oregon. **Anne Simons, M.D.,** Coauthor, *Before You Call the Doctor;* Family Practitioner, San Francisco Department of Public Health; Family Practitioner and Assistant Clinical Professor, Family and Community Medicine, University of California San Francisco Medical Center, San Francisco, California. **Harold Zimmer, M.D.,** Obstetrician and Gynecologist, Bellevue, Washington.

●Bunions

Relief for

Painful Feet

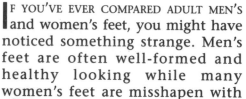

IF YOU'VE EVER COMPARED ADULT MEN'S and women's feet, you might have noticed something strange. Men's feet are often well-formed and healthy looking while many women's feet are misshapen with painful bunions, corns, and curled toes. In fact, women seek help from podiatrists and orthopedic surgeons for foot problems five times more frequently than men. Why? Ill-fitting shoes.

Men's shoes usually are long enough and wide enough to accommodate their feet comfortably. Women's shoes, even flat dress shoes, tend to feature pointed toe boxes that pinch the toes and have no arch support. Add high heels that rock the body's weight onto the balls of the feet, shorten the Achilles tendon, and shift the pelvis forward, and you've got all the ingredients for bunions and other foot problems.

A bunion, called hallux valgus (Latin for "turning outward of the first toe") by doctors, is a swelling on the foot, usually at the joint of the big toe. A bony protrusion forms at the outside edge of the big toe and often forces it to overlap with one or more other toes. There is also inflammation of the bursa (fluid-filled sac) that acts as a cushion for the joint.

SYMPTOMS

Bunions may be acute or chronic. Acute bunions are a type of bursitis, or inflammation of a bursa. With an acute bunion, the bursa covering the big toe joint becomes inflamed from friction at the joint and can cause considerable pain. In chronic or long-term bunions, the swelling develops into an inflexible bony protrusion.

Over time, continued pressure on the big toe can cause the other toes to misalign and overlap. The result is often the development of corns—hard, thickened areas of dead skin—and other foot problems. Shoe friction can also cause "bunionettes," small bunion-type bumps that form on the outside of the foot near the little toe.

CAUSES

Bunions are usually caused by friction or pressure on the joint, often from poorly fitting shoes. With the preponderance of uncomfortable, pointed, and high-heeled women's shoes on the market, it's no wonder that three times as many women as men suffer from bunions.

Bunions can also be caused by inherited abnormal bone structures in the foot. In a normal foot, the two main bones of the big toe align to fit together. However, some feet have loose joints that allow the big toes to point toward the other toes (metatarsus varus). This inherited tendency isn't a problem until the foot is encased in a shoe. The shoe forces the big toe inward while forcing the big toe joint outward, forming an unattractive bump known as a bunion. As the joint rubs against the inner surface of the shoe, the bursa, or fluid-filled sac, that protects the big toe joint becomes inflamed, and the overlying skin toughens and thickens into a callus.

Other times, bunions develop as a result of changes in the bony structures of the feet caused by fallen arches (flat feet). Bunions may also be caused by arthritis, cerebral palsy, or other diseases that cause joint destruction.

AT-HOME TREATMENT

Once you've developed a bunion, at-home remedies can't cure the problem. They can only reduce the pressure and help alleviate the pain. For a permanent cure, surgery is required to realign or make other structural changes in the big toe and foot. However, many doctors recommend at-home treatments rather than surgery for older women with bunions.

Wear loose shoes. Make sure your shoes are large enough, especially across the widest part of the foot, to accommodate your foot and its bunion. When the weather permits, wear open shoes that don't cause friction to the big toe joint.

Barefoot it. Shoes only aggravate your bunion. Whenever it's safe to do so, go barefoot.

Go for support. Make sure your shoes provide good arch support, especially if your foot problems come from fallen arches. Unfortunately, most women's shoes have little arch support built into them. If you buy shoes large enough, you can purchase off-the-shelf arch supports and add them to your shoes. Or you can talk with your podiatrist, orthopedist, or chiropractor about custom-made supports called orthotics that can help properly support and align your feet.

---

9 STEPS TO AVOID BUNIONS

- Buy round-toed shoes.
- Purchase shoes that are wide enough for your feet.
- Shop for shoes in the afternoon.
- Wear low heels.
- Wear flat shoes whenever possible.
- Add padding and arch supports to your shoes.
- Buy shoes with thick heels.
- Wear sandal-type shoes.
- Shop in stores that sell "comfortable" shoes.

Pad it. If your bunions haven't become too large, sometimes bunion pads that provide a cushion between the joint swelling and your shoe can offer some relief. Look in the foot care section in pharmacies.

Apply ice. When your bunions cause pain, apply ice to the area. While the ice won't change the condition, it can provide temporary pain relief and help reduce inflammation.

Try OTC pain relievers. Aspirin, ibuprofen, and acetaminophen are available over the counter and can also help provide temporary relief from the pain caused by bunions.

PREVENTION

Prevention is the key with bunions. Once bunions develop, they are self-perpetuating and progressively get worse if left untreated. Since bunions can be an inherited condition aggravated by ill-fitting shoes, the first thing to do is look at your family's feet. If there's a family tendency, it's important for you to wear only comfortable, well-fitting shoes with wide toe boxes.

Comfortable shoes are crucial to prevention. Follow these shoe tips to prevent bunions:

Go for the round look. Buy shoes that are more rounded in the toe area. Avoid pointy shoes that pinch the toes.

Buy wide. Make sure shoes are wide enough. Your shoes should feel comfortable even across the ball area, the widest part of your foot.

Be a P.M. shopper. Shop for shoes in the afternoon, when your feet are slightly swollen.

Keep it down. Wear the lowest heel you can find. The body can tolerate about a one-inch heel without problems. Unfortunately, convention dictates that in many settings, especially in business, women are expected to wear higher heels. But this fashion statement can have unhappy results for your health. In addition to bunions, the weight-forward position that high heels force women into can cause tendinitis, back pain, joint irritation and dys-

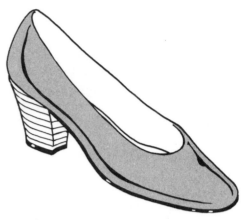

function, and eventual postural accommodations that can permanently alter the upper back.

Bring your lunch shoes. Wear lower-heeled or flat shoes to and from work and during lunch.

Add support. Buy shoes large enough to add padding or an arch support.

Look for stability. Buy the thickest heel possible for the greatest stability.

Let your toes breathe. Whenever possible, wear open, sandal-type shoes that don't pressure the big toe joint.

Try specialty stores. Look for stores that advertise "comfortable" shoes. Often these are specialty stores that sell to hard-to-fit customers. Their shoes are usually a bit more expensive, but they can often find you a heeled dress shoe that won't put undue pressure on your big toe.

Sources: Kathleen Galligan, D.C., President, Oregon Chiropractor's Association, Portland, Oregon. **Anne Simons, M.D.,** Coauthor, *Before You Call the Doctor;* Family Practitioner, San Francisco Department of Public Health; Family Practitioner and Assistant Clinical Professor, Family and Community Medicine, University of California San Francisco Medical Center, San Francisco, California.

6 WAYS TO EASE THE PAIN

- Wear loose shoes.
- Go barefoot whenever practical.
- Try arch inserts or custom orthotics.
- Use bunion pads.
- Apply ice.
- Try nonprescription pain relievers.

Soothing

Strategies for

the Soreness

USUALLY YOU DISCOVER IT WITH YOUR tongue. It's a rough area about the size of a pencil eraser that hurts like the devil when you eat or drink. You've got a canker sore.

The good news is that canker sores aren't dangerous or catching, and the misery they produce is usually pretty short-lived.

First, you have to determine whether you really have a canker sore or if you have its second cousin, a cold sore (also called a fever blister). If you have a cold sore, you'll usually see a cluster of tiny blisters that eventually become one or more larger blisters. Once the blisters begin to dry, they form a scab. You'll usually find them on the lips and face and they hang around for seven to ten days.

In contrast, a canker sore usually travels alone. It appears in the mouth, often inside the lip or cheek and sometimes on the gum or tongue. It appears as a small, red crater with a grey or yellow center. Canker sores can be painful and make talking and eating difficult.

CAUSES

One out of every five people develops canker sores, but unlike highly contagious cold sores, you can't pass canker sores from one person to another. Doctors don't know what causes canker sores, but stress and other resistance-lowering influences such as poor diet and menstruation seem to be a factor. Minor mouth injuries like the jab of a toothbrush can also precipitate a canker sore. Some researchers believe that certain foods, such as spicy dishes and citrus fruits that irritate the mouth's tissues, also may be to blame.

Women appear to develop more canker sores than men. Some report they get canker sores at certain times during their menstrual cycle.

AT-HOME TREATMENT

While there's no cure for canker sores, home remedies can provide some relief. Canker sores can take up to two weeks to heal. If one sticks around longer than that, see your dentist.

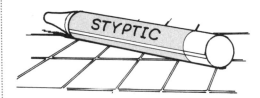

Styptic it. Styptic pencils, used by barbers to stem bleeding from minor cuts, can numb a canker sore's nerve endings and give temporary pain relief.

Try milk of magnesia. Mix together equal amounts of milk of magnesia or Kaopectate and Benylin or Benadryl and apply the mixture to the canker sore with a cotton swab. Don't swallow it! (It can numb the reflex that closes the windpipe when you swallow.) Milk of magnesia and Kaopectate contain ingredients that coat wet tissues, and Benylin and Benadryl act

6 WAYS TO SOOTHE A SORE

- Use a styptic pencil.
- Try a "milk of magnesia bandage"(see text).
- Apply an over-the-counter anesthetic gel.
- Take aspirin.
- Eat cool foods.
- Avoid alcohol and smoking.

as mild topical anesthetics and also as antihistamines that reduce inflammation.

Go for the OTC anesthetic gels. Over-the-counter products like Anbesol or Orabase numb the pain and cover the surface of the sore, which helps prevent secondary infection.

Take aspirin. Aspirin, acetaminophen, or ibuprofen can help relieve pain. If aspirin or ibuprofen upsets your stomach, try an enteric coated brand. Pregnant women or women with a history of ulcers should not take aspirin or ibuprofen without a doctor's approval.

Cool it. Stick to cool foods. Foods that are spicy or hot from the oven burn and sting tender canker sores.

Give up the booze and smokes. Both alcohol and cigarettes irritate canker sores.

Take a gentle approach. Take it easy with the toothbrush to avoid irritating the canker sore. And stay away from rough, scratchy foods like chips.

PREVENTION

There's no surefire way to guarantee you'll never get another canker sore. But you can take steps to reduce your chances.

Keep a canker sore diary. If canker sores are a chronic problem, consider keeping a diary. Note the foods you eat, events that may be stressful, the timing of your menstrual cycle. Then look for patterns that may precipitate an outbreak of canker sores.

Nix spicy and acidic foods. Try an experiment: If you seem to develop canker sores after eating spicy foods or acid products like tomatoes or citrus fruit, eliminate them from your diet and see if your incidence of canker sores is reduced.

Improve your diet. Some researchers believe that people who develop canker sores have deficiencies in iron, folic acid, zinc, and vitamin B_{12}. Eat a variety of foods and be sure to get plenty of fresh fruits and vegetables and whole grains.

Relax. Since canker sores have been associated with stress, consider adopting some relaxation strategies. You might try meditation, regular aerobic exercise, listening to music, progressive relaxation, or biofeedback.

---

4 PREVENTION STRATEGIES

- Keep a canker sore diary.
- Improve your diet.
- Avoid spicy or acid foods.
- Learn to relax.

Sources: Becky DeSpain, R.D.H., M.Ed., Director of the Caruth School of Dental Hygiene, Baylor College of Dentistry, Dallas, Texas. Robert P. Langlais, D.D.S., M.S., Spokesperson for the American Academy of Oral Medicine; Professor, Department of Dental Diagnostic Science, University of Texas Health Science Center at San Antonio School of Dentistry, San Antonio, Texas. Alan S. Levy, D.D.S., Clinical Instructor, University of Southern California School of Dentistry, Los Angeles, California. Richard Price, D.M.D., Consumer Advisor/Spokesperson, American Dental Association.

•CARPAL TUNNEL SYNDROME

Wrist Relief

at Last

Y OU MAY HAVE NOTICED IT AT FIRST AS a bothersome tingling or numbness in your hands. Now pain and burning radiate from your wrists to your fingertips. You have another long report to type this afternoon, and you're dreading the moment when you have to sit down at the keyboard. What is going on with your hands and wrists?

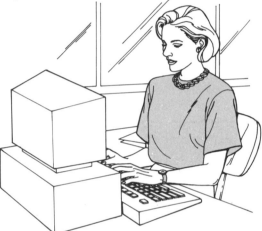

If you work at any job where you have to use your hands in a rapid, repetitive motion—word processing, punching cash register keys, operating a jackhammer, tightening bolts on an assembly line—you may be at risk for developing a painful condition called carpal tunnel syndrome (CTS). Painful symptoms can appear in the hand, fingers, and wrist when the median nerve in the wrist is compressed.

While the problem has been around for decades, CTS didn't become a household term until the 1980s, when personal computers came to dominate many workplaces. Suddenly, millions of people began using their hands in rapid, repetitive motions on computer keyboards for hours at a time. According to the Bureau of Labor Statistics, cumulative trauma disorders such as carpal tunnel syndrome account for more than half of all occupational illnesses in the United States. Not surprisingly, CTS is most prevalent among women in their 30s, 40s, and 50s who use word processors or computer terminals. But it can also affect musicians, factory workers, and others who use their hands in repetitive motions.

SYMPTOMS

Carpal tunnel syndrome is not really a disease in itself, but a collection of symptoms that most often includes tingling, numbness, burning, weakness, and pain from the wrists to the fingers. It usually begins with feelings of numbness, burning, or "pins and needles" in the thumb, index, or middle finger or on the inner side of the ring finger. Some people report aching pain traveling up the forearm and even into the shoulder, neck, and chest.

The pain from CTS may be constant or it may come and go. One or both hands may be involved. Pain often increases with manual work or work that involves flexing the wrist or palms. Many people report that the pain is worse in the morning and evening.

In the later stages of CTS, it may be difficult to make a fist, the fingernails may deteriorate, and the skin over the affected areas may become dry and shiny. Another late-stage symptom is weakness of the fingers, which occurs as muscles waste away (atrophy). If left unchecked, permanent damage to the muscles and nerves can result.

CAUSES

Inside the wrist, the hand (median) nerve travels through a narrow opening, called the carpal tunnel, formed by the wrist bones (carpals) and a tough membrane that holds them together. This narrow wrist passageway is only about the size of a postage stamp, but it's packed with nerves, blood vessels, and nine different tendons that control finger movement. As in a busy freeway tunnel at rush hour, if anything blocks the tunnel, everything gets backed up. If the tissues around the carpal tunnel swell, the tunnel narrows; this decreases blood supply to the thumb, index, and middle finger and compresses the median nerve, causing a "traffic jam" of CTS symptoms. (The little finger isn't involved in carpal tunnel syndrome because its nerve supply bypasses the crowded carpal tunnel.)

The most common cause of swelling in the carpal tunnel area is repetitive motion of the hands and fingers. But the tissues surrounding the tunnel can also become swollen due to hormonal changes. Women are especially susceptible to CTS because the hormonal changes triggered by pregnancy, menopause, and menstruation can cause tissue swelling and result in CTS.

Injury or disease can also cause localized swelling around the carpal tunnel. A sprain, dislocation, or fracture of the wrist sometimes precipitates CTS symptoms. Rheumatoid arthritis can cause the coverings of the wrist tendons to swell and compress the median nerve. People who suffer from diabetes or low thyroid function (hypothyroidism) also have a greater risk of developing CTS. Other possible CTS causes include wrist joint inflammation, noncancerous tumor, tuberculosis, amyloidosis (a disease characterized by abnormal deposits of the protein amyloid), and acromegaly (overgrowth of connective tissue).

AT-HOME TREATMENT

If you're already experiencing the tingling, numbness, and pain associated with CTS, you may be able to prevent further damage and promote healing by making a few simple changes in your lifestyle. While the following suggestions can help you reduce your CTS symptoms, if your symptoms become severe, or if they don't resolve after two weeks of self-care, see your doctor.

Give yourself the CTS test. It may be difficult to tell whether or not your symptoms are caused by carpal tunnel syndrome or other health conditions, such as arthritis in the neck. To give you an idea if your problem really is CTS, try this simple test: Place the backs of your hands together, fingers pointing straight down, wrists at a 90 degree angle so that your elbows point straight out to the sides. Hold this position for one or two minutes. If your symptoms develop within one minute, there's a good chance you have CTS.

Take a break. If you've started experiencing tingling, numbness, and pain, try stopping your repetitive finger movements for several days and see if your symptoms improve. If you feel better, explore the possibility of arranging your life so that you don't have to spend so much time doing tasks that predispose you to CTS. With all the recent publicity surrounding carpal tunnel syndrome, many employers are sensitive to the problem and are willing to reassign people who develop the condition or at least restructure or rotate jobs to lessen the problem.

Mobilize early. Pay attention to the early warning signs of CTS: morning stiffness in the hands or arms, clumsiness, inability to make a fist, and thumb weakness. Don't wait until symptoms become acute. Take preventive and self-care action immediately.

Shake it off. Some people experience CTS pain up the forearm and even into the shoulder, neck, and chest. Shake the hand vigorously or dangle the arm loosely from its socket to relieve this type of pain.

Try ice. You can reduce swelling and inflammation from carpal tunnel syndrome with ice. Place an ice pack on the affected wrist and forearm for five to fifteen minutes, two to three times a day.

Nix the heat. In contrast to ice, heat can increase inflammation, swelling, and pain from CTS. Heat may soothe sore muscles, but it should never be used with irritated nerves.

Reach for the aspirin/ibuprofen. To reduce pain and inflammation, try aspirin or ibuprofen. If these drugs upset your stomach, ask your pharmacist for an "enteric coated" brand, which dissolves in the intestine rather than in the stomach. Pregnant or breast-feeding women and

---

8 SELF-CARE STRATEGIES

- **Do a CTS test.**
- **Take a break from repetitive tasks.**
- **Pay attention to early warning signs and take action.**
- **Shake out your hands and arms to relieve pain.**
- **Try ice.**
- **Stay away from heat.**
- **Try aspirin or ibuprofen.**
- **Use a splint.**

---

those with a history of ulcers should not take aspirin or ibuprofen without a doctor's permission.

Splint it. Wrist splints—braces that hold the wrist in a slightly cocked-back position with the thumb parallel to the forearm—can help provide relief. Available from medical supply houses, pharmacies, and physicians, these splints keep the wrist in a position that allows the tunnel to be as open as possible. Splints can be worn during the day or at night. Doctors caution that some over-the-counter splints can be too flimsy and allow the wrist to move around. They also warn against wearing the splint so often that muscles shrink (atrophy). Consult your physician before purchasing a splint from a pharmacy or from another source.

AT THE DOCTOR'S

The doctor will usually first try conservative CTS treatments such as splinting and exercises. If those strategies don't work, and inflammation of the wrist is causing the symptoms, he or she might inject cortisone into the carpal tunnel.

If these treatments are ineffective, surgery may be necessary to release the transverse ligament to relieve pressure on the nerve and prevent further damage. Symptoms usually subside shortly after surgery, and strength gradually returns to the hands. However, if surgery has been delayed for too long, the muscles may have become severely deteriorated and full strength may not return. Recurrence of CTS is a possibility.

12 STRATEGIES TO PROTECT YOUR WRISTS

- Strengthen hands and wrists.
- Change your work routine.
- Alter your sleeping position.
- Modify or rotate your job.
- Keep your wrists in a "neutral" position.
- Don't rest your wrists on desk or table edges.
- Slow down and apply only the force you need.
- Operate vibrating tools at the "smoothest" speeds.
- Grip with the entire hand.
- Change hands often.
- Try ergonomics.
- Use hand exercises.

PREVENTION

Carpal tunnel syndrome is such a painful and potentially debilitating condition, the best advice is to avoid it in the first place. Try these strategies.

Keep the blood flowing. A body whose circulatory and immune systems are in good working order is less likely to suffer injury. Get exercise, and practice good nutrition. A balanced diet should contain a wide variety of foods, including plenty of fresh fruits, vegetables, whole grains, and legumes. Get adequate sleep (six to eight hours for most people). Avoid cigarette smoking (it decreases circulation to all areas of the body).

Strengthen your wrists and hands. Exercise regularly to increase the flexibility and strength in your wrists, hands, and fingers. While exercise can't guarantee you won't develop CTS, it will decrease your chances.

Break it up. Fatigue is a warning sign that you need to change your pattern of work. As soon as you feel tired or stiff, get up and change your activity. Even better, don't wait until you feel fatigued. Schedule a one- or two-minute break every 20 to 30 minutes and a longer break every hour.

Watch your sleeping position. Many people find they are bothered more by CTS symptoms at night. Doctors suggest that this may be because the fluid in the body is redistributed when you lie down, so that more of it accumulates in the wrists. Many people also cause wrist compression by sleeping with one hand tucked under the head. If you are one of them, alter your sleeping position to keep your wrist from being bent or compressed. You might also try wearing a wrist splint just at night to protect the area.

Modify your job. It may not be possible for you to change professions, but you may be able to modify your job so that you rotate duties. Talk with your supervisor or union about altering your job routine so that you can switch tasks frequently or combine tasks. The key is to avoid doing the same thing over and over for extended periods. Once your employer realizes that job rotation can reduce stress and minimize production losses, he or she will probably be open to making some changes.

"Neutralize" your wrists. The most natural and comfortable position for the wrists is a "neutral" position, one that is straight, not cocked. Rearrange the level of your keyboard so that you don't have to strain, reach, or bend your wrists. The wrists should always be in a straight line with your forearms. Also check to ensure that your computer screen is at eye level and your work is within your "comfort zone," not too close or too far away.

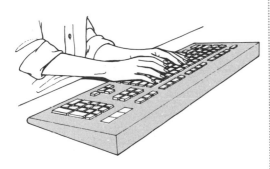

Keep your wrists off the edge. A common problem for typists and computer operators involves resting the wrists on the edge of the table or desk while working. This can cause pressure on the wrists. Check your workstation and adjust it to keep your wrists off the edge.

Conserve energy. Powerful, high-speed movements cause the most CTS problems. Relax and conserve your energy. Slow down and apply only the force needed to get the job done.

Watch the vibes. People who use vibrating tools like saws, sanders, and jackhammers for long periods of time are at risk of developing CTS symptoms. If you have to operate vibrating tools, take frequent breaks and, whenever possible, operate the tool at the speed that causes the least vibration.

Check your grip. It's common to grip with only the thumb, index, and middle fingers. This places undue pressure on the wrist. Instead, when gripping or twisting something, use your whole hand, not just your fingers.

Change hands. Often, it's the dominant hand that suffers from CTS symptoms. Whenever possible, use the other hand.

Try ergonomics. There's a whole new technology, called "ergonomics," that focuses on the creation of furniture and equipment specially designed for ease of human use. "Ergo" tools and workstations cause less stress on the body. Some tools have been redesigned to work with less force, while others have better grips and handles. Look for items that reduce strain on your wrists and hands. But don't be fooled by expensive "miracle" devices that claim to cure carpal tunnel syndrome.

Exercise those hands. Many times, initial problems with the wrist are actually tendon problems that haven't yet involved the nerves. These exercises, suggested by the National Safety Council, can help relieve tendon problems before they become CTS. Perform them two to four times a day or whenever you need a break. Stop doing any exercise, however, if it makes your symptoms worse.

1) *Wrist circles.* With palms down and hands out, rotate both wrists five times in each direction.

2) *Thumb stretch.* Hold out your right hand and grasp your right thumb with your left hand. Pull the thumb out and back until you feel a gentle stretch. Hold for five to ten seconds and release. Repeat three to five times with each thumb.

3) *Five-finger stretch.* Spread the fingers of both hands far apart and hold for five to ten seconds. Repeat three to five times.

4) *Finger-thumb squeeze.* Squeeze a rubber ball tightly in one hand five to ten times. Afterward, stretch the fingers. Repeat with the other hand.

Do the following exercises using small, hand-held weights to strengthen the wrist tendons. Don't use weights heavier than five pounds, as too much weight can traumatize the wrists.

5) *Palm-up wrist curls.* Rest your forearms on a table, with your palms facing upward and your hands held straight out over the edge of the table. With a light weight (one to two pounds) in each hand, flex your wrists up ten times. Over the course of several weeks, gradually build up to 40 repetitions. Increase the weight of the dumbbells each week by one pound to a maximum of five pounds.

6) *Palm-down wrist curls.* Adopt the same position as in the previous exercise, but have your palms facing downward. Flex your wrists up ten times. Gradually increase the number of repetitions over several weeks.

7) *Arm curls.* Stand and hold the weights at your sides, palms facing forward. Slowly curl your arms up, keeping your wrists straight. Start with ten curls. Over several weeks, build up to 40.

Sources: **Michael Martindale, L.P.T.,** Physical Therapist, Sports Medicine Center, Portland Adventist Medical Center, Portland, Oregon. **David Rempel, M.D.,** Assistant Professor of Medicine, Director, Ergonomics Laboratory, University of California at San Francisco, San Francisco, California. **Anne Simons, M.D.,** Coauthor, *Before You Call the Doctor;* Family Practitioner, San Francisco Department of Public Health; Family Practitioner and Assistant Clinical Professor, Family and Community Medicine, University of California San Francisco Medical Center, San Francisco, California. **Mark Tager, M.D.,** Coauthor, *Working Well;* President, Great Performance, Inc., Beaverton, Oregon.

Strategies for

Soft Hands

EVERYONE GETS DRY HANDS ONCE IN A while. But some of us—especially people like nurses, day-care workers, hairstylists, and new parents who find themselves constantly washing their hands—end up with chapped skin. So-called "dishpan hands" are red, rough, scaly, and sometimes even cracked and bleeding.

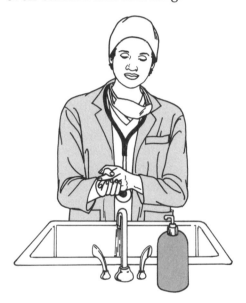

CAUSES

To understand how hands can become badly chapped, let's take a look at the skin itself. The skin's top layer, the stratum corneum, is made up of six to twelve layers of cells. These layers contain lipids, or fats, that act as a barrier to keep you from losing your body's moisture. Since the outside air is drier than inside the body, your skin acts like a giant sack, keeping you from losing water from the inside out.

This lipid-filled barrier works quite well until you repeatedly wet and dry it. Constantly wetting and drying the skin removes the protective oils that seal in the body's moisture. Dryness from moisture loss can damage the skin and make it subject to infection. When you combine loss of the skin's protective oils with moisture loss, you can quickly wind up with painful, chapped skin.

The amount of moisture in the air is directly related to dry skin. The drier the air, the greater the loss of moisture from the skin. People in hot, dry climates often find they have to frequently use moisturizers and creams to keep their skin from drying out.

Winter is an especially dangerous time for skin. Forced-air heat dries the indoor air and helps pull moisture from the skin. Outdoor cold and wind further rob the skin of moisture. Even winter sun and high altitude can add to the drying effect.

Age is a factor in dry, chapped skin, too. As we age, the oil (sebaceous) glands in the skin shrink and produce less protective oil.

Not only does dry, chapped skin tend to be less attractive and more wrinkled, it can actually be dangerous to your health. Badly chapped skin can become vulnerable to secondary bacterial infections and irritation from substances like harsh detergents.

AT-HOME TREATMENT

The good news is that with a few lifestyle changes, you can protect your skin from drying and chapping. If your hands are already chapped, these home-care remedies can help you repair the damage.

Put on warm gloves. Your mother was right—you should wear gloves or mittens outside in the winter cold. Every time you head for the door, grab your gloves. It's also a good idea to carry an extra pair in your car during the winter months.

11 WAYS TO SOFTEN CHAPPED HANDS

- Wear gloves.
- Choose vinyl, not rubber, gloves.
- Wear sunscreen.
- Use petrolatum.
- Apply moisturizers often.
- Don't use products with expensive additives.
- Keep your hands out of water.
- Avoid fragrances.
- If you use soap, use superfatted soaps or liquid cleaners.
- Stay out of hot water.
- Use a humidifier to increase moisture in indoor air.

Let vinyl do the job. If you have to expose your hands to harsh chemicals or detergents, protect your skin with vinyl gloves. Get into the habit of wearing gloves for routine tasks like washing dishes and scrubbing the bathroom. Always wear gloves when you're working with chemicals like paint thinner or acetone, which in addition to drying the skin can cause severe allergic reactions. Gloves may feel awkward at first, but your skin will thank you for it. When choosing gloves, opt for vinyl instead of rubber ones, which are more likely to cause allergic reactions. Also look for vinyl gloves with cotton liners, which will help draw away perspiration and keep your hands dry (perspiration can irritate chapped skin). For "dry" work, such as dusting, wear thin cotton gloves to cut down on friction and reduce exposure to harsh chemicals.

Nix suntans. Many women love to sunbathe, but your golden brown tan is not great for dry skin. The sun's ultraviolet light dries skin cells and can increase the risk of potentially deadly skin cancer (malignant melanoma). Whenever you're out in the sun, wear a sunscreen with a sun protection factor (SPF) of at least 15 on all exposed skin, including your hands.

Bring on the petroleum jelly. OK, it's heavy, "gunky," and messy, but petrolatum, or petroleum jelly, is one of the best and least-expensive treatments for dry, chapped hands. Many of the thinner lotions billed as "moisturizers" or "skin creams" are made mostly of water. For the greatest protection, you want a product that has more oil and less water. Petrolatum is all oil; it acts to seal in the skin's natural moisture. Unlike other moisturizers that tend to sit on top of the skin, petrolatum actually penetrates the top layers of skin cells and replaces the missing lipids or fats. It works best when it's applied as soon after the damage occurs as possible.

Here's an effective way to use petrolatum without the mess: Apply a thick layer all over your hands and then put on cotton gloves for several hours. This is especially effective overnight. Try it for a week.

Moisturize, moisturize. If you can't stand the heavy greasiness of petrolatum, use a cream moisturizer like Nivea, Eucerin, Lubriderm, or Moisturel. The heavier and creamier the product, the more oil it has and the better it will protect your skin from drying and chapping. Apply moisturizers several times a day, especially after washing or bathing.

Don't fall for the hype. Many skin products claim to include ingredients like mink oil or vitamins A, E, or C. Save your money. None of these ingredients has been found to work more effectively than petrolatum or cream-type moisturizers. Many dermatologists say the higher the price, the less likely the product is useful.

Stay high and dry. You'd think that water would be good for moisturizing your skin. But it's exactly the opposite. Water, especially hot water, actually pulls moisture from the skin. Repeated exposure to water leaches important proteins from the skin that normally keep it moist. That's why people like doctors, who must wash their hands repeatedly, often develop chapped hands. As much as possible, keep your hands out of water. When you must expose them to water, protect them with gloves.

Nix the fragrances. A single fragrance can contain a large number of chemicals, many of which can have drying effects on the skin. Fragrances also increase the risk of allergic reactions and can cause severe rashes in some people.

Go mild. Soaps tend to dry out the skin and can actually damage its outer layer. Stay away from deodorant soaps. Instead use a superfatted soap or a liquid cleanser such as Dove, Basis, Eucerin, Aquanil, or Moisturel. Many skin specialists recommend the mild skin cleaner Cetaphil for problem skin.

Go warm, not hot. There's nothing like soaking in a steamy, hot bath—that is, for removing moisture and natural oils from your skin. Instead of long, hot soaks, opt for short, warm showers. Avoid exposing your skin to really hot water. You'll save on energy bills and you'll save your skin, too.

Get humid. During some of the seasons, you may need to increase the humidity in the air of your home or office with a humidifier. The added moisture in the air will help prevent moisture loss from your skin.

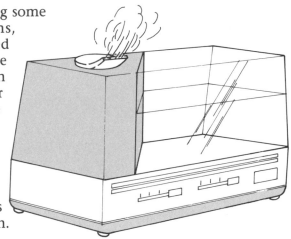

Sources: Ruby Ghadially, M.D., Assistant Clinical Professor, Department of Dermatology, University of California at San Diego, San Diego, California. **Albert Kligman, M.D., Ph.D.,** Emeritus Professor of Dermatology, University of Pennsylvania School of Medicine, Philadelphia, Pennsylvania. **Paul Lazar, M.D.,** Professor of Clinical Dermatology, Northwestern University School of Medicine, Chicago, Illinois. **Jerome Z. Litt, M.D.,** Author, *Your Skin: From Acne to Zits*; Assistant Clinical Professor of Dermatology, Case Western Reserve University School of Medicine, Cleveland, Ohio. **Frank Parker, M.D.,** Professor and Chair, Department of Dermatology, Oregon Health Sciences University, Portland, Oregon. **James Shaw, M.D.,** Chief, Division of Dermatology, Good Samaritan Hospital and Medical Center; Associate Clinical Professor of Medicine, Oregon Health Sciences University, Portland, Oregon.

CHAPPED LIPS

Tips for More

Kissable Lips

IF THE THOUGHT OF PUCKERING UP sounds horrifying, chances are you've got chapped lips. Rough, red, cracked, sensitive lips can make kissing definitely out of the question and leave you with little to smile about. While chapped lips aren't life threatening, they can make you miserable. Fortunately, they're one of life's little annoyances that you don't have to put up with.

CAUSES

Normally, natural skin oils keep the lips smooth, moist, and soft. But dry, cold, windy conditions or mucus-drying drugs like antihistamines can interfere with the lips' moisturizing process and leave them dry, cracked, and irritated. People who habitually lick their lips may suffer from chronic chapping. Those suffering from nasal congestion due to allergies or a head cold who have to breathe through the mouth often find that their lips become dried and chapped. Even using some brands of lipstick or toothpaste and mouthwash can cause irritation of the lips and chapping among some women.

Chapped lips aren't just a cosmetic problem. When the skin's surface is dry, chapped, or fissured, chemicals and bacteria can penetrate more easily, causing irritation or even infection. Cold sores, bacterial infections, and other problems are more likely to strike lips that are already damaged by chapping. When lips are dry, sometimes inflamed and painful cracks develop in the corners of the mouth. Often these cracks don't readily heal because they become infected with yeast.

AT-HOME TREATMENT

In most cases, chapped lips can be effectively treated with home remedies. However, if you develop signs of infection (redness, swelling, weeping) or if your chapping doesn't respond to home care, see your dermatologist.

Nix the licks. Frequent exposure of the skin to water causes it to lose moisture. When you repeatedly lick your lips, you're exposing them to moisture over and over and drying out the skin. If your lips are already chapped or dry, licking your lips may make you feel better, but you're doing more harm than good.

Balm it. Lip balms are wax-based or grease-based products that act to seal moisture in the lips with a protective barrier. They're relatively inexpensive and available over the counter. Try several to find one you like and will use frequently.

Pull out the petrolatum. One of the best skin protectors and moisturizers is petrolatum, or petroleum jelly. It's inexpen-

9 SOOTHING TIPS FOR CHAPPED LIPS

- Don't lick your lips.
- Use lip balm frequently.
- Try petroleum jelly.
- Wear lipstick.
- Avoid prolonged exposure to dry, cold, windy conditions.
- Protect your lips from the sun.
- Change toothpaste/mouthwash brands.
- Avoid irritating foods and alcohol.
- Try over-the-counter antifungal creams.

sive, goes on easily, and provides instant relief. Unlike some barrier skin products, petrolatum penetrates the top layer of skin cells and replaces lost lipids, or fats.

Color 'em. If you enjoy the look and feel of wearing lipstick, go right ahead. It might actually help keep your lips from becoming chapped. Lipstick provides some moisturizing properties and acts as a screen against the sun's drying rays. Be wary of cosmetic products made outside of the United States, however, because their purity may vary widely. Also, if you develop any redness, irritation, itching, or flaking, stop using the product immediately; you may be allergic to one of the ingredients.

Avoid cold, windy conditions. When possible, avoid prolonged exposure to cold, windy conditions. If you must be in dry, cold, windy weather, use lip balms to prevent the problem before it starts.

Bring on the sunscreen. The sun's ultraviolet rays can dry and damage skin anywhere on the body, particularly the sensitive skin of the lips. Unlike other skin, the lip skin doesn't contain melanin, the brown pigment, or coloring, that can help protect against the sun's burning rays. In fact, the lips are a common site for skin cancer (malignant melanoma). This form of cancer is particularly serious on the lips because it has a tendency to spread to other parts of the face. When

you must be in the sun, wear a hat or visor to protect your lips and face and a lip balm that contains a sun protection factor (SPF) of at least 15.

Watch the toothpaste. Some people will develop chronically chapped lips due to an allergic reaction to their toothpaste or mouthwash. If you're suffering from chronically dry, chapped, irritated lips, try switching toothpaste and mouthwash brands and see if the problem resolves.

Give sensitive lips a break. Be careful not to irritate chapped lips further with spicy or salty foods or alcohol.

Try antifungal creams. If your mouth develops cracked corners try applying an over-the-counter antifungal cream (miconazole or clotrimazole) two or three times a day. At night, apply zinc oxide ointment.

Sources: **Ruby Ghadially, M.D.,** Assistant Clinical Professor, Department of Dermatology, University of California at San Diego, San Diego, California. **Albert Kligman, M.D.,** Ph.D., Emeritus Professor of Dermatology, University of Pennsylvania School of Medicine, Philadelphia, Pennsylvania. **Paul Lazar, M.D.,** Professor of Clinical Dermatology, Northwestern University School of Medicine, Chicago, Illinois. **Jerome Z. Litt, M.D.,** Author, *Your Skin: From Acne to Zits;* Assistant Clinical Professor of Dermatology, Case Western Reserve University School of Medicine, Cleveland, Ohio. **Anne Simons, M.D.,** Coauthor, *Before You Call the Doctor;* Family Practitioner, San Francisco Department of Public Health; Family Practitioner and Assistant Clinical Professor, Family and Community Medicine, University of California San Francisco Medical Center, San Francisco, California.

CHRONIC FATIGUE SYNDROME

Strategies for

Dealing with

the Symptoms

ABOUT TEN YEARS AGO, A STRANGE SET of symptoms began afflicting young, healthy men and women. They complained of extreme fatigue, muscle aches, sore throat, general malaise (feeling bad), low-grade fever, joint pain, and swollen lymph glands. Some thought it was the flu. The media lightly dubbed the mysterious ailment the "yuppie flu" since it seemed to attack young, affluent, hard-driven individuals. Others said it must be mononucleosis or some other infectious disease.

The mysterious illness is chronic fatigue syndrome (CFS), also unofficially called chronic fatigue and immune dysfunction syndrome. It's a collection of flulike symptoms that has left its sufferers frustrated and doctors baffled. The symptoms mimic a bad case of the flu or even mononucleosis, but unlike those ailments, CFS can persist for months or even years.

Most people who develop CFS are sickest during the first year or two, usually before they're diagnosed. Some people spontaneously recover, while the illness lingers indefinitely in others.

Like many who suffer chronic illnesses, some people with chronic fatigue syndrome experience emotional problems. Depression can go hand-in-hand with CFS's flulike symptoms, or depression can be absent or mild in CFS. In addition, many sufferers experience cognitive problems such as confusion, forgetfulness, and sleep disorders.

CAUSES

Unfortunately, after more than ten years, no one knows what causes CFS. At one time, researchers called the syndrome "chronic Epstein-Barr syndrome" because many early sufferers were infected with the Epstein-Barr virus, the same agent that causes mononucleosis. However, many other people who complain about the fatigue, aches, swollen glands, and fever of CFS show no trace of Epstein-Barr infection. Ninety percent of the public show evidence of having had the Epstein-Barr virus in the past.

Although no one has come up with a definitive answer about the causes of chronic fatigue syndrome, there are a number of theories. Some researchers suggest that stress might trigger the syndrome. Others believe it's a virus or some kind of dysfunction of the immune system.

Researchers don't believe chronic fatigue syndrome is contagious. In fact, it may be something within the person (what doctors call the "host factor"), rather than an infectious agent, that allows the condition to occur.

IS IT CFS?

Even diagnosing CFS isn't clear-cut. There's no blood test or X ray that will confirm a CFS diagnosis. Chronic fatigue syndrome symptoms mimic a wide range of other health problems such as anemia, multiple sclerosis, thyroid disorders, lupus, and even cancer. In fact, chronic fatigue as a symptom is one of the most common complaints doctors hear from patients. A diagnosis of CFS comes only through a sometimes long, tedious, and expensive process of eliminating a host of other possible illnesses.

In 1988, guidelines were established for CFS research diagnosis. According to the guidelines, to have chronic fatigue syndrome, you must have suffered from debilitating fatigue that has reduced your activities by 50 percent for at least six months and have had other possible conditions excluded through review of your history, physical examination, and laboratory examination. You must also have at least eight of the following symptoms:

- Mild fever or chills.
- Sore throat.
- Generalized muscle weakness.
- Fatigue that lasts at least 24 hours after exercise that's normal to the individual.
- Headaches that differ from those before the illness began in their type, severity, and pattern.
- Joint pain without swelling or redness.
- Forgetfulness, confusion, or inability to concentrate.
- Sleep problems, such as insomnia.
- Painful lymph nodes.
- Muscle pain.
- Rapid onset of symptoms, usually within a few hours or days.

AT-HOME TREATMENT

You've learned that there's no known cause and no cure for chronic fatigue syndrome. It isn't fatal and it's not usually progressive, but it makes you feel terrible. Doctors can't even say how long you'll be ill, but they know it can last for months or even years. Now what do you do?

You learn to cope with the illness. Like many others who live with chronic health conditions, you can learn how to make yourself feel as good as you are able to both mentally and physically. The coping strategies offered here are from doctors, psychotherapists, and patients who have dealt extensively with the condition. With your doctor's advice

24 STRATEGIES FOR COPING

- **Develop a partnership with your health-care providers.**
- **Learn everything you can about chronic fatigue syndrome.**
- **Accept that you have a chronic illness.**
- **Let yourself feel and express all your emotions without guilt or shame.**
- **Don't go on a guilt trip.**
- **Educate your friends and family about CFS.**
- **Join a support group.**
- **Consider seeing a psychotherapist.**
- **Ration your energy.**
- **Set attainable goals.**
- **Live more efficiently.**
- **Rest when you need it.**
- **Set priorities.**
- **Adapt to how you feel at the moment.**
- **Control your schedule.**
- **Eat a balanced, low-fat diet.**
- **Be sure to include play and social time in your life.**
- **Don't overdo exercise.**
- **Keep a journal.**
- **Stay sexually active.**
- **Reclaim control by exercising the choices you have.**
- **Lighten up and laugh.**
- **Don't fall for so-called "miracle" products or treatments.**
- **Live one day at a time.**

and care, you can learn to live successfully with CFS.

Develop a partnership. You need experienced, caring, and empathetic health-care providers to help you deal with CFS. Take time to build a health-care team that will meet both your physical and emotional needs. Interview your physician and ask questions such as the following:

- What experience do you have with CFS? What experience do you have with other chronic ailments that would help in dealing with CFS?

• Do you take phone calls? Do you charge for them? How soon do you usually return calls?

• What do you see as your responsibility in my health care? What do you see as my responsibility?

• How do you feel about answering my questions?

• How do you feel about my having someone else with me (spouse, friend, relative, or other patient advocate) during exams or consultations?

The specific answers to the questions the physician gives you are less important than how you feel about his or her answers. Trust your "gut level" or intuitive reactions. If necessary, interview several doctors until you find one you feel is a good match. Go through the same process with a psychotherapist and any other health-care provider who will play a significant role in your care.

Become involved. This isn't the time to be a passive patient. Get involved and learn all you can about your disease, possible treatments, and coping strategies. Ask questions. Read current articles or books on the topic. A good place to start is with the National Chronic Fatigue Syndrome and Fibromyalgia Association, 3521 Broadway, Kansas City, Missouri 64111. Staying well-informed about CFS will help you feel more in control and maybe lead you to the strategies that work for you.

Accept your condition. Denial is a common reaction to being diagnosed with a chronic health problem. Try to accept the fact that you have a chronic illness and grieve for what you've lost. That means you'll have to give up, at least for a time, some aspects of your old life and accept new realities. Concentrate on preserving the best of your "old self" as you adjust to your situation.

Feel your feelings. Chronic ailments like CFS bring up a wide range of emotions—anger, sadness, guilt, loss, and grief. Let yourself feel all of those feelings and express them.

Give up the guilt. There's a dangerous concept going around that somehow people "bring on" or "attract to them" certain illnesses or problems. Another party line says, you can overcome anything if you just work hard enough. This kind of thinking leaves people feeling guilty and ashamed. Let it go. You are not responsible for your illness. You are responsible only for your reactions to your illness.

Inform your friends and family. Support from those closest to you is important during any difficult time. Unfortunately, CFS is widely misunderstood and many sufferers complain that their friends and family think they are faking, malingering, or "neurotic." Get some literature from the National Chronic Fatigue Syndrome and Fibromyalgia Association and educate them.

Try a support group. Talking with other people who are also coping with CFS helps alleviate feelings of isolation, provides a forum for sharing coping strategies and information about new treatments, and gives you another source of support besides your friends and family. Contact local mental health agencies or the National Chronic Fatigue Syndrome and Fibromyalgia Association for referrals to groups in your area.

Consider a therapist. If you're like most CFS sufferers, you're going to experience a wide range of emotions, some of them conflicting and difficult. Many sufferers experience chronic depression. It may be tough at times to distinguish between feelings of tiredness and the helplessness and hopelessness of depression. The support of a skilled psychotherapist can help you work through your situation.

Ration your energy. Fatigue is one of the biggest symptoms of CFS. Sufferers simply don't have much energy. You have to learn to spend the energy you do have wisely on things that are really important. Energy can be deceptive. You might think you are fine, then suddenly find yourself depleted. Expect to feel depleted at times.

Take a "power rest." When you have CFS, you need to rest and "recharge" your batteries frequently. Instead of exhausting "power lunches," try "power rest periods" or "power naps."

It's critical that you have rest periods before and after activities. Learn to tune in to your body and listen to what it says. If you're tired, rest.

Go for efficiency. Think of ways to be more efficient. When you go downstairs to do the laundry, take a book and plan to read until the laundry is done so you don't have to climb up and down the stairs several times. If you're chopping food or stirring a pot, sit on a stool rather than standing. Get a handicapped parking sticker to save you walking long distances. Use an electric shopping cart or consider having your groceries delivered. Hire someone to clean your house and mow your lawn.

Set reachable goals. You can't expect to accomplish as much as you could before you developed CFS. Set goals that you can reasonably attain. If you are having a particularly difficult day, lower your expectations and rethink your goals for the day. Instead of doing the grocery shopping, perhaps you should only wash the dishes.

Prioritize. There's nothing like a chronic illness to make you rethink your priorities and get in touch with what's really important. Remember you only have a limited amount of energy. You want to spend it on activities that are important to you. One way to prioritize is to make a list of what you must do, what you would like to do, and what really doesn't matter. Then focus on what's really important.

Stay flexible and adapt. You're going to have to pay attention to how you feel at the moment and adapt to your situation. For example, if you've agreed to go to a movie with a friend and you're too tired, ask the friend to bring over a video to watch on the VCR. Too tired to go out to eat? Order in! The key is to stay flexible and aware and to adapt as necessary.

Watch your scheduling. Try not to schedule more than one big event in a day. Keep your work and home schedules on the same calendar so you don't end up with a big sales presentation and your child's third birthday party on the same day.

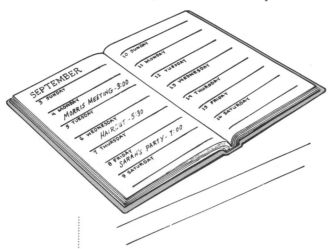

Eat right. There's no evidence that dietary changes alter the course of the illness, but you may as well give your body the best fuel available. Eat a low-fat, high-fiber diet and choose your foods from a varied menu.

Balance work and play. Both work and recreation are important in your life. While you may not be able to play in the same way with friends, don't shut them out. Make time in your schedule and budget your energy to include social time.

Don't overdo exercise. It's important to exercise as much as your energy allows. But listen to your body and don't overdo it. Walk instead of running, and if you're still too tired, stroll instead of walking.

Write down your thoughts and feelings. A journal can give you a place to vent your feelings and provide a focus for your thoughts. Rereading it will reveal the up-and-down pattern of your illness and remind you on your toughest days that it does get better.

Keep sexually active. CFS doesn't mean you have to give up sexual activity. Schedule lovemaking when you have the energy and feel good. Morning or afternoon is probably better than evening. Don't limit your sexuality to intercourse. Consider exploring a variety of ways of pleasuring one another.

Exercise your choices. Too often, people with chronic fatigue syndrome feel as though they have no control and that their choices have been stripped from them. Not true. While some choices (mountain climbing, perhaps) aren't possible right now, others are open to you. By exercising your choices, you can reclaim control over your life and fight feelings of depression.

Use laughter. It's tough to feel like laughing when you have a chronic illness and are facing a serious challenge just coping with day-to-day living. But laughter is, in fact, wonderful medicine. It will make you feel better and may even boost your immune function. Rent comedy movies, listen to humorous albums, read funny books, or catch a comedy act at a local club. Laughter will also help you take yourself and your situation less seriously.

Have patience. Recovery from CFS can be a long process, but some people may turn a corner in their recovery within 12 to 24 months and begin to regain their old energy. While that recovery might take a while, having patience and trusting in the process will go far towards making your journey tolerable.

Be wary of "miracle" claims. Any time there isn't a definitive treatment for an illness, a flood of "miracle cures" appear. People with CFS or any debilitating, chronic illness are vulnerable to hucksters selling unproven treatments. Hundreds, perhaps thousands, of CFS sufferers have been taken in by ineffective treatments like vitamin shots, hair analysis, oral doses of hydrogen peroxide, fasting diets, liquid potassium supplements, bee pollen, and others. Desperate CFS sufferers tell of spending thousands of dollars over the years on a wide range of CFS "treatments." Your pocketbook may not be all that suffers when you fall for these scams. Some "cures" may worsen your condition or be dangerous to your health. For example, the herb ginseng can actually increase fatigue. Be suspicious if:

• The claims sound too good to be true. If it sounds too good to be true, it probably is.

• The product claims to "cure" CFS. To date, there is no cure.

• The product relies on testimonials rather than scientific evidence to prove its worth. Even when testimonials appear to be sincere, keep in mind that CFS may spontaneously go into remission or the person may feel better due to the product's placebo effect (a beneficial effect that occurs but cannot be attributed to any special property of the substance).

• The advertisements use words like "secret," "little known," or "exclusive," or if you're told, "You're one of the few, lucky people to know about this product." If it's so good, why don't more people know about it? Why don't the hundreds of researchers working on CFS know about it?

• The product has been used in the past to "treat" other ailments. Many products and treatments, which were touted

•CHRONIC FATIGUE SYNDROME

as cures for cancer, arthritis, or AIDS, have been recycled and are now the newest "cure" for chronic fatigue syndrome.

• The promoter or advertising literature warns you against telling your doctor about it.

• The product is sold through a multilevel, "pyramid" marketing scheme.

• The ads claim the product "cleanses toxins," "oxygenates the tissues," or "detoxifies your system."

• If the physician or practitioner is obviously profiting from the treatment. For example, if he or she offers you supplements from his office or insists you buy from a particular pharmacy.

Live one day at a time. Many of the 12-step recovery programs advise people to "live one day at a time." That's good advice for all of us and especially for people with CFS. It's difficult to live with the unknown. Will you feel worse or better tomorrow? Will there be a breakthrough in treatment or a cure next week or next month? Not knowing can make you feel out of control. You can maximize the known by living for today. If you feel good, terrific. Make the most of it. Live in the now.

AT THE DOCTOR'S

It may be difficult to find a doctor who is knowledgeable and sympathetic to symptoms as vague and perplexing as those of chronic fatigue syndrome. But if you've been suffering from fatigue and other CFS-like symptoms for more than a month or two, you need to consult a physician for proper diagnosis. CFS symptoms can mimic other illnesses, some quite serious. Your physician needs to eliminate them as a cause of your symptoms.

You can help your doctor determine the cause of your symptoms by writing down the answers to these questions before you go for your appointment. Then take your written answers with you.

• When did your symptoms first begin?

• What symptoms exactly do you have?

• Do certain things make you feel better or worse?

• Are you having any difficulties in your job? Your relationships? With friends or family? Other personal problems?

• Does anyone in your family suffer from chronic fatigue syndrome?

• What, if any, prescription or over-the-counter medications, vitamins, and/or food supplements are you taking?

Sources: Judy Basso, President, Chronic Fatigue Syndrome Association of Minnesota, Minneapolis, Minnesota. **James F. Jones, M.D.,** Professor, Pediatric Medicine, University of Colorado School of Medicine; Staff Member, National Jewish Center for Immunology and Respiratory Medicine, Denver, Colorado. **Brian Lutterman,** CFS patient, Author, *Long Night's Journey: Coping With Chronic Fatigue Syndrome.* **Kobrin Pitzele,** author *We Are Not Alone: Learning to Live with Chronic Illness.* **Orvalene Prewitt,** President, National Chronic Fatigue Syndrome and Fibromyalgia Association, Kansas City, Missouri. **John H. Renner, M.D.,** President, Consumer Health Information Research Institute, Kansas City, Missouri; Board Member, National Council Against Health Fraud. **Anne Simons, M.D.,** Coauthor, *Before You Call the Doctor;* Family Practitioner, San Francisco Department of Public Health; Family Practitioner and Assistant Clinical Professor, Family and Community Medicine, University of California San Francisco Medical Center, San Francisco, California. **Meredith Titus, PhD.,** Senior Psychologist, The Menninger Clinic, Topeka, Kansas.

Strategies to

Help You Feel

Better

Ⓨou feel stuffy and your nose runs constantly. Your throat is raw from a hacking cough. You feel feverish, achy. Your head hurts and your eyes itch. Welcome to the wonderful world of the common cold.

It may be comforting to know you're not alone in your cold misery. Most adults contract two to four colds a year; children up to 12 colds a year. Over a lifetime, we spend more time sick with colds than with all other diseases combined. Colds are so common, in fact, that we spend $5 billion annually on doctor visits and various cold remedies. Unfortunately, since there is no cure for a cold, it's often money poorly spent.

Causes

A cold is actually an infection of the upper respiratory tract, which includes the nose, throat, and sinuses. It can be caused by any one of more than 200 viruses. Technically, each virus produces a "unique" cold with various combinations of the symptoms we associate with the common cold.

The body has an amazing system for defending against colds. Cold viruses reproduce best at about 90 degrees Fahrenheit. To keep viruses from reproducing in the body, the nose warms and moistens incoming virus-laden air. Additionally, the mucus that lines the nose and throat traps virus particles, and the microscopic hairs (cilia) in the throat push the virus-filled mucus into the stomach where they are destroyed.

Sometimes, however, this front-line defensive system breaks down. Virus particles penetrate the mucus layer of the nose and throat and attach themselves to cells there. The virus punches holes in the cell membranes, allowing viral genetic materials to enter the cells. Within a short time, the virus takes over and forces the cells to produce thousands of new virus particles.

The body responds to the viral invasion: The nose and throat release chemicals to trigger the immune system; the injured cells produce chemicals called prostaglandins, which trigger inflammation and attract infection-fighting white blood cells; tiny blood vessels stretch, allowing spaces to open up to allow blood fluid (plasma) and specialized white cells to enter the infected area; as the plasma is released, the body temperature increases, enhancing the immune

---

WARNING!

Most colds can be effectively treated with home care. However, call your doctor if:

- **You have a headache and stiff neck with no other cold symptoms. (Your symptoms may indicate meningitis.)**
- **You have a headache and sore throat with no other symptoms. (Your symptoms may indicate strep throat.)**
- **You have cold symptoms and significant pain across your nose and face that doesn't go away. (You may have a sinus infection that requires antibiotics.)**
- **Your fever is above 101 degrees Fahrenheit (adults), you've taken aspirin, and it doesn't go down. Your child has a fever above 102 degrees.**
- **Your cold symptoms seem to be going away, but you suddenly develop a fever. (This may indicate pneumonia, which tends to set in toward the end of a cold.)**
- **You develop a "dry" cough (one that doesn't bring up phlegm and debris) for more than ten days.**
- **You cough up blood.**
- **You have nasal congestion that lasts longer than three weeks or causes severe ear pain or hearing loss.**

---

response; and histamine is released, increasing nasal mucus production in an effort to trap viral particles.

Then the body brings out its big guns: specialized white blood cells called monocytes and lymphocytes; interferon, the "body's own anti-viral drug"; and 20 or more proteins that circulate in the blood plasma and coat the viruses and infected cells, making it easier for the white blood cells to identify the invaders and destroy them. The cold symptoms you experience are not caused by the viruses, but by these bodily responses to their invasion. It takes about a day after the viral attack for you to feel like you have a cold coming on.

AT-HOME TREATMENT

There's an old saying in medical circles, "Treat a cold and it'll last a week. Leave it alone and it'll last seven days." Colds are "self-limiting," which means that if you do nothing they run their course and eventually go away. No cure exists for the common cold and there's little your doctor can do to help ease your cold misery. So when you catch a cold, there's no wonderful pill to make it all go away. But simple prevention measures and effective home remedies can help you come down with fewer colds and, when you do catch one, hasten your recovery. Here's what to do when the cold bug bites:

Drink, drink, drink. Fluids keep the mucus thin, which helps move virus particles out of the body. Additionally, colds tend to dehydrate you, so drink at least eight ounces of fluids every two hours.

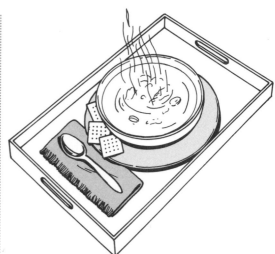

Go with grandma's advice. She was right: Chicken soup helps ease cold symptoms. Doctors at Mt. Sinai Hospital in Miami Beach studied the effects of sipping hot fluids and cold water on the clearance of mucus. To their surprise, chicken soup was the most effective, hot water the next, and cold water came in a distant third. Chicken soup and other hot liquids also have a decongestant, throat-soothing, and cough-suppressing action.

Take a load off. Doctors disagree about whether or not you should take a day or two off work when you come down with a cold. They do agree that extra rest helps speed recovery. From a prevention standpoint, your coworkers will appreciate your not spreading your virus around the office, especially during the first couple of days when your cold is most contagious. At home, resist the urge to get some chores done. Take a nap. Read a good book. Forego your regular exercise routine, as well.

Keep the chill off. While getting chilled won't give you a cold, it's a good idea to stay inside and stay warm once you've caught one.

Try salt water. Recent evidence shows that you can use a salt-water wash to actually wash out molecules called cytokines, or lymphokines that cause inflammation and swelling in the nose and reduce fluid production. Fill a nasal spray bottle with diluted salt water (one level teaspoon of salt to one quart of water) and spray each nostril three or four times, five to six times a day.

Gargle. Warm salt water (¼ teaspoon of salt to four ounces of water) also makes a great gargle for soothing sore throats and loosening mucus.

Try vitamin C. Research has been mixed on vitamin C as a cold remedy. It's not the sure cure that some have claimed it to be in the past. However, some studies seem to indicate that taking vitamin C may lessen the severity of symptoms but not the duration of the cold.

Don't overdo it with vitamin C, however. It's relatively safe up to 10,000 mg daily, but some people have found that 10,000 mg or more causes diarrhea. The safest way to increase your vitamin C intake is probably to choose vitamin C-rich foods more often. Since you need more fluids when you have a cold anyway, consider filling some of that requirement with orange juice.

Bring out your vaporizer. Vaporizers can loosen mucus, especially if you have thick sputum. They can also slightly raise the humidity in rooms where the air is dry from artificial heat.

Kick the nicotine habit. Colds are a great reason to quit smoking. Cigarette smoke irritates the throat and bronchial tubes. Smokers have been shown to have longer colds than non-smokers, perhaps because smoking depresses the immune system.

Nix the hot toddies. Almost everyone has a recipe for an alcohol-laden "hot toddy." While it may sound inviting when

18 TACTICS FOR FIGHTING THE COLD WAR

- Drink plenty of fluids.
- Try chicken soup or other hot liquids.
- Rest.
- Stay warm.
- Use a saltwater nasal wash.
- Gargle with warm salt water.
- Take vitamin C.
- Use a vaporizer.
- Stop smoking.
- Forego alcohol.
- Stand in a hot shower.
- If you use over-the-counter cold medicines, choose "single-action" ones.
- Don't overdo decongestants.
- Avoid antihistamines.
- If you have a mild fever, don't suppress it.
- For a sore throat, suck on hard candies or anesthetic lozenges.
- Forget antibiotics.
- Stay positive.

you're feeling achy and stuffy, alcohol actually increases mucous membrane congestion.

Go for "single action" cold remedies. If home care remedies aren't enough, you can ease your symptoms with the myriad over-the-counter cold "remedies" available. Many people opt for multi-action cold remedies, but cold experts recommend against them because they tend to overmedicate and are more expensive than single-action ones. Cold symptoms occur serially, not all at once. Why pay for cough medicine when all you have is a sore throat? And why risk the side effects from medications you don't even need?

If you need a decongestant, look for products like Sudafed that contain the ingredient pseudoephedrine. This ingredient effectively shuts down the swelling and fluid production and promotes drainage. People who have high blood pressure or heart disease, however, should avoid pseudoephedrine. Women who are pregnant should not take any drugs, even over-the-counter ones, without consulting their doctor. To loosen thick sputum and make it easier to cough up, choose a cough syrup with glyceryl guaiacolate (not dextromethorphan).

Steam it up. When you're feeling congested, stand in a hot shower and breathe the steamy vapors. Or boil hot water in a pan, let it cool a bit, and breathe in the steam (be careful not to get scalded). The steam will loosen your congestion and help the mucus flow so you don't feel so stuffy.

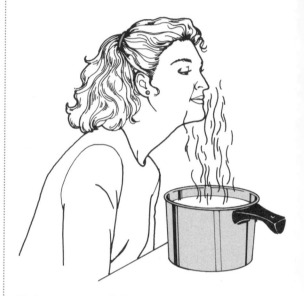

Take care with decongestants. Over-the-counter decongestant pills or sprays can provide congestion relief too, but don't overdo them. Don't use sprays for longer than three days or you may experience "rebound congestion"; in other words, you can end up with even worse congestion than when you started.

Decongestant pills won't cause the rebound effect, but they can cause side effects such as insomnia, restlessness, irritability, anxiety, and feelings of "speediness." Don't take over-the-counter decongestants if you have diabetes, high blood pressure, glaucoma, heart disease, or a history of stroke or if you may be pregnant.

Don't take antihistamines. These drugs work fine for allergies, but they do nothing for the common cold. They may stop the release of histamine and halt the runny nose, but they also dry up mucous membranes that are already irritated, thicken the nasal mucus, and cause an irritated cough and drowsiness. Antihistamines are often an ingredient found in multi-symptom cold formulas. Read labels and avoid those that contain them.

Let it burn. Cold experts say that a mild fever (below 102 degrees) actually enhances the body's ability to fight the cold virus. If you develop a mild fever, don't take aspirin or acetaminophen to lower it. (If you're over 60 or if you have heart disease or any immune-compromising condition, however, contact your physician at the first sign of fever.)

Give yourself a pep talk. Some doctors are still skeptical about the mind-body connection, but many suggest that a positive I-can-beat-this-cold attitude may actually stimulate your immune system and speed your recovery. Unfortunately, cold symptoms—headaches, stuffy nose, aches, cough—tend to bring on the blues. Researchers do know that negativity suppresses the immune system, causing longer, more severe colds. Whether or not a positive attitude can boost your immunity, it certainly can't hurt your cold or your mood to try to think positive.

Try hard candies or throat lozenges. If a sore throat is one of your cold symptoms, suck on hard candies or mild, throat-numbing lozenges.

Forego antibiotics. At the first sign of a cold, many people run to their doctor and request antibiotics. Antibiotics kill bacteria, not viruses, so they're ineffective against the common cold. If you develop a bacterial complication to your cold, such as pneumonia or a sinus infection, for example, antibiotics are appropriate.

PREVENTION

While there's really no surefire way to guarantee you won't contract a cold, you can decrease your risk with these tips:

Boost your immune system. No one is really sure why the body is able to fend off cold viruses one week and fall prey to the invaders the next. Some believe it may be related to how well the immune system is working. Many people, for example, find they contract more colds when

5 TIPS TO PREVENT A COLD

- Boost your immune system with a healthy lifestyle.
- Avoid contact with people who have a cold.
- Use Lysol to kill cold viruses on inanimate objects.
- Raise the humidity in the air with a humidifier.
- Use disposable paper tissues.

they're under stress and their immune system is compromised. Some women say they're more vulnerable to catching colds during their periods.

How do you keep your immune system in tip-top

shape? Live a healthy lifestyle. Eat a balanced diet, get enough rest, and exercise regularly. Effectively manage your stress with meditation, biofeedback, progressive relaxation, or any number of stress reduction techniques.

Avoid exposure. People who travel frequently or who have a high number of close contacts outside their community are more likely to encounter new cold viruses. While you can't quit your job or become a hermit just to avoid cold viruses, you can try to stay away from people with colds.

Cold authorities now say that cold viruses are spread by two methods: by viral-filled droplets from the nose being inhaled by others, which is the so-called "aerosol method," or by direct contact. A person with a cold blows her nose, which contaminates her fingers with the virus. When you shake hands with her, the virus is passed to you. Then you rub your eyes or touch your nose (people unconsciously touch their nose several times an hour) and catch the cold. Cold viruses can also live on inanimate objects such as telephones, doorknobs, and cloth handkerchiefs. No one is sure exactly how long they live. If you must shake hands or be in close contact with many people, try to wash your hands regularly and don't touch objects handled by people with a cold.

Bring on the Lysol. Wipe countertops, doorknobs, telephones, and so on with Lysol disinfectant to kill any cold viruses that may be lurking.

Humidify the air. If the air is too dry, the mucous membrane in the nose and throat can become dried out and vulnerable to viral invasion. Keep indoor humidity at home and in the office in the "comfort zone" of 50 to 60 percent with a humidifier.

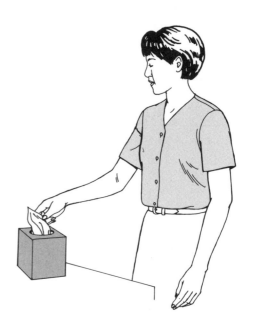

Use paper tissue. When you do have a cold, don't pass it on. Use paper tissues rather than cloth handkerchiefs, which reinfect your fingers.

Sources: **Michael Castleman,** Former Editor, *Medical SelfCare* magazine; Author *Cold Cures.* **David N. Gilbert, M.D.,** Director, Chiles Research Institute; Director, Department of Medical Education, Providence Medical Center, Portland, Oregon. **Donald Girard, M.D.,** Head, Division of General Medicine, Oregon Health Sciences University, Portland, Oregon. **Stephen Jones, M.D.,** Chief of Medicine, Good Samaritan Hospital and Medical Center; Associate Professor of Medicine, Oregon Health Sciences University, Portland, Oregon.

Relief from

Painful Lips

YOU WANT TO LOOK YOUR BEST FOR that important upcoming appointment—the meeting with your boss, lunch with your future mother-in-law, a photo shoot with the local paper. Then you feel the tell-tale tingling. Within hours, your lip has exploded into dozens of tiny white blisters and then a painful, unsightly sore. Once again, you've gotten a cold sore when you need it least.

Cold sores, also called fever blisters, are fluid-filled blisters that appear on the lips and on or around the nose. They often appear in association with a cold—hence the name. Some people experience no initial symptoms, while others feel a numbness, tingling, or tenderness (prodrome) a few hours before blisters appear. In one to two weeks, the blisters crust over, dry up, and heal.

CAUSES

Cold sores are caused by one of two closely related and highly contagious viruses, herpes simplex Type 1 and Type 2. The herpes virus is quite common and most people are exposed to it very early in life. Once exposed, you have it for life. Most experts believe the virus lies dormant in certain nerve cells in the mouth or nose. Then when you're stressed or the body's capacity to fight infection is compromised, the virus is reactivated. It overruns the body's protective system back along the nerve to the site of the original infection, and a cold sore develops.

Some people only experience one cold sore in their lives. Their bodies then effectively fight off any recurrence. Others suffer recurrences every few weeks or whenever their immune systems become compromised. Any number of things can precipitate an outbreak—a fever, a cold, emotional stress, skin injury from dental work, too much exposure to sun or wind. Many women find they are subject to cold sore outbreaks at certain times during their menstrual cycle or during pregnancy.

AT-HOME TREATMENT

There's no cure for cold sores. Doctors have used the prescription drug acyclovir for both cold sores and genital herpes, but it's more effective against genital herpes.

While you can't cure cold sores, you can ease their discomfort and avoid passing them along to others with these tips.

Avoid irritating foods. Once you develop a cold sore, don't irritate it further with salty or acidic foods.

Kill pain with aspirin or ibuprofen. These over-the-counter pain relievers can reduce pain and inflammation. Forego acetaminophen; it has no anti-inflammatory action. If aspirin

---

4 TIPS FOR DEALING WITH SORES

- Avoid irritating foods.
- Use aspirin or ibuprofen.
- Try creams with benzocaine.
- Don't pass it on.

---

or ibuprofen upsets your stomach, ask your pharmacist for "enteric" coated brands. Pregnant or lactating women or those with a history of ulcers should not take aspirin or ibuprofen unless it is recommended by a doctor.

Try benzocaine. For the pain of a cold sore, try a local anesthetic ointment that contains benzocaine.

Avoid passing it on. Herpes viruses are highly contagious even before blisters break out. Don't share cups or towels and avoid skin-to-skin contact (including kissing) until your lesions have completely cleared.

7 WAYS TO AVOID COLD SORES

- Manage your stress.
- Live a healthful lifestyle.
- Try not to catch colds.
- Avoid skin-to-skin contact with someone who has a cold sore.
- Use sunscreen.
- Protect your lips from the cold.
- Avoid injuring your lips.

PREVENTION

You can reduce your chances of getting cold sores with these tips.

Protect with petroleum jelly. Protect your lips when you go out in cold weather. Apply a coating of petroleum jelly or some other lip protectant.

Manage stress. Researchers have found that stress decreases the body's ability to fight infection. To prevent stress-related outbreaks of cold sores, adopt a stress-reducing regimen. Take particularly good care of yourself when you know your body is under stress, such as just before or during your period.

Live healthfully. A healthy lifestyle can help keep your immune system working at peak efficiency. Eat a healthful diet that contains plenty of fresh fruits and vegetables, whole grains, and legumes. Get enough rest (six to eight hours of sleep for most people). Exercise regularly; regular moderate exercise boosts the immune system. Manage your stress and don't smoke.

Try not to catch colds. Avoid close contact with people who have colds. Wash your hands frequently. Wipe counters and inanimate objects with Lysol disinfectant to kill cold viruses.

Avoid lip injuries. You can injure your lips by bumping into things. Lip injuries make you vulnerable to a cold sore.

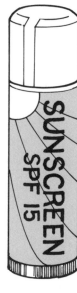

Avoid skin-to-skin contact. Herpes viruses are highly contagious. Avoid any skin-to-skin contact with anyone who has a cold sore.

Use sunscreen. Exposure to the sun can bring on an outbreak of cold sores. Apply sunscreen with a sun protection factor (SPF) of 15 or higher to your lips and nose.

Sources: Evan T. Bell, M.D., Infectious Disease Specialist, Lenox Hill Hospital, New York, New York. **Marcia Kielhofner, M.D.,** Clinical Assistant Professor of Medicine, Baylor College of Medicine, Houston, Texas. **Anne Simons, M.D.,** Coauthor, *Before You Call the Doctor*; Family Practitioner, San Francisco Department of Public Health; Family Practitioner and Assistant Clinical Professor, Family and Community Medicine, University of California San Francisco Medical Center, San Francisco, California.

•CONSTIPATION

How to Get

Regular and

Stay Regular

CONSTIPATION IS JUST ANOTHER OF life's little inconveniences— right up there with ink stains on a new silk blouse, plumbers who keep you waiting all day, and taking your car to the dealer for service. It's not life-threatening or horribly painful; just annoying and uncomfortable. It also doesn't make for polite cocktail conversation. But almost everybody has suffered from it at least once or twice in a lifetime and none of us has enjoyed it.

SYMPTOMS

It's important to remember that, when you're thinking about constipation, "regularity" is a relative term. People's natural rhythms differ greatly. Normal bowel habits can range anywhere from three bowel movements a day to three a week. The reality is that the definition of constipation has a lot to do with a person's comfort level.

A doctor will usually describe the symptoms of constipation as fewer than three bowel movements per week, a marked change in bowel patterns, straining and difficulty while trying to pass a movement, and the production of unusually hard stools. These symptoms are often accompanied by gassiness, bloating, and stomach distension.

CAUSES

Constipation can be caused by just about anything: stress, quitting smoking, not enough fiber, a lack of exercise, you name it. The condition is usually nothing to worry about. With the home treatments mentioned in the next section, you can expect that it will probably go away within a few days.

Occasionally, however, constipation can be a symptom of a more serious problem, such as an underactive thyroid, irritable bowel syndrome, or cancer, to name a few. If you notice a major change in your bowel pattern, blood in your stool, or unusual stomach distension or you have severe pain during bowel movements, skip the home treatments and head for your doctor's office. Likewise, if your constipation lasts longer than a few weeks, it's wise to give the physician a call.

AT-HOME TREATMENT

For the occasional bout of constipation, here are some tips to get you back on track:

Stay active. Exercise seems not only to boost your fitness level but also to promote regularity. It is not uncommon for athletes to become constipated when they take a few days off from their workouts. This may be because a lack of activity gives the bowels a signal to rest along with the rest of the body.

Low activity levels may be partially responsible for the tendency of older people to become constipated. The same goes for those who are bedridden. If you've been remiss in the activity department, consider starting a program of regular walking.

Drink to regularity. Upping your fluid intake may help alleviate

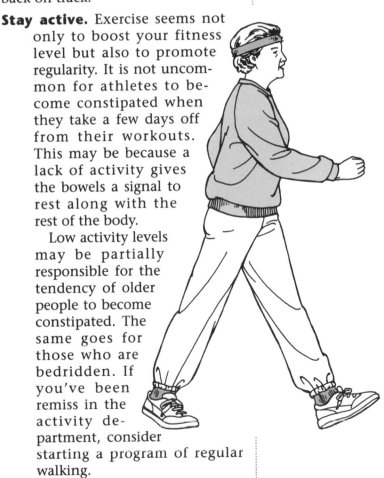

85

constipation or prevent it from happening in the first place. The reason for this is simple: If you are dehydrated, your stools will be dry, too. And dry stools are harder to pass. However, there's no need to go overboard: Excess fluid will only be passed out as urine. For people who are otherwise in good health, a good rule of thumb is to drink eight cups of fluid a day. (This rule does not apply if you suffer from a kidney or liver problem or from any other medical condition that may require you to restrict your intake of fluid.) Drink even more when it's hot or when you're exercising. Some dietitians suggest that athletes weigh themselves before and after a workout. Any weight lost during the activity reflects water loss. To replace it, they should drink two cups of liquid for every lost pound of body weight.

All liquids are not created equal, as far as treating constipation is concerned. Water, seltzer, juice, and milk are good choices. Limit alcohol consumption and avoid drinking a lot of caffeinated drinks. Caffeine acts as a diuretic, taking fluid out of your body when you want to retain it.

Listen to nature's call. People often suppress the need to move their bowels because they are busy, have erratic schedules, or just don't want to use public rest rooms. Over time, ignoring nature's call can block the urge so that it doesn't come at all. If at all possible, head for the bathroom in a timely manner.

Retrain yourself. Babies are born with a reflex to defecate a short time after they're fed. As we are socialized (and toilet trained), we learn to control our bladders and bowels, inhibiting this natural reflex. You may be able to revive it by choosing one mealtime a day and trying to move your bowels after eating. Younger people usually have more success with this method than the elderly.

Suspect your medications. Several prescription and over-the-counter medications can throw your system out of whack, causing constipation. Among the drugs that can cause constipation are calcium-channel blockers taken for high blood pressure, beta-blockers, some antidepressants, narcotics and other pain medications, antihistamines (to a lesser degree), and certain decongestants. Antacids that contain calcium or aluminum can also cause constipation. When choosing an antacid, remember that the names of many aluminum-containing antacids start with the letter "a." Those that start with the letter "m" usually contain magnesium, which does not constipate. If you are unsure of a product's ingredients, check the label or ask your pharmacist. If you are currently taking any medication, you might want to ask your doctor or pharmacist whether it could be responsible for your constipation.

Just add fiber and serve. The typical, highly refined, nutrient-deficient American diet is conspicuously low in fiber. And often, a good amount of fiber and roughage is all that's needed to ensure regularity. Fiber, the indigestible part of plant foods, adds mass to the stool and stimulates the colon to push things along. Fiber is found in fruits, vegetables, whole grains, and beans. It is almost completely absent from meats, chicken, fish, and fats.

The current recommendation for dietary fiber is to consume between 20 and 35 grams per day. Most of us get only 10 to 15 grams, so there's plenty of room for improvement. Fiber supplements may be helpful, but most doctors and dietitians agree that it's preferable to get your fiber from food.

Don't overwhelm your system. If you're switching from a low-fiber to a high-fiber diet, do it slowly. Your system will become accustomed more easily to these foods if you add them in gradually, eating small amounts of one high-fiber food at a time. Wait a couple of days before adding in the next high-fiber food. It's also important to drink generous quantities of fluids with high-fiber foods, to avoid a rebound constipation effect. (It's simple physics: A big, dry mass of fiber will be hard to move through the intestines.)

Increase your intake of fruits and vegetables. Aim for at least five servings of fruits and vegetables

---

12 TIPS TO TREAT AND PREVENT CONSTIPATION

- Start an exercise program.
- Drink eight cups of fluid a day (coffee, tea, cola, and alcohol don't count).
- Don't put off going to the bathroom.
- Try to get into a routine of going to the bathroom after a particular meal each day.
- Ask your doctor or pharmacist if your medication could be causing your constipation.
- Avoid antacids that contain calcium or aluminum.
- Increase your fiber intake.
- Add high-fiber foods into your diet gradually.
- Eat five servings of fruits and vegetables and six to eleven servings of grains every day.
- Learn to love beans.
- Substitute whole foods for processed and refined foods whenever possible.
- Don't use laxatives as a quick fix.

---

each day. This is also the number of servings government researchers are recommending to help prevent a variety of different cancers and other diseases.

One serving equals a half-cup of cooked vegetables, a half-cup of fruits such as berries or grapes, one piece of fruit, half a banana, or a cup of raw vegetables. If you eat a variety of fruits and vegetables, you'll be covering all your nutritional bases. Good choices are potatoes (white and sweet), apples, berries, apricots, peaches, pears, oranges, prunes, corn, peas, carrots, tomatoes, broccoli, and cauliflower.

Go for grains. Six to eleven servings of grains a day—in addition to the five servings of

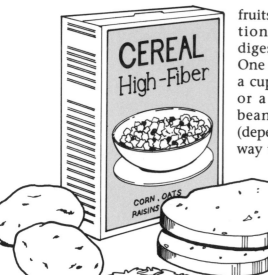

fruits and vegetables just mentioned—will also help your digestive system stay regular. One serving equals half a bagel, a cup of pasta, a slice of bread, or a half-cup of corn, peas, beans, potato, rice, or cereal (depending on the cereal). One way to get a good chunk of the fiber you need in the day is to start the morning with a high-fiber cereal. Check the labels on cereal boxes—anything with more than five or six grams of fiber per serving qualifies as high fiber. If you don't like any so-called "high-fiber" cereals, the best thing to do is to check the labels of the cereals you would be willing to eat and pick the one with the most fiber for your breakfast.

Labels are also helpful when choosing breads. Just because a bread is brown doesn't mean it contains a lot of fiber. Find a bread that has at least two grams of fiber per slice. Watch the portion size, too, when looking for high-fiber foods. Sometimes the package will list a very large portion size that's unrealistic for one serving.

Take a tip from your vegetarian friends. While animal-based sources of protein, such as meats and dairy products, contain almost no fiber, dried beans and legumes are excellent sources of roughage. This goes for pinto beans, red beans, black-eyed peas, lima beans, navy beans, and garbanzo beans. Many peo-

ple don't like beans because eating them may cause gassiness, but proper cooking can make this a problem of the past. Here's a tried-and-true technique for cooking dried beans to make them a little less "explosive": Soak the beans overnight, then dump the water out. Pour new water in and cook the beans for about half an hour. Throw that water out, put in new water, and cook for another 30 minutes. Drain the water out for the last time, put new water in, and finish cooking.

Don't take the fiber out of high-fiber foods. Compare the following: A glass of orange juice provides 0.1 grams of fiber, while eating an orange gives you 2.9 grams. A serving of white rice has 0.5 grams of fiber; a serving of brown rice contains 2.4. And while a serving of potato chips has only 0.6 grams of fiber, a serving of popcorn supplies 2.5 grams. The moral of the story? Processing and refining takes the fiber out of foods.

Bump up your fiber intake by switching to less-refined foods whenever possible. Switch from a highly processed cereal to a whole-grain cereal, move from heavily cooked vegetables to less-cooked vegetables, and choose whole-grain products over products made with white flour.

The rule is that as soon as you start juicing something or straining it or taking the pulp out, you're taking out the fiber. So try roughing it for regularity.

Don't fall into the laxative trap.
In our quick-fix society, we tend to want to take a pill for whatever ails us. However, while laxatives may seem like an easy solution for constipation woes, they can cause many more problems than they solve. Indeed, these tablets, gums, powders, suppositories, and liquids can be habit-forming and may produce substantial side effects if used incorrectly.

Laxatives work in many different ways, each with its own problems. Some lubricate, others soften the stools, some draw water into the bowel, and still others are bulk-forming. One real danger present with most types is that people can become dependent on them, needing ever-increasing amounts to do the job. Eventually, some types of laxatives can damage the nerve cells of the colon until the person can't evacuate anymore. Some laxatives inhibit the absorption or effectiveness of medications. Those with a mineral-oil base can prevent the absorption of vitamins A, D, K, and E. Still others can damage and inflame the lining of the intestine.

Some physicians believe that laxatives should be avoided in most cases and, when they are used, taken only under a doctor's care. In the long run, they say, you'll be much better off if you depend on exercise, adequate fluid intake, and a high-fiber diet to keep you regular.

Sources: **Peter A. Banks, M.D.,** Director, Clinical Gastroenterology Service, Brigham and Women's Hospital; Lecturer on Medicine, Harvard Medical School, Boston, Massachusetts. **Mindy Hermann, R.D.,** Spokesperson for the American Dietetic Association. **Marvin Schuster, M.D.,** Professor of Medicine with Joint Appointment in Psychiatry, Johns Hopkins University School of Medicine; Chief, Division of Digestive Diseases, Francis Scott Key Medical Center, Baltimore, Maryland. **Elyse Sosin, R.D.,** Supervisor of Clinical Nutrition, Mount Sinai Medical Center, New York, New York.

CORNS AND CALLUSES

How to Relieve

the Discomfort

IT'S ONLY NOON, BUT ALREADY THE CALlus on the ball of your left foot is killing you. It's been like this for a week now, and you're fed up. You can't wait until the weekend, when you can put on your comfy slippers and leave those uncomfortable high heels in the closet.

Corns and calluses are the most common foot ailments. Both are patches of toughened skin that form to protect sensitive foot tissue against repeated friction and pressure.

Corns are small, round mounds of firm, dead skin that form on or between the toes and, sometimes, on the bottom of the foot. Their hard, waxy core bores down into the skin and presses on the underlying tissue and nerves. Hard corns appear on the tops of the toes or on the outer sides of the little toes, where the skin rubs against the shoe. Soft corns develop between the toes, where moisture keeps them from getting as firm as the hard corns.

Calluses generally form over a flat surface. They usually appear on the weight-bearing parts of the foot—the ball or the heel. Sometimes a hard corn may form on the ball of the foot beneath a callus.

SYMPTOMS

Corns are usually rounded. They can be white, gray, or yellow in color. They most often form on the outside of the first or fifth toes, since that is where pressure most often occurs. When a shoe or another toe puts pressure against the corn, the tip can hit sensitive underlying tissue, causing pain. When a corn occurs on the bottom of the foot beneath a callus, a sharp, localized pain may occur with each step.

Calluses vary in size and shape, depending on where they grow and on how much skin is affected. Sometimes, calluses grow so thick and irregular in shape that the hardened skin cracks. When calluses occur on the bottom of the foot, each step presses the toughened area against the underlying tissue and may cause aching, burning, or tenderness, but rarely sharp pain. When pressure is relieved (by taking off your shoes and putting your feet up, for example), the pain usually subsides.

CAUSES

The skin buildup present with both corns and calluses results from excessive friction or pressure against the surface of the skin. As the pressure against the skin surface mounts, dead skin cells accumulate and the skin thickens. Since corns and calluses often follow blisters on the same site, they are considered to be the body's way of shielding the affected area against further injury. Wearing high heels and tight shoes can promote the growth of corns and calluses by increasing pressure on certain parts of the feet.

AT-HOME TREATMENT

The good news is that there are some things you can do to relieve the discomfort associated with these two conditions. Try the tips that follow to take the pressure off those sore spots. If, despite these self-help strategies, your corn or callus continues to cause you discomfort, see a podiatrist. If you have atherosclerosis, diabetes, or any other disorder that affects circulation, do not attempt to self-treat any foot problem; see your podiatrist right away.

Uncover the problem. Corns and calluses develop to protect certain spots on the feet from excess pressure and friction. So the best remedy for corns and calluses is to uncover and eliminate whatever is causing the problem. It may be a certain pair of shoes or heels that are too high.

Choose well-fitting shoes. When it comes to corns and calluses, it's important to go for practicality over vanity. Shoes that don't fit properly or that put excessive pressure on certain parts of the foot can cause corns and calluses.

Here are some guidelines for getting a better fit:

• Ask the salesperson to measure each foot twice every time you shop for shoes. Don't ask for a certain size just because it's the one you have always worn; the size of your feet can change.

• Try on both the left and the right shoe. Stand during the fitting process, and check to see that there is adequate space (three-eighths to one-half inch) for your longest toe at the end of each shoe. If one foot is slightly larger than the other, buy the shoes for the larger foot and use padding, if necessary, for a better fit on the smaller foot.

• Check to be sure that the shoe fits snugly at the heel. A heel that is too loose can chafe the foot, making corns and calluses more likely to form. In addition, make sure the ball of your foot fits snugly into the widest part of the shoe.

• Do your shoe shopping at the end of the day. Your foot can swell by as much as a half-size as the day goes by.

• Don't fall into the "Oh, they'll stretch out" trap. If the shoes don't feel right in the store, they may never fit comfortably.

• Talk a stroll around the store in the shoes to make sure they fit and they feel comfortable with each step.

• If possible, try the shoes out on a hard surface. Feet will not spread as much on carpeting.

• When buying shoes for everyday use, look for ones with fairly low heels.

• Choose shoes that have uppers made of soft, pliable material.

• Check into the store's refund policy. If possible, bring the shoes home and wear them around the house for an hour. If they don't feel comfortable, take them back.

• Have more than one pair of shoes, so that you do not wear the same pair day after day.

Since not all feet are created equal, finding comfortable shoes can be a difficult proposition. But don't give up; you'll be doing your feet a big favor. Also, do not allow other people to borrow your shoes. They may stretch them out in odd areas, ruining the fit.

Stay perfectly pedicured. Toenails that are trimmed correctly protect the toes from injury. However, if a toenail is too long, the pressure of a shoe can force the joint of the toe to push up against the shoe, forming a corn. To ease the pressure, keep your toenails trimmed. Trim them by cutting straight across so that they don't extend beyond the tip of the toe (cutting rounded corners may make ingrown toenails more likely to develop). After trimming, file each toenail to smooth any rough edges.

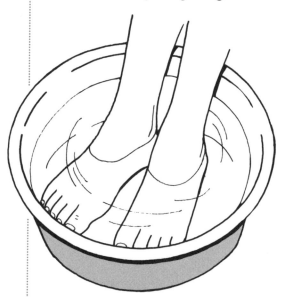

Take a foot bath. Here is a recipe for temporarily relieving the sharp pain of a corn: Soak the affected foot in a solution of Epsom salts and warm water, then smooth on a moisturizing cream. Wrap the foot in a plastic bag and rest for a couple of hours. Then remove the bag and gently rub the corn in a sideways motion with a pumice stone.

Try an ice pack. For a hard corn that is painful and swollen, apply an ice pack to the area for about 20 minutes to reduce swelling and discomfort.

Resist the urge to try home surgery. Skip the paring and cutting tools sold to remove corns and calluses. Cutting into your skin is always dangerous. You may end up contracting an infection or causing uncontrollable bleeding.

Cushion your step. Padding will transfer the pressure of the shoe from a painful spot to an area that is free of pain. Nonmedicated corn pads surround the corn with material that is higher than the corn itself, thus protecting the area from contact with the shoe. Use a similar technique when padding a callus. Cut a piece of moleskin (available at your local drugstore or camping-supply store) into two half-moon shapes and place the pieces on opposite sides of the area to protect it from further irritation.

Give your toes some space. You can help to relieve the pain of soft corns that form between toes by keeping the toes separated with lambswool or cotton. You can also use a small felt pad, like those sold for hard corns.

Keep it dry. A little cornstarch or baby powder sprinkled between toes will help absorb moisture and protect the skin from breaking down.

Use a home-brewed callus treatment. You can mix up your own callus softener by making a paste consisting of five or six crushed aspirin tablets and a tablespoon of lemon juice. Apply to the callus, wrap your foot in a plastic bag, and place a warm towel around the bag. Wait ten minutes, then unwrap the foot and gently rub the callus with a pumice stone.

Try a lube job. If you're going to be doing an unusual amount of walking or running, spread a little petroleum jelly on your toes to reduce chafing.

Use an over-the-counter treatment. Salicylic acid—the main ingredient in aspirin—is the only over-the-counter drug that the Food and Drug Administration (FDA) has deemed safe and effective for treating calluses and hard corns. For medicated disks, pads, or plasters, the recommended concentration of salicylic acid is 12 to 40 percent. A concentration of 12 to 17.6 percent is recommended for liquid corn and callus removers.

Keep in mind, however, that many podiatrists advise against the use of these products as home remedies, mainly because the active ingredient is an acid that can burn the healthy skin that surrounds the dead skin of a callus or corn. If you do decide to try one of these products, follow the package directions carefully and be sure to apply the product only to the area of the corn or callus, avoiding the surrounding healthy tissue (one way to do this is by spreading petroleum

---

11 Corn and Callus Helps

- Find out what's causing the corn or callus and come up with a way to eliminate the problem.
- Choose well-fitting shoes.
- Keep your toenails trimmed.
- Try a warm soak or an ice pack to relieve corn pain.
- Do not cut or pare a corn or callus.
- Use padding to relieve pressure and friction.
- Separate your toes with cotton or lambswool.
- Apply powder or cornstarch between your toes.
- Make a callus-softening paste out of five or six crushed aspirin and a tablespoon of lemon juice.
- Lubricate your toes with a little petroleum jelly.
- Use an over-the-counter treatment containing salicylic acid.

---

jelly in a ring shape around the corn or callus). If your corn or callus does not improve within two weeks, stop using the product and see a podiatrist. If you are diabetic or have any medical condition that hinders circulation, do not attempt to treat any foot problem at home; you should see a podiatrist at once.

Don't bother trying the following ingredients, which are not generally recognized as being safe and effective for removing corns and calluses, according to the FDA: iodine, ascorbic acid, acetic acid, allantoin, belladonna, chlorobutanol, diperodon hydrochloride, ichthammol, methylbenzethonium chloride, methyl salicylate, panthenol, phenyl salicylate, and vitamin A.

Sources: Joseph C. D'Amico, D.P.M., Podiatrist, New York, New York. Suzanne M. Levine, D.P.M., Podiatrist, New York, New York. Mary Papadopoulos, D.P.M., Podiatrist, Alexandria, Virginia.

●DANDRUFF

Get Rid of the

Flakes Fast Y OU'VE SEEN THE TELEVISION COMMER-cials. He's interested. He's obviously flirting with her. He finds her really attractive—until he spots those telltale flakes on her shoulders. Horrors! She's got dandruff!

Everyone experiences some degree of dandruff, skin scaling, and flaking on the scalp. One in five of us sheds enough scalp flakes to consider dandruff a problem. Dandruff has nothing to do with cleanliness. It isn't a precursor to baldness. And it isn't caused or cured by changes in your diet.

CAUSES

Dandruff is part of a natural and important process of shedding skin cells that goes on continuously all over the body. Every hour, your skin sheds millions of dead skin cells. In fact, every 27 or 28 days, all the old cells have been replaced and you have a brand new suit of skin. It's an important process because if you didn't shed these cells, your skin would become tremendously thick. In most cases, you don't notice the tiny flakes of skin continuously dropping off your arms and legs.

For unknown reasons, this natural skin shedding process is even more pronounced on the scalp. Instead of floating away like the dead skin cells do on other parts of the body, the tiny scalp flakes become trapped by the hair. Oil from the hair and scalp causes the flakes to clump together into larger, visible flakes. These more conspicuous lumps are called dandruff.

Doctors don't yet understand why some people's scalps shed more than others. A number of researchers blame a microscopic fungus called *Pityrosporum,* which normally lives on the scalp and other oily parts of the skin. People who suffer from large amounts of dandruff have unusually large numbers of *Pityrosporum.* Other skin experts believe problem dandruff is caused when the scalp sheds skin cells faster than normal. Whatever the cause, doctors don't yet have a cure.

AT-HOME TREATMENT

Anyone who has gone to a job interview or an important date wearing dark clothes covered with scalp flakes knows that dandruff is a cosmetic problem rather than a danger to one's health. Luckily, while it can't be cured, it can be easily controlled.

Shampoo every day. Often, the only treatment you need to control dandruff is a daily washing with your regular brand of shampoo. By shampooing the hair and scalp every day, you get rid of excess oils and flakes.

Try a dandruff shampoo. If your regular shampoo isn't holding off the flakes, try washing your hair with an antidandruff shampoo available over the counter in many grocery stores and pharmacies. The Food and Drug Administration recognizes five different agents that are effective against dandruff: coaltar extract, selenium sulfide, sulfur preparations, salicylic acid, and zinc pyrithione. Read shampoo labels and select one that has one or more of these ingredients.

Have patience. Antidandruff shampoos don't work right away. It may take a few weeks of regular shampooing to see results. The antidandruff effect of medicated shampoos lasts only two or three days, so be sure you're lathering with these shampoos at least every other day. If you wash your hair more often, use a regular shampoo in between.

Lather twice. Once is good, but twice is better, say many dermatologists. The first lather and rinse gets rid of loose flakes and excess oil; the second really goes to work on the scalp.

Leave it on. To be effective, the antidandruff medication must be in contact with the scalp for several minutes before rinsing. This gives the medication a chance to penetrate the skin cells and do what it's supposed to do. Lather and rinse the first time. Then lather and rinse a second time, leaving the suds on for at least five minutes.

Keep switching. Often the body builds up resistance to the antidandruff ingredient in a shampoo. If this happens to you, switch to another brand. Or, better yet, have several brands with different active ingredients on hand and rotate them every month.

Beat the tar out of it. If antidandruff shampoos aren't working, try one that contains tar. These shampoos are considered the "big guns" in the antidandruff war. They've been used effectively against dandruff for more than 200 years. The tar not only washes away excess flakiness and oil, it decreases cell turnover. Tar shampoos are

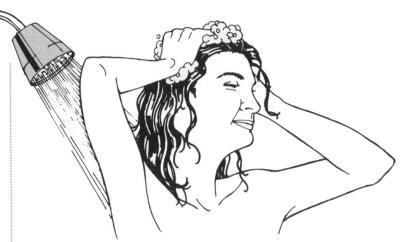

effective, but they do have their drawbacks: They have a strong odor, they can stain light-colored hair, and they can irritate the skin. If you find tar shampoos irritate your scalp and inflame your hair follicles, discontinue use immediately.

Rinse with lemon. If you're using a tar-based shampoo, try rinsing your hair with lemon juice to remove any lingering odor.

Try the shower cap. For persistent cases of problem dandruff that don't improve with routine antidandruff shampooing, try lathering and covering the sudsy scalp with a plastic shower cap; wait 30 minutes to two hours, and rinse.

Condition it. Many antidandruff shampoos are harsh. They tend to stiffen the hair and make it less manageable. To tame your tresses, use a conditioner after shampooing.

Resist the urge to scratch. A dry, flaky scalp can itch like crazy. Don't scratch it. You may end up causing wounds on the scalp that can make it vulnerable to infection. If you do

14 TIPS FOR TREATING THE FLAKES

- Shampoo every day.
- Try dandruff shampoo.
- Have patience. Antidandruff shampoos may take a few weeks to work.
- Lather twice.
- Leave antidandruff shampoo on your scalp for at least five minutes.
- Switch shampoo brands.
- Try tar-based shampoos.
- Rinse your hair with lemon juice.
- For persistent dandruff, wear a shower cap over lathered hair.
- Use a conditioner.
- Don't scratch.
- Shampoo out sweat.
- Use hairdressing products sparingly.
- Manage your stress.

scratch your scalp and cause lesions, discontinue using antidandruff shampoos and switch to a mild one like baby shampoo until the scalp heals.

Get rid of the sweat. Like other parts of the body, the scalp sweats. This perspiration can irritate the scalp and speed the flaking of skin cells. After exercise or strenuous work that makes you sweat, shampoo your hair as soon as possible to get rid of perspiration.

Go more natural. Sticky gels, sprays, and mousses may make your hairstyle look great, but they can contribute to flaky skin buildup. Most dermatologists advise cutting down and using them less often.

Relax. No one is quite sure why, but stress contributes to a number of skin conditions, including the proliferation of skin cells.

People under great stress seem to have more dandruff. Adopt an effective stress management program and find ways to relax and let off steam.

AT THE DOCTOR'S

Persistent dandruff that doesn't respond to home remedies may require a doctor's prescription for a stronger medication. Or it may indicate health problems other than simple dandruff.

If you have scaling and inflammation of the scalp and sometimes other body parts like the eyebrows, sides of the nose, the ears, and chest, you may be suffering from seborrheic dermatitis. If you notice scaly patches, you may have psoriasis, which is caused by an unusually rapid turnover of skin cells.

Prescription medications can control both of these conditions. Psoriasis, seborrheic dermatitis, and a number of other scalp inflammations can mimic dandruff. If the home remedies don't work or if you suspect your problem may be something other than dandruff, consult your doctor.

Sources: **Joseph P. Bark, M.D.,** Chairman of Dermatology, St. Joseph Hospital, Lexington, Kentucky; Author, *Retin-A and Other Youth Miracles* and *Skin Secrets*. **Fredric Haberman, M.D.,** Author *The Doctor's Beauty Hotline* and *Your Skin: A Dermatologist's Guide to a Lifetime of Beauty and Health*. **Andrew Lazar, M.D.,** Assistant Professor of Clinical Dermatology, Northwestern University School of Medicine, Chicago, Illinois. **Paul S. Russel, M.D.,** Past Officer, American Academy of Dermatology; Clinical Professor of Dermatology, Oregon Health Sciences University, Portland, Oregon. **Anne Simons, M.D.,** Coauthor, *Before You Call the Doctor*; Family Practitioner, San Francisco Department of Public Health; Family Practitioner and Assistant Clinical Professor, Family and Community Medicine, University of California San Francisco Medical Center, San Francisco, California.

•DENTURE DISCOMFORT

Strategies to

Soothe Sore

Gums

IF YOU WEAR DENTURES, YOU'RE IN GOOD company. More than 20 million Americans wear complete upper and lower dentures. Experts estimate that, by age 40, one in four people wears complete dentures.

Dentures have come a long way since George Washington's time. Back then dentures fit so poorly and so loosely, many denture wearers actually took out their dentures to eat. Today, denture wearers have a wide range of choices. There are full dentures and partial dentures. You may choose dentures that can be removed or those that are implanted into the bone and become much like your own teeth.

Dentures today are more lifelike, more durable, less bulky, and less porous (less likely to emit an offensive odor) than ever before. Refinements in dental techniques have made fitting them more precise, so that they fit properly both on the gums and in the "bite," the proper relation between the upper and lower jaws when they are closed.

Of course, there's nothing like your natural teeth. But if they become weak, decayed, broken, cracked, severely worn, or misaligned, your teeth can cause you misery. In fact, damaged teeth can become badly infected and cause serious health problems. For some people, dentures are a definite improvement over their own teeth.

However, new dentures can cause discomfort, especially during the initial "adjustment" phase. And well-used dentures can become uncomfortable years later when they have worn down and no longer fit properly. That's when the age-old problems come back—sore mouth, difficulty eating and talking, and "slipping" dentures.

CAUSES

It's poor fit that causes most denture wearers' problems. Dentures fit over the bony ridge of gum and bone. It may take a while for new dentures to be adjusted properly to fit exactly on the gum ridge. More likely, it'll take some time for you to become accustomed to the feel of the dentures. During this time, it's common to develop some soreness.

Even dentures you've had for several years can become a problem. When teeth are extracted, the bony ridge that's left no longer gets stimulation from the teeth. Without that stimulation, over the years, the bone is reabsorbed into the body. The plastic denture, of course, stays the same and begins to fit badly.

As the bony ridge shrinks, the dentures can slip, move around, and rub, causing sore areas. Too often, people try to refit loose dentures with commercial denture adhesives. While these products can temporarily solve the problem, using too much adhesive changes the relationship of the denture to the soft tissue and can result in even more soreness. Sometimes the body itself tries to refit the dentures by overgrowing tissue.

TREATMENT

While your dentures may never feel as comfortable as your own teeth, there are plenty of things you can do to ease denture discomfort.

Clean 'em up. It's vitally important when your teeth are first extracted that you keep your new dentures clean. Excess bacteria can retard the gums' healing process. Once you've grown accustomed to your new dentures, be sure to clean them at least twice a day. You can use a toothbrush with toothpaste or a special denture cleaner. Some people prefer cleaning their dentures with plain old soap and water. Just remove the dentures and scrub them with a hand brush and soap and water.

Keep the gums healthy. It's important to keep the underlying gum tissue healthy. Use a soft brush and gently brush them twice a day. This will stimulate the tissue and remove excess bacteria. While you're at it, brush your palate and tongue, too. This will stimulate the tissues, increase circulation, reduce bacteria, and remove plaque.

Try salt water. Diluted salt water (one half teaspoon of salt to four ounces of warm water) is an astringent that can both soothe and toughen gum tissue. It also helps clean out bacteria. During the adjustment period, or any time you develop a sore area in your mouth, rinse your mouth with salt water every three or four hours.

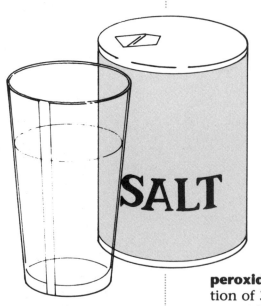

Go for the hydrogen peroxide. A half-and-half solution of 3 percent oral hydrogen peroxide (available at pharmacies) and water can also help clean out bacteria. Swish with the solution once a day for 30 seconds or so (don't swallow) and then spit it out.

Take it easy. It's not easy adjusting to the compression created by new dentures. Take your time and baby your mouth so you don't injure tender gums. During this adjustment period, eat soft foods. You'll be able to eat normally as soon as your gums have healed and your dentist is able to make the fine adjustments to your dentures. However, you may want to continue avoiding some foods like apples or corn on the cob. These hard foods can traumatize the gums of the upper jaw. You may be wise to be kind to your gums; remember to cut up your apples and take the corn off the cob.

Ease the pain. Your mouth will probably feel sore during the denture break-in period. Aspirin, acetaminophen, or ibuprofen can ease minor discomfort. If your pain is severe or if you've had your dentures for several years and pain develops, see your dentist.

Give your gums a break. It's OK to remove your dentures if your mouth gets sore. If you're feeling uncomfortable, you've probably got a little soft-tissue damage. Take the dentures out for an hour, then put them back in.

If you develop a sore, red spot, remove your dentures for up to 24 hours. If the soreness doesn't go away or if it returns when you start using the dentures again, see your dentist.

Massage your gums. Healthy gums need good circulation. One way to promote circulation and give your gums a healthy firmness is to regularly massage them. Place your thumb and index finger over your gums (thumb inside) and massage gently. You can do this several times a day.

Practice talking. It often feels awkward to talk with new dentures. It takes time for the tongue and lips to become adjusted to their contact with your new teeth. Practice by reading aloud and by speaking slowly and deliberately.

Don't play dentist. Avoid the temptation to play dentist and adjust your own denture with a pocketknife or other tool. Cutting or filing your dentures can cause them to break down, change the "bite," and alter their fit against the gums. If dentures are fitting loosely, don't try to fill the space between the denture and the gums with extra, over-the-counter adhesive. Dentures that slip or fit poorly can be adjusted or relined by your dentist.

Take 'em out. It's important to give your gums time to recover from the trauma caused by dentures. Many dentists say you should wear your dentures no more than 50 percent of the time. Whenever possible, especially when you go to sleep, take them out.

Seek help. You can often handle minor denture discomforts yourself. But see your dentist if:

---

11 WAYS TO TREAT YOUR CHOMPERS

- **Keep your dentures clean.**
- **Brush your gums, tongue, and palate.**
- **Eat softer foods.**
- **Take aspirin, acetaminophen, or ibuprofen for pain.**
- **Remove your dentures if soreness develops.**
- **Rinse with salt water.**
- **Rinse with 3 percent hydrogen peroxide diluted in water.**
- **Massage your gums.**
- **Practice talking.**
- **Avoid "readjusting" your dentures yourself.**
- **Wear dentures only half the time.**

- You develop soreness that doesn't improve within a week.
- You have an area on the gum that bleeds or is filled with pus.
- There's extra tissue growing, especially between the upper lip and the gum.
- You have a white sore for more than one week.
- You have a sore that doesn't heal completely within ten to 14 days.

Sources: Jack W. Clinton, D.M.D., Associate Dean of Patient Services, Oregon Health Sciences University School of Dentistry, Portland, Oregon. **Sandra Hazard, D.M.D.,** Managing Dentist, Willamette Dental Group, Portland, Oregon. **Ken Waddell, D.M.D.,** Dentist, Tigard, Oregon. **Ronald Wismer, D.M.D.,** Past President, Washington County Dental Society, Beaverton, Oregon.

●DEPRESSION

Self-Help for

Battling the

Blues

IN BED, YOU TOSS AND TURN, UNABLE TO get a good night's sleep. You feel anxious and worried. There's plenty to do, but the work piles up because you feel listless and tired. You don't even want to do anything fun. Friends tell you to "pull yourself together," but you feel helpless and hopeless. You have difficulty concentrating and making decisions. When you look in the mirror, you hate yourself. You are definitely in one of life's valleys—you are depressed.

Everyone gets the blues once in a while. Emotional lows and highs are a normal part of life. The blues become depression when you feel so lethargic and listless you can't function normally in everyday life.

WARNING!

People who are depressed are at risk for suicide. Friends and loved ones should always take hints or threats about suicide seriously. If you're having feelings or thoughts about suicide, see a mental health professional immediately. You or someone you know may be at greater risk for suicide when any of the following risk factors are present:
- **Recent death of a loved one**
- **Recently diagnosed serious illness**
- **Lack of a strong support system**
- **Previous history of suicide attempts**
- **Drug or alcohol abuse**

SYMPTOMS
If you're feeling depressed, you're probably having some of these symptoms:
- Crying spells.
- Feelings of guilt: "It's all my fault."
- Self-condemnation or self-hatred: "I can't do anything right."
- Trouble falling asleep or staying asleep.

- Extreme fatigue.
- Difficulty concentrating.
- Feelings of helplessness and hopelessness: "It doesn't matter. Nothing matters."
- Difficulty making decisions.
- Changes in appetite and/or noticeable weight changes.
- Periods of being in frenzied activity, followed by periods of total lethargy.
- Loss of interest in sex or sudden excessive interest in sex.
- Suicidal thoughts.
- Thoughts about dying.
- Physical symptoms such as headaches, backaches, digestive upsets, or other problems.

Depression often follows a stressful life event such as the death of a loved one, the breakup of a relationship, or the loss of a job. Other factors that can add to depression are poor nutrition, particularly skipping meals, eating junk food, and drinking alcohol; medications or street drugs; seasonal changes in light; or holidays, which remind people of times past or of loved ones no longer present.

Many people think of depression as a "women's problem," probably due to the emotional swings that can be caused by hormonal fluctuations during the menstrual cycle, pregnancy, and menopause. Others speculate that the problems many women have with low self-esteem and depression relate to the fact that most women have to juggle numerous roles—wife, mother, worker, housekeeper—while having less status and fewer opportunities in a "man's world." Some mental health experts say that women are at two to three times greater risk for depression than men. However, even these statistics may be questionable because women tend to seek help from mental health professionals more readily than men do. For this reason, there are more "depressed" women available to count.

Depression has plagued both men and women for ages. It transcends sex, race, religion, and socioeconomic class. Early Babylonians believed depression was a form of demonic possession. This theme resurfaced during medieval times when so-called possessed "witches" were drowned or burned at the stake for behaviors psychologists now say were most likely symptoms of depression. Even famous leaders like Abraham Lincoln and Winston Churchill suffered the "black dog."

If you suffer from depression, you're not alone. Depression is so common, some mental health authorities call it the "common cold of mental health." They tell us that at least 30 million Americans feel so depressed they don't feel pleasure and are unable to function in their daily lives.

IS IT REALLY DEPRESSION?

For many women, depression tends to be a catchall term for a wide range of feelings. Since it's "acceptable" in our culture for women to experience depression, it may serve as a disguise for other, less socially acceptable feelings like anger or sadness. Some mental health professionals believe depression is anger turned inward. Others say that any time feelings like sadness, guilt, or regret are repressed and go unexpressed, depression can develop.

Unhappy feelings aren't necessarily bad. In fact, some are downright healthy. For example, when someone you care about dies, mourning is a healthy form of sadness, a natural reaction to loss. Over time (sometimes a year or more), these feelings of grieving progress from bad to better.

The "downs" most people feel from the normal stresses of life usually last a few days to a week, and then resolve. With effective home remedies, these feelings can often be resolved even faster. In depression, however, a person often becomes stuck in the blues. There is no progression of feelings. Emotions become trapped in a repeating loop. If you feel depressed for more than a couple of weeks or if your depression interferes with your daily life, you should seek professional assistance.

Mental health professionals have categorized several types of depression, each with its own treatment. Reading the following descriptions may help you identify your situation and the treatment that is best for you.

Reactive depression. This type of depression is a reaction to stressful events—divorce, death of a loved one, a chronic illness, or any personal tragedy. The person is unable to recover normally from the feelings associated with the event. Common feelings include self-pity, pessimism, and loss of interest in life. It affects people of all ages.

Seasonal Affective Disorder (SAD). If you live in the northern latitudes and suffer depression during the winter months, you may suffer from seasonal affective disorder caused by a lack of exposure to sunlight. Doctors aren't sure exactly what physio-

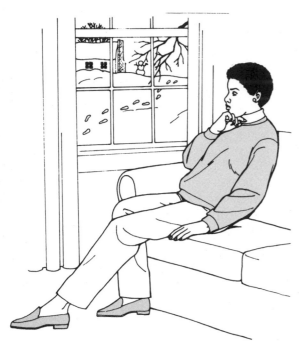

logical mechanisms are at work in SAD, but they speculate that depressed feelings and other symptoms may be due to an increase in the release of the hormone meltonin. SAD sufferers feel lethargic and irritable. They may also suffer from chronic headaches, increased appetite, weight gain, and an increased need for sleep. For unknown reasons, SAD is truly a "woman's depression," in that it affects women six times more frequently than men. Since about half of all SAD sufferers have relatives who also suffer from SAD or other emotional problems, researchers speculate that the problem may be inherited. If you think SAD is your problem, read the SAD profile in this book.

Biochemical depression. Doctors aren't sure why, but some people develop a biochemically based depression sometime during midlife. It's likely that this type of depression is caused by biochemical problems within the brain. The problem usually responds well to antidepressant medication. You may be more likely to develop this type of chemical depression if other members of your family have also suffered from this problem.

A special class of biochemical disorder is manic depression, known as bipolar disorder. The person experiences severe mood swings and intense, alternating periods of activity and despair. This requires professional intervention.

Postpartum depression. It is common for women to feel down a few days after giving birth. This is often referred to as the "baby blues." New mothers may be weepy, insecure, and confused, wondering how they could be feeling this way when they are simultaneously so happy about having had the baby. The "blues" pass in a few days. Postpartum depression, in contrast, may begin days or even weeks after a baby is born and is a potentially more serious condition. A woman may become very withdrawn, anxious, and agitated. She may have frightening thoughts about hurting herself or her baby and may be afraid to tell anyone what she is feeling. Whenever a woman has any of these frightening feelings, she should seek help immediately. Current medical treatments for postpartum depression are very effective.

Doctors say there are several reasons why so many new mothers experience this after-pregnancy depression: a sudden shift of hormones after birth that affects one's moods; a sense of anticlimax after the excitement of pregnancy and birth; fatigue from the rigors of late pregnancy and birth; fear and insecurity about one's ability to handle the duties of motherhood; and feelings that one's horizons have shrunk, especially if the woman has previously worked outside the home.

Disease or drug-related depression. Some diseases such as AIDS, hepatitis, stroke, chronic pain, and hypothyroidism can cause depression. In hypothyroidism, the thyroid gland malfunctions, leading to too little or no thyroid hormone circulating in the bloodstream. In addition to depression, other symptoms of hypothyroidism include fatigue, weakness, weight gain, impaired memory, constipation, and shortness of breath. Fortunately, the depression and other symptoms of hypothyroidism can be effectively treated with adequate doses of thyroid hormone.

Certain drugs such as alcohol, tranquilizers, and heart and blood pressure medications, as well as withdrawal from some street drugs like cocaine, can cause drug-related depression. Some women who take birth control pills find the drugs make them irritable, anxious, and depressed.

WHEN ARE YOU MOST AT RISK?

There are certain times in a woman's life when she's more vulnerable to developing depression. Some are related to the reproductive cycle; others involve life transitions or losses. By developing an awareness about when you are most vulnerable, you can learn when you need to use home remedies to take special care of yourself and avoid falling victim to severe depression.

The premenstrual period. The mood shifts, tension, anxiety, irritability, and depression many women feel during the week or days before the onset of menstruation are related to a woman's shifting hormones. Fortunately, the dark moods of women's premenstrual periods are transitory and usually lift with the first menstrual blood. This type of cyclical depression is not related to

"clinical" depression that generally requires medical intervention.

The postpartum period. As we said earlier, this is a period of doubts, anxiety, and sadness that many women experience a few days after having a baby. These "new baby blues" are generally mild and disappear fairly quickly. A small number of women, however, become more severely depressed for periods of up to six months. These women are more at risk for developing clinical depression that requires a mental health professional's care. Women with family histories of depression or postpartum depression are more likely to experience the postpartum blues.

The reproductive period. There's some evidence that taking birth control pills is related to depression. Some women report feelings of anxiety, sadness, and lethargy when they use certain types of the Pill.

The menopausal period. Menopause does not necessarily mean you're going to be plunged into depression. Research does not support that women are at greater risk for depression during menopause. However, some women do experience depressive feelings around the menopausal period. Mental health and aging experts speculate that this may be due to negative feelings some women have about aging and loss of fertility rather than to hormonal changes.

The grieving period. Grief, with its wide range of feelings—including sadness, anger, regret, guilt, relief—is a natural response to the loss of a loved one. Death and dying experts say that the mourning period usually lasts one year, sometimes several years. "Successful" grief means accepting the loss, feeling all the accompanying feelings, and eventually going on with your life.

Periods of change. Any life transition can be stressful and may precipitate feelings of depression. Even so-called "positive" changes such as moving into a bigger house, getting a promotion, or leaving an unhappy marriage can cause some people to feel depressed.

Periods of relationship difficulties. With divorce rates in the United States hovering around 50 percent, it's not surprising that marital disruptions are the cause of many women's depression. But it's not only divorce that can lead to depression. Any marital discord can cause feelings of depression. Relationship experts say that depression about marital difficulties often masks feelings of frustration, failure, hopelessness, anger, and unmet needs.

AT-HOME TREATMENT

When you're depressed, you wonder whether you'll ever feel good again. You can often beat mild to moderate feelings of depression with home remedies.

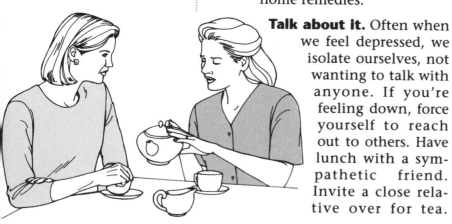

Talk about it. Often when we feel depressed, we isolate ourselves, not wanting to talk with anyone. If you're feeling down, force yourself to reach out to others. Have lunch with a sympathetic friend. Invite a close relative over for tea.

Talking out your feelings is cathartic, can make you feel less isolated and alone, and can help you gain new insights into your situation.

If friends or relatives can't provide enough support, seek out a qualified mental health therapist or pastoral counselor, or look for a support group. Various support groups are available (many of them free) for a wide range of needs, including bereavement and chronic illness.

Get out and move. When depression knocks on your door, it's easy to want to pull up the covers and hide in bed all day. That's the worst thing you can do. Mild to moderate exercise is one of the best home remedies available for fighting the blues. It's been shown to be as effective against certain types of depression as antidepressant medications (without the side effects). Regular exercise releases endorphins, the body's own "feel good" chemicals, and can also help you feel more empowered and in charge. Any exercise helps, but aerobic exercise that gets your pulse up to between 70 and 80 percent of the maximum recommended for your age group (220 minus your age, multiplied by .7 or .8), four or five times a week, works best. If you haven't been exercising before, start with a brisk 15 or 20 minute walk three times a week. Even if you can't do that much, just get out and do something.

Try a change of scenery. Depression caused by being stuck in a routine or by stressful life events can often be eased by taking a vacation for a few days. Don't think of a change of scenery as running away from your troubles. Instead, consider it a way to give yourself a much-needed break from your obligations and perhaps get a fresh perspective on your problems.

Don't junk out. Often when we're stressed, we eat high-fat, high-sugar junk foods. Experts disagree about whether deficiencies in vitamins B_6, B_{12}, and folic acid contribute to depression. In any case, it can't hurt to make sure you get your RDA of these vitamins. Perhaps more importantly, foods that run down your physical condition certainly won't help your depression. Eat a balanced, low-fat, high-fiber diet.

Accept and feel your feelings. Often we feel depressed because we resist negative feelings like sadness. In order for healing to take place, mental health experts say we have to be willing to accept a loss and experience all the accompanying feelings without shame or guilt.

Get a balance of rest. People who are depressed either sleep too much or have difficulty sleeping and become exhausted, which can further contribute to depression. If you find yourself oversleeping, set your alarm, get up, and exercise instead of sleeping late. If you're having difficulty sleeping, stay away from caffeinated beverages, don't exercise right before bedtime, and try a soothing nightcap such as hot milk or an herbal tea (not alcohol).

Write it down. There's something powerful about writing down how you feel. It gives you an outlet for your emotions and can help you to assess your fears, feelings, and options a little more objectively.

Say goodbye. One of the difficulties of losing a loved one is accepting the death and saying goodbye. Death and dying experts suggest writing letters to departed loved ones, telling them everything you wanted to say when they were here. Another healthy way to say goodbye and honor loved ones is with private rituals of commemoration on the anniversary of their death or at other special times like holidays. It doesn't matter how small the ceremony is. Light a candle. Say a prayer. Write a poem. Give yourself permission to re-experience those feelings of grief and say goodbye as many times and in as many ways as you need.

Reconsider your birth control. If you're taking birth control pills and you think your depression may be related to them, ask your physician for a different formulation or try another form of birth control. If you change your birth control and you're still feeling depressed, you may want to seek professional help.

Use laughter. Of course, the last thing you feel like doing when you're depressed is laughing.

---

14 TIPS TO HELP YOU BEAT THE BLUES

- Talk about it.
- Exercise regularly.
- Take a vacation.
- Eat a balanced diet.
- Keep a journal.
- Get enough rest (but don't overdo it).
- Accept and feel all your feelings.
- Allow yourself to say goodbye if a loved one has died.
- Re-evaluate your birth control.
- Expose yourself to comedy.
- Try relaxation techniques.
- Ask for help with a new baby.
- Try SAD lights.
- Consider professional support.

But research has shown that laughter is a powerful antidepressant. Rent funny movies, listen to comedy albums, or check out a comedy club.

Nix the alcohol. Many people reach for an alcoholic drink when they feel down. Resist the urge! Alcohol makes you feel worse, since it's a depressant.

Go for the relaxation. Try stress-reducing techniques like meditation, deep "belly" breathing, progressive relaxation, biofeedback, etc.

Ask for practical help. If you've just given birth and you find

yourself feeling depressed and overwhelmed, get help coping with the new baby. When friends and family aren't available, consider hiring some professional help, especially at first.

Try SAD lights. If your problem is winter depression, high-intensity, full-spectrum lights have been shown to be very effective for eight out of ten SAD sufferers. Individuals who are exposed to these special lights usually experience relief within seven to ten days. You can purchase or lease these lights through mental health professionals; use them only under a professional's care.

Consider professional support. While mild to moderate depression can often be helped with home remedies, it's important to get help when you need it. If you've tried self-care strategies and they haven't helped, if your depression lasts for several weeks, or if you're having suicidal thoughts or fantasies, don't be afraid to get professional help.

Sources: Wendy Davis, Ph.D., Therapist, Portland, Oregon. Sadja Greenwood, M.D., Author, *Menopause Naturally*; Assistant Clinical Professor, Department of Obstetrics, Gynecology, and Reproductive Services, University of California at San Francisco, San Francisco, California. Anne Simons, M.D., Coauthor, *Before You Call the Doctor*; Family Practitioner, San Francisco Department of Public Health; Family Practitioner and Assistant Clinical Professor, Family and Community Medicine, University of California San Francisco Medical Center, San Francisco, California. Susan Woodruff, B.S.N., Childbirth and Parenting Education Coordinator, Tuality Community Hospital, Hillsboro, Oregon.

•DERMATITIS AND ECZEMA

How to Beat

the Itch

ALMOST EVERYBODY HAS SUFFERED from an itchy insect bite or a 24-hour case of heat rash at one time or another. However, if you've got a scaly, itchy rash that doesn't seem to go away after a day or so and is actually getting worse, it is probably some form of dermatitis or eczema.

The term "dermatitis" simply means that your skin is inflamed—itchy, red, swollen, just plain irritated. "Eczema," too, is often employed as a catchall term for a persistent, itchy rash. Some experts use the term interchangeably with dermatitis; others consider eczema to be a type of dermatitis. However, under these two broad headings are several types of itchy skin irritations, all of which have different symptoms, causes, treatments, and prevention strategies.

Many types of dermatitis can be successfully treated at home. However, because there is such a bewildering variety of skin diseases, and because some can be dangerous if neglected, it's probably a good idea to see a physician if your condition doesn't clear up within several days.

CAUSES AND SYMPTOMS

Dermatitis can be caused by a number of different irritants and ailments, all with their own characteristic symptoms. The following is a breakdown of several recognized types, as well as their causes and symptoms:

Contact dermatitis. A skin inflammation caused by a substance that has touched the skin. When the reaction is caused by repeated exposure to harsh chemicals, it is called irritant contact dermatitis. When it is caused by an allergy, it is called allergic contact dermatitis.

How can you tell the difference between allergic and irritant contact dermatitis? Soap, for example, can cause either one. But it's repeated exposure to soap that causes irritation. In contrast, an allergic reaction can be triggered by a brief exposure to the perfume, or an antibacterial agent in the soap can set off an allergic reaction.

Irritant contact dermatitis may be caused by numerous industrial chemicals, as well as household soaps, detergents, oven cleaners, and bathroom cleaners. Allergic contact dermatitis is a bit more complicated. Sometimes it appears soon after contact with the substance. Other times, it may not develop until five or six days after the contact. In rare cases, the reaction shows up only after years of repeated use. There are also cases in which a substance, such as a shaving lotion or cosmetic, produces a "photoallergic" reaction—that is, a rash develops when the skin under the substance is exposed to sunlight.

The most common cause of allergic contact dermatitis is poison ivy, which causes reactions in about half the people exposed to it. The next most common allergen that causes this type of dermatitis is nickel, a metal commonly used in costume jewelry. Nickel can be hard to avoid, since even 14-karat gold jewelry contains some (24-karat, or pure, gold does not). Up to ten percent of the population may suffer from a nickel allergy.

Some other possible causes of allergic contact dermatitis include: Neomycin, a topical antibacterial drug; benzocaine, which is found in

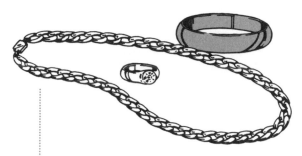

topical anesthetics; leather; formaldehyde, which is used in shampoo, detergent, nail hardeners, waterless hand cleaners, and mouthwashes; cinnamon flavor in toothpaste and candies; PABA, the active ingredient in some sunscreens; chemicals found in hair dyes; and the preservatives found in some cosmetics.

Latex is another common source of allergic contact dermatitis. With the advent of the AIDS epidemic, more and more people are using latex condoms in their practice of safe sex. Indeed, some 500 million condoms were sold in 1986. Likewise, more health-care professionals are routinely wearing latex gloves. As a result, more people are showing signs of being allergic to latex. Included in this group is approximately ten percent of all health-care workers. Between one and two percent of the general population has a latex allergy.

Some people may react to a protein in the rubber itself, others to some of the antioxidizing chemicals contained in the rubber (these help keep the rubber from breaking down), and still others to the preservatives, such as paraben, used in the "wet" condoms. (Most of the lubricated condoms in the United States use a silicone-based lubricant that's dry.)

Symptoms of "condom dermatitis" may include vaginal burning, redness and swelling in the groin, and an eczema-like rash on the inner thighs. If you have a reaction to the dentist's latex gloves, you might develop a rash around your mouth. The rubber dam used by some dentists can also cause allergies. If you're allergic to latex, you may also notice problems when you visit the doctor. For example, you may experience a vaginal itch after you see the gynecologist, because of the gloves the doctor uses during the exam.

You can test yourself by wetting your hand, then wearing a latex glove (or just the fingers of the glove) for 15 to 30 minutes and then looking for any reaction. If you react to latex on your hands, any part of your body will react to latex.

Eczema. An inflammation of the skin, marked by small blisters, redness, oozing, scales, crusts, scabs, burning, itching, and dryness. The skin at the back of the knee and the top of the elbow are common targets. When eczema is caused by allergies, it is often called atopic dermatitis (*see below*).

Atopic dermatitis. This condition, which is characterized by intense and miserable itching, takes its name from atopy, the term for an inherited condition that can show up as dermatitis, as allergies to certain airborne substances, or as asthma. If any other family members have any one of these conditions, you may be at risk for atopic dermatitis.

Infants and children are most likely to be plagued by atopic dermatitis. However, a majority of these cases subside by adulthood. If you or your child suffers from this chronic rash, you'll need the care of a physician, most likely a dermatologist or an allergist. Certain foods (such as wheat, milk, and eggs) and other substances (such as pollen and fur) often bring on symptoms.

Localized neurodermatitis. A condition in which thick, sharp-bordered, scaly breaks appear on the skin, occasionally with little blisters. This form of dermatitis may be caused by habitual scratching of an insect bite or other irritation. It usually disappears when the scratching is stopped.

In the case of an itch in the area around the openings of the vagina and colon, however, other ailments, such as warts, pinworms, hemorrhoids, or infections, are usually to blame.

Nummular dermatitis. A dermatitis characterized by coin-shaped patches of blisters, which later ooze and crust over, as well as dry skin and itching. Most often, it appears on the legs and sometimes on the buttocks and trunks of middle-aged people.

Seborrheic dermatitis. This condition causes dandruff in adults and cradle cap in infants. Symptoms may include scaling and inflammation of the scalp and sometimes the face or other body parts.

Stasis dermatitis. This stubborn skin inflammation of the lower legs is usually the result of poor blood return from the area. There is redness, mild scaling, and brown discoloration of the skin. If the condition is neglected, the skin swells and may become infected or ulcerated. This type of dermatitis should be treated by a doctor.

The symptoms of any kind of dermatitis may create a vicious cycle: Your skin itches, so you scratch it. It becomes red and swollen, and then tiny, red, oozing bumps appear that eventually crust over. You keep scratching, because the itching is unbearable, so the rash gets even more irritated and perhaps even infected.

AT-HOME TREATMENT

No matter what type of dermatitis you're suffering from, some general rules apply when you're searching for relief. These are outlined below. However, remember that the tips that follow offer only symptomatic relief from itching and irritation. With dermatitis, the only real "cure" is preventing it from recurring. So once your itch has calmed down enough that you can concentrate, read the next section on prevention strategies.

Chill out. Cool compresses can calm the itch and the swelling of many types of dermatitis. You can make one out of a clean handkerchief or thin towel. Dip the cloth into cool water or Burow's solution (available at your local pharmacy) and place it on the rash for 10 to 15 minutes every hour. Use wet compresses on weeping, oozing blisters, because the water will dry up the rash.

If it's late at night and you can't get to the drugstore for Burow's solution, you can dip your cloth into whole milk and apply it to the rash. The protein in the milk may help relieve the itching.

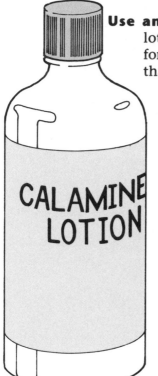

Use an old standby. Calamine lotion is an excellent remedy for itching. Apply it thinly, so that you don't seal the pores, two to three times a day. The one drawback with this remedy is that you end up walking around with visible pink patches on your skin. At least one manufacturer, however, has created a version of calamine lotion that's a little less noticeable. Ask your pharmacist for a recommendation.

Try using hydrocortisone cream. The one-percent formulation of hydrocortisone cream (available over the counter) is effective for the itch of allergic contact dermatitis, but it will not work as well for irritant dermatitis. It also won't help if you have a bacterial or fungal infection (two other common rash causes).

Avoid topical anesthetics and antihistamines. Topical anesthetics, especially the ones whose names end in "caine," are well-known for causing allergies in sensitive individuals. These products are often sold to soothe the pain of scrapes and burns. Likewise, topical antihistamines often cause allergic reactions. They may provoke dermatitis or significantly worsen an existing case.

Take an allergy pill. Over-the-counter oral antihistamines, such as Benadryl or Chlor-Trimeton, can help relieve itching. These medications cause drowsiness, but that side effect may actually be an asset at night, when itching may be severe enough to keep you from sleeping. If you take an antihistamine during the day and it makes you drowsy, avoid driving and operating heavy machinery.

Leave it alone. Dermatologists warn that scratching the itch can break the skin and cause a secondary infection. If you are going completely crazy with the itching, try rubbing the skin—gently—with your fingertips instead of scratching with your nails.

Bathe your itch. A soothing bath with warm, not hot, water can temporarily relieve an itch. Adding oatmeal or baking soda to bathwater will make it even more effective. Purchase an over-the-counter colloidal oatmeal bath treatment (the oatmeal is ground up so that it dissolves better) or add a cup of baking soda to the warm bathwater.

PREVENTION

The following are prevention strategies for allergic contact dermatitis, irritant contact dermatitis, and atopic dermatitis, the three types of dermatitis that are most treatable at home (for tips on treating seborrheic dermatitis, or dandruff, see the chapter on dandruff). However, if you feel that you are suffering from another type of dermatitis, if your rash becomes very uncomfortable, or if it persists for more than a week or so, it's probably a good idea to call your doctor.

Allergic Contact Dermatitis. It seems obvious: The best way to prevent allergic contact dermatitis is to find out what's causing the reaction and avoid it. For example, if you suffer from "condom dermatitis," you may be able to switch to another brand of condom for relief. Another option: Use a condom made of processed sheep's intestine. (This type, however, does not protect against the AIDS virus. To better protect against infection, try layering the latex condom with one of sheep's intestine. The order they're worn, of course, depends on which partner suffers from the allergy.)

The trouble is that uncovering the cause of allergic contact dermatitis is not always easy. First of all, we use so many products on our skin every day that it may be difficult to sleuth out which caused the problem (the average woman uses 17 different products on her scalp, head, and face each morning!). Another difficulty is the delay that can occur between exposure to the allergen and the development of the rash.

If you're having trouble pinning down the cause of your irritation, a dermatologist or allergist may be able to help. Either can do a test for common allergens (called a patch test) and ask you the right questions to detect the culprit.

Here are some prevention tips:

Keep your cool while wearing jewelry. The combination of hot, humid weather and jewelry that contains nickel may worsen the allergic reaction because perspiration leaches out some of the nickel. So before you start turning up the heat,

7 WAYS TO BEAT AN ITCH

- Apply a cool compress.
- Use calamine lotion.
- Try hydrocortisone cream, especially for allergic contact dermatitis.
- Don't use topical anesthetics or antihistamines.
- Take an oral antihistamine.
- Don't scratch.
- Take a warm bath.

remove any nickel-containing jewelry.

Be wary of all products. The term "hypoallergenic" on a label is very ambiguous. The only requirement for its use is that the product must have been tested on 200 rodent ears and not caused a reaction.

Paint on a protective coating. If you must wear jewelry containing nickel, paint the surfaces that come in contact with your skin with clear nail polish.

Cover up. Protect your skin when you're working in the garden, for example, by wearing work gloves and a long-sleeved shirt.

Irritant Contact Dermatitis. With this type of dermatitis, there is only one sure prevention strategy: Avoid exposure to the irritant. Until you manage to do that, you'll keep subjecting your skin to the irritant, and the rash will continue. If exposure to household cleansers is the problem and your hands are suffering, wear vinyl gloves, rather than those made of rubber, when doing household chores. (Almost no one is allergic to vinyl.) Wearing cotton liners with the gloves will help keep perspiration from further irritating your skin, although this can be a bulky combination.

Atopic Dermatitis. The key to preventing bouts of atopic dermatitis is to reduce irritation to the skin. The following tips will help you do just that:

Wash away the irritant. Before wearing new clothes, wash them to help remove formaldehyde and other potentially irritating chemicals that are used to treat fabrics and clothing. It's also wise to rinse your clothes twice to make sure that all the soap is removed, even if you use a mild laundry detergent.

Don't wear polyester. Choose loose-fitting, open-weave cotton or cotton-blend clothing to allow your skin to "breathe."

Avoid abrupt temperature changes. Your skin may be irritated by quick changes from hot to cold and vice versa, so try to keep temperatures as consistent as possible in your home. Maintaining constant humidity levels can help, too.

Skip the dragon-lady manicure. Keep your fingernails trimmed short. This will make it more difficult for you to scratch effectively and therefore harder to cause further damage to your irritated skin.

Go jump in a tub. Skip the hot water and instead slip into a warm bath or shower. Bathe for at least 15 minutes. Avoid the use of a washcloth (except for cleaning the genital area), because it's abrasive.

Don't dry out your skin with soap. Choose a gentle cleansing bar, such as Dove, Oiltum, Alpha Keri, Neutrogena, Purpose, or Basis; a nonsoap cleanser, such as Aveeno or Emulave; or a liquid cleaner, such as Moisturel, Neutrogena, or Dove. Rinse thoroughly, gently pat away excess moisture, and then apply moisturizer to your skin while it is still damp to help lock in moisture. Your best bet for an after-bath sealant is petroleum jelly.

Moisturize. Using a moisturizer is extremely important. Some good products to try are Aquaphor ointment, Eucerin cream, Moisturel cream or lotion, D.M.L. cream or lotion, Lubriderm cream or lotion, Neutrogena emulsion, Eutra, Vaseline dermatology lotion, or LactiCare lotion.

No tanning, please. The sun's rays will only act as a further irritant to your skin. Use a high-powered sunscreen (at least SPF 15) whenever you go out.

Rinse off the chlorine. After swimming, take a shower and use a mild soap all over. This will help rinse away chlorine and other chemicals found in most swimming pools—substances that can irritate your skin. Reapply your moisturizer after you've patted yourself dry.

Be a diet detective. The connection here is still up for debate. Some physicians believe that food allergies may play a role in atopic dermatitis, while others remain unconvinced. If you suspect that a certain food aggravates your rash, omit it from your diet for a few weeks. If your rash clears up and then returns when you eat the food again, you should probably avoid that food.

Sources: Col. Ernest Charlesworth, M.D., Assistant Chief of Allergy and Immunology, Wilford Hall U.S. Air Force Medical Center, San Antonio, Texas. Alexander A. Fisher, M.D., F.A.A.D., Author, *Contact Dermatitis*; Clinical Professor of Dermatology, New York University Medical Center, New York, New York. Paul Lazar, M.D., Professor of Clinical Dermatology, Northwestern University School of Medicine, Chicago, Illinois. Jerome Z. Litt, M.D., Author, *Your Skin: From Acne to Zits*; Assistant Clinical Professor of Dermatology, Case Western Reserve University School of Medicine, Cleveland, Ohio. Alan N. Moshell, M.D., Director, Skin Disease Program, National Institute of Arthritis and Musculoskeletal and Skin Diseases, National Institutes of Health, Bethesda, Maryland. Noreen Heer Nicol, M.S., R.N., F.N.C., Dermatology Clinical Specialist/Nurse Practitioner, National Jewish Center for Immunology and Respiratory Medicine; Senior Clinical Instructor, University of Colorado Health Sciences Center School of Nursing, Denver, Colorado.

18 WAYS TO PREVENT DERMATITIS

ALLERGIC CONTACT DERMATITIS:
- Find out what's causing the reaction and avoid it.
- Avoid wearing jewelry containing nickel in hot, humid weather or while exercising.
- Be wary of labels that say "hypoallergenic."
- Paint parts of nickel-containing jewelry that touch your skin with clear nail polish.
- Wear work gloves and a long-sleeved shirt when working in the garden.

IRRITANT CONTACT DERMATITIS:
- Avoid exposure to the irritant.
- Wear vinyl gloves, rather than latex gloves, when doing household chores.
- Try gloves with cotton liners to avoid the irritation that perspiration can cause.

ATOPIC DERMATITIS:
- Wash new clothes before wearing.
- Double-rinse your laundry.
- Avoid synthetic fabrics. Instead, wear loose-fitting, cotton clothing.
- Keep the temperature and humidity in your home as consistent as possible.
- Keep your nails short.
- Take a warm bath or shower.
- Choose a nonsoap cleanser or a gentle cleansing bar.
- Use a good moisturizer.
- Always wear sunscreen with an SPF of at least 15 when you go out during the day.
- Take a shower to wash off the chlorine after you get out of a swimming pool.

●DIABETES

Strategies for a

Full and

Healthful Life

Diabetes is more common than many people think. Doctors estimate that at least 12 million Americans have this chronic disease. Only about half of those who have diabetes know it; the rest go undiagnosed. With proper management, most people who have diabetes can live full, productive, healthful lives. However, some forms can result in blindness, kidney disease, blood vessel damage, infection, heart disease, high blood pressure, stroke, limb amputation, and even coma and death.

Doctors call it *diabetes mellitus,* Latin for "flowing honey," after the sweet-smelling urine produced by people with the disease. Diabetes is a malfunction of the way the body processes carbohydrates, the body's major source of energy. Normally, when we eat sugars and starches, they are converted into a form of sugar called glucose. The glucose is carried by the bloodstream until the blood-sugar levels rise to a certain point and the pancreas, a large gland located behind the stomach, goes to work. The pancreas produces insulin, a hormone that signals the body's cells to absorb the glucose from the blood. Once in the cell, the glucose is then converted to energy in the form of heat or is stored as fat for use at a later time.

That's what *should* happen. When you have diabetes, however, the body stops producing insulin or becomes unable to use the insulin it does produce. Without insulin, the glucose can't enter the cells and be used as fuel. Instead, this sugar builds up in the bloodstream, eventually ending up in the urine. In short, the blood sugar rises while the cells go hungry.

There are two types of diabetes: Type I, or "insulin-dependent," diabetes and Type II, or "non-insulin dependent," diabetes (also called "adult-onset" diabetes). About ten percent of people diagnosed with diabetes have the more serious Type I variety, most of them children and young adults. Because people with Type I diabetes produce little or no pancreatic insulin, they require daily insulin injections to control blood sugar.

Type II, or non-insulin dependent, diabetes usually doesn't require daily insulin injections. It can often be controlled with lifestyle changes such as diet, weight control, and regular exercise. Sometimes, oral medications are also needed to control blood sugar.

Symptoms

The high sugar content of the blood draws water out of the body and causes the diabetic to urinate frequently and feel excessively thirsty. The condition also causes the blood vessels throughout the body to narrow, decreasing circulation. As less blood is carried to vital areas, more complications can arise: kidney disease, slow wound healing, and foot and eye problems. Diabetes also alters how the body metabolizes fat and increases the risk of heart attack from atherosclerotic plaque ("hardening of the arteries").

Early warning signs of Type I diabetes include:
• Frequent urination
• Excessive thirst
• Extreme hunger
• Rapid weight loss
• Fatigue and weakness
• Irritability
• Nausea and vomiting

Early warning signs of Type II diabetes are often mild and may be ignored. See your doctor if you experience any of these warning signs:
- Frequent urination
- Excessive thirst
- Blurred vision or changes in vision
- Tingling or numbness in the legs, feet, or fingers
- Slow healing of cuts or bruises
- Drowsiness
- Vaginitis (or erectile dysfunction in men)
- Unsteady gait

CAUSES

Diabetes is still something of a mystery to researchers. Although experts aren't sure what causes Type I diabetes, recent research has suggested that it is an autoimmune disease in which something goes awry with the immune system which usually protects the body from disease. The immune system attacks the pancreatic cells that produce insulin. The "trigger" for this error may be a viral infection such as the flu or chicken pox.

Doctors aren't sure what causes Type II diabetes either, but it is typically associated with obesity. In people who have this condition, the body continues to produce the needed insulin, but for some reason is unable to use it properly.

Both Types I and II may also have a genetic component. It's not unusual for members of the same family to develop diabetes. For unknown reasons, women appear to be at greater risk for developing Type II diabetes than men. However, the risk for developing diabetes doubles for both women and men with every decade after age 40.

About 60,000 women annually develop a temporary form of diabetes during pregnancy called gestational diabetes. Women who are overweight and over the age of 35 are at greatest risk. The condition usually doesn't require taking insulin, but because gestational diabetes affects metabolism and can pose risks to the fetus, mothers-to-be with pregnancy-related diabetes must be strictly monitored and control their blood sugar carefully with diet. Although gestational diabetes usually resolves within 24 hours after delivery, women who develop this form of diabetes and deliver babies weighing ten pounds or more have a greater risk of developing Type II diabetes later in life.

AT-HOME TREATMENT

If you have diabetes, it's important that you be diagnosed and treated as early as possible to prevent serious complications. If you become pregnant, the American Diabetes Association recommends you get tested for gestational diabetes during the 24th to the 28th week of pregnancy.

Diabetes requires the ongoing care of your doctor and your own active participation in your treatment. You play an integral role in managing your condition and minimizing complications.

Watch your diet. The goal of dietary intervention in Type I diabetes is to normalize blood sugar in order to minimize complications. In Type II diabetes, the goal is to achieve and maintain normal weight.

Your diet must be adjusted with your doctor's or dietitian's advice to meet your individual needs. However, these guidelines from the American Diabetes Association can help:

• Carbohydrates should make up more than half your total daily calories. Each gram of carbohydrate provides four calories.

• Protein intake should not exceed 12 to 20 percent of your total daily calories. A gram of protein also provides four calories.

• Fat should make up 30 percent or less of your total calories. Substitute polyunsaturated or monounsaturated fat for saturated varieties in your diet (saturated fats come from animal products, such as butter). Each gram of fat provides nine calories—twice as many as a gram of carbohydrate or protein.

• Include plenty of fiber in your diet. Good sources of fiber include whole grains, legumes, and fresh fruits and vegetables.

Go for the complex carbos. Traditional wisdom says that diabetics should only eat complex carbohydrates like grains, potatoes, beans, and peas, while simple sugars like table sugar are forbidden. That's because complex carbohydrates raise the blood-sugar level less and raise it more slowly than simple sugars. While it's true that most of the carbohydrates in your diet should be complex ones, different foods affect blood sugar differently in different people. New evidence indicates that sucrose (table sugar) may not be strictly off the list for some Type II diabetics. However, before you begin munching on chocolates or bon bons, talk with your doctor and have your blood-glucose response tested with a wide range of foods.

Fill up with fiber. Fiber, the indigestible parts of plants, may be the reason that complex carbohydrates raise blood sugar more slowly than simple sugars do. In addition to helping control your blood sugar, fiber-rich foods make you feel full faster and can help you control your weight.

Lose excess weight. Eight out of ten people with Type II diabetes are obese. Being overweight can accelerate the onset and progression of diabetes and bring on serious complications,

19 WAYS TO COPE WITH DIABETES

• **Watch your diet.**
• **Go for complex carbohydrates.**
• **Fill up with fiber.**
• **Lose excess weight.**
• **Don't "crash" diet.**
• **Eat smaller meals more often.**
• **Take care of your feet.**
• **Adopt an exercise program.**
• **Choose your exercises carefully.**
• **Avoid dehydration.**
• **Set realistic exercise goals.**
• **Monitor your glucose level.**
• **Practice good oral hygiene.**
• **Don't ignore ill-fitting dental appliances.**
• **See your eye doctor yearly.**
• **Don't give up on having children.**
• **Maintain your sex life.**
• **Get support.**
• **Be prepared for an emergency.**

such as stroke and heart disease. The good news is that losing even modest amounts of weight can make a difference in your disease: High insulin levels drop, the liver secretes less glucose into the bloodstream, and peripheral muscle tissues begin to more effectively take up the insulin when you lose excess weight.

For many people with Type II diabetes, *losing weight is the cure for their condition.* Once they lose the excess weight, their disease disappears. If you're over your ideal weight, lose the excess pounds by eating a low-fat diet that is high in complex carbohydrates and by exercising regularly.

Forget crash diets. Severe "crash" diets can cause dangerous swings in blood sugar and can damage hormonal control. In addition, most people who rapidly lose weight regain it just as quickly. If you go on a very low-calorie diet, do so only under a doctor's guidance and only for a short time. Avoid nonprescription appetite suppressants containing phenylpropanolamine (PPA).

Eat less, more often. An excellent way to keep your blood sugar from dropping dangerously low and then spiking is to graze on several small meals throughout the day. Try for at least three small meals, plus two or three snacks in between and you'll find it will be easier for your insulin to handle. Just be careful not to go over your calorie limit for the day.

Watch your feet. People with diabetes often suffer from neuropathy, or damage to the nerves, especially in the feet and legs. Symptoms of neuropathy include burning, pain, and numbness. This condition can be particularly dangerous because with loss of feeling, minor injuries and sores can go unnoticed and become seriously infected, potentially leading to gangrene and even amputation. Here's how to take care of your feet:
• Examine them often. Before retiring, look your feet over to make sure you haven't developed a sore, blister, cut, scrape, or any problem that could become more serious. Women with vision problems should have someone else examine their feet. When you go to the doctor, remind him or her to examine your feet carefully and thoroughly.
• Keep them clean. Keep your feet scrupulously clean and dry to lower your susceptibility to infection.
• Don't perform surgery on yourself. Never use a razor or caustic agents on corns or calluses. Even pumice stones, which normally would be safe, are dangerous for you. Have your podiatrist or general practitioner take care of your corns and calluses.

117

• Don't ignore little problems. If you develop any cut, scrape, blister, burn, or other injury, take care of it immediately. Wash the lesion with soap and water to remove any foreign material and then cover it with a protective, sterile dressing. Be careful using adhesive tape, which can weaken the skin when it's pulled off. A better choice is paper or cloth-type tape. If the sore isn't healing, or if you notice signs of infection (redness, swelling, pain, or pus), see your podiatrist immediately.

• Never go barefoot. Your feet need the protection of shoes at all times.

• Buy shoes that fit. If you suffer from neuropathy, you may not be aware of the pain caused by ill-fitting shoes. Be especially careful that the shoes you buy fit correctly and are wide enough, have plenty of room in the toe box, and don't slip at the heel.

Exercise regularly. Exercise tones the heart and other muscles, strengthens bones, lowers blood pressure, improves the respiratory system, helps raise HDL ("good") cholesterol, provides a sense of well-being, decreases tension, and helps control weight. A program of regular exercise is important for everyone, but it's especially important for people suffering from diabetes. In addition to helping diabetics control their weight, a program of regular exercise promotes the movement of sugar from the blood-stream into the cells. It also helps your cells' ability to respond to insulin. Exercising in water will help you protect your feet from stress injuries.

Choose your exercise carefully. Some types of exercise are better than others for people with diabetes. For example, because many diabetics have neuropathy, jogging and high-impact aerobics that could damage nerve endings in the feet aren't good choices. Better activities might be brisk walking, bicycling, or swimming. If you're over 40, you should have a physical examination before beginning an exercise program. Talk with your physician about which exercise program is right for you.

Avoid dehydration. People with diabetes are particularly sensitive to dehydration. Once you start your exercise program, be sure to stay adequately hydrated by drinking plenty of water before, during, and after exercise.

Set realistic exercise goals. After your doctor gives you the go-ahead to begin exercising, set yourself up for success, not failure. Set realistic goals to avoid too-high or too-low blood sugar levels or other problems associated with doing too much too soon. Start slowly and build up your stamina.

Monitor your glucose level. If you keep your blood sugar levels as close to normal as possible, you'll be less likely to develop serious complications. At-home glucose monitors are now available that allow you to quickly and easily get an accurate reading on your blood sugar and enable you to adjust your diet, exercise, and/or medication dosage to keep your glucose at the right level.

Practice good oral hygiene. Because diabetics have increased risk of infection, it's important to prevent tooth decay and gum disease. Maintain a program of careful brushing and flossing after every meal and before bedtime, as well as regular professional cleanings and checkups.

Watch those dentures. Sores in the mouth caused by ill-fitting dentures or bridgework aren't pleasant for anyone, but for diabetics they can spell real trouble. Don't ignore sore spots or dental appliances that slip or move around. See your dentist right away.

See your eye doctor. Eye damage caused by diabetes (diabetic retinopathy) can lead to blindness. However, regular eye exams and laser surgery can help control the problem. See your eye doctor at least once a year.

Don't give up on having children. It used to be gospel that women with diabetes couldn't have children. Some diabetic women can't, but many with well-controlled diabetes can. Realize that diabetes does complicate pregnancy. Talk with your doctor about the pros and cons of having children.

Stay sexual. Some women with diabetes find they enjoy sex less because they have difficulty with vaginal lubrication and chronic vaginal infections. Estrogen replacement therapy can be helpful for older women with lubrication problems. Younger women might want to try lubricants like K-Y Jelly or bland vegetable oil (not Vaseline). Vaginal infections can be minimized with good blood sugar control.

Diabetes causes erection difficulties in some men. If your partner has this problem, have him ask his physician for a referral to a certified sex therapist. Studies have shown sex therapy to be helpful in aiding many diabetic men to achieve and maintain erection.

Get support. Having any chronic illness can leave a woman feeling frustrated, angry, powerless. It's helpful to talk with others who share your disease. Call the American Diabetes Association at 1-703-549-1500 or an ADA local chapter in your area to find a support group.

Be prepared. It's a good idea to keep quick "blood sugar" foods with you (fruit, peanut butter and crackers, hard candies, etc.), as well as some blood testing supplies. If you are insulin-dependent, bring along extra insulin and sy-

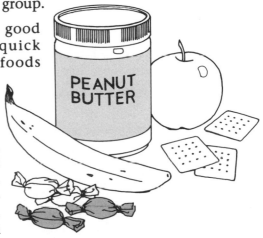

ringes. Regardless of the type of diabetes you have, always wear a Medic-Alert bracelet or necklace to let others know what should be done in case of an emergency.

PREVENTION

There are no guarantees that you won't develop Type II diabetes sometime in your life. However, you *can* reduce your chances by taking some preventive steps.

Know your risk factors. You should become familiar with your risks of developing diabetes. You are at greater risk of diabetes if:
• You have a family history of diabetes.
• You've had gestational diabetes.
• You're over age 40.
• You're of African American, Hispanic, Native American, or Asian Indian ethnic heritage. (Anyone can develop diabetes, but these ethnic groups appear to be at greater risk.)
• You're overweight.

5 TIPS FOR PREVENTING DIABETES

• Know your risk factors.
• Keep your weight under control.
• Be aware of your body type.
• Exercise regularly.
• Manage your stress.

Keep your weight under control. Type II diabetes appears to be directly related to being overweight. If you carry excess poundage, lose it with a low-fat, high-carbohydrate diet and regular exercise.

Be aware of your body type. You're at greater risk if you have an "apple-shaped" body and carry your extra weight around your waist and stomach rather than your hips, buttocks, and legs.

Exercise regularly. Regular, moderate exercise can help keep off the excess weight. It also promotes movement of blood sugar from the bloodstream into the cells, where it is burned for energy, and it improves the cells' ability to respond to insulin.

Manage your stress. No one claims that stress causes diabetes, but recent evidence suggests that stress could bring on symptoms in someone who may be prone to diabetes. The chemicals released in the body's "fight or flight" stress response may make the body less responsive to insulin in people who are predisposed to Type II diabetes.

Sources: Andrew Baron, D.D.S., Clinical Associate Professor, Lennox Hill Hospital, New York, New York. John Buse, M.D., Ph.D., Assistant Professor, Department of Medicine, Section of Endocrinology, University of Chicago; Director, Endocrinology Clinic, University of Chicago, Chicago, Illinois. Joseph C. D'Amico, D.P.M., Podiatrist, New York, New York. Ira J. Laufer, M.D., Clinical Associate Professor of Medicine, New York University School of Medicine; Medical Director, The New York Eye and Ear Infirmary Diabetes Treatment Center, New York, New York. Harold E. Lebovitz, M.D., Professor of Medicine, Chief of Endocrinology and Diabetes, Director, Clinical Research Center, State University of New York Health Science Center, Brooklyn, New York. Anne Simons, M.D., Coauthor, *Before You Call the Doctor*; Family Practitioner, San Francisco Department of Public Health; Family Practitioner and Assistant Clinical Professor, Family and Community Medicine, University of California San Francisco Medical Center, San Francisco, California.

Ways to Win

the Battle

MAYBE IT'S A FLU BUG OR THE ANTIBIotics you're taking. There could be many causes, but the result is that you feel miserable. You have the sudden urge to go again and again. When you do, your stools are watery and you may also have painful cramps, nausea, or vomiting. Diarrhea can be caused by intestinal flu, viral infection, or food poisoning, among other causes.

The most common symptom of diarrhea, of course, is loose, watery stools that can be mild (three or four times a day) to intense (10 to 20 times a day). The severity of the diarrhea depends on what's causing it and the overall health of the person who has it.

In most cases, diarrhea isn't serious. A day or two of diarrhea once or twice a year for healthy adults is common. In fact, intestinal problems are second only to the common cold in causing adults to call in sick for work. However, if diarrhea becomes chronic; if it affects the very young, the elderly, or people who are already seriously ill; or if there is blood present, it can be a real problem. Also, if you fail to drink enough fluids during your bout with diarrhea and you become dehydrated, you can turn a common, harmless situation into a more serious problem.

CAUSES

In situations where diarrhea lasts only a couple of days, the reason for it usually remains unknown. Most cases of diarrhea are caused by the following:

Viral or bacterial infections. Viruses or bacteria invade the intestine, causing it to absorb excessive fluid, which leads to watery stools. These "bugs" cause food poisoning, viral gastroenteritis, and traveler's diarrhea (also called "Montezuma's Revenge," "Delhi belly," or the "Turkey Trot," among other colorful names). If you visit a developing country in Asia, Africa, or Latin

---

WARNING!

While most cases of diarrhea can be self-treated, there are times when diarrhea is a clear signal to call your doctor. Diarrhea may be an early symptom of serious illnesses like Crohn's disease, gastrointestinal ulcers, diabetes, scleroderma, hyperthyroidism, ulcerative colitis, pancreatitis, cancer, and even AIDS. Or it may be a symptom of a mysterious and apparently stress-related condition called irritable bowel syndrome that causes alternating constipation and diarrhea. You should call your doctor if the following occur:

- **Diarrhea in infants or young children.** The smaller the body, the smaller the blood volume and the sooner dehydration can occur. Dehydration from diarrhea can occur in minutes in infants; hours in young children. Call the doctor at the first sign of diarrhea in an infant. Although diarrhea is less serious in children over 18 months, it still warrants a call to the doctor. He or she should be able to tell you how to treat your baby and what to give him or her to prevent dehydration and electrolyte imbalance. Once children reach eight years of age, follow the recommendations listed in this chapter for adults.
- **Diarrhea in the elderly.** Older people can't afford to lose much fluid because of age-related changes in their circulatory systems. Insufficient fluid in the blood due to diarrhea-induced dehydration increases the risk of stroke, heart attack, and kidney failure in older people.
- **Diarrhea in anyone who is chronically ill.** Diarrhea may be a sign of a change in their condition.
- **Blood (red or black) appears in the stool.**
- **Signs of dehydration appear.** These include dizziness on standing; scant, deep yellow urine; increased thirst; and dry skin.
- **Fever or shaking chills accompany diarrhea.**
- **Diarrhea lasts 48 to 72 hours.**

America, you've got a 30 to 50 percent chance of developing traveler's diarrhea. If you're in countries such as southern Spain, Italy, Greece, or Turkey, your chances of developing diarrhea drop to ten to 20 percent. The lowest risk areas are Canada and northern Europe.

Children in day-care centers are commonly infected by a large number of viruses and bacteria. Young children are notoriously unaware of good hygiene and commonly contaminate their hands with microorganisms in fecal material. They put their hands in their mouths or other children's mouths or touch food, and there's an outbreak of diarrhea, abdominal cramping, fever, and fatigue.

If members of a family all get diarrhea at different times, it's likely the problem is a viral infection. If you develop diarrhea on a trip out of the country or if several of you eat out and six hours later you all develop diarrhea, chances are good that bacteria is the culprit.

Intestinal parasites. These are less common than viral or bacterial infections and cause amebiasis (amebic dysentery) or giardiasis (giardia). Intestinal parasites are protozoa found in contaminated food and water that enter the gastrointestinal tract and try to set up housekeeping.

Amebic dysentery—which can cause no symptoms or stomach upset, flatulence, fever, abdominal cramping, and bloody diarrhea—used to be encountered only in the tropics, but the disease is becoming more common in temperate climates.

Giardia lamblia is the protozoan that causes the persistent diarrhea, abdominal distress, belching, headache, and fatigue of giardiasis. Giardia organisms are now widespread among mammals in North America and their feces have contaminated virtually all water sources, including those in remote, high elevations. This is of particular concern to campers who may drink from these sources.

Drugs. Diarrhea can be a side effect of a number of drugs, including some antibiotics, high doses of vitamin C, some prescription heart and cancer drugs, magnesium-based antacids such as Maalox or Mylanta, and laxative abuse. Some herbs, such as cascara sagrada, also have a laxative effect.

Lactose intolerance. Many adults and some children lack the ability to digest lactose, the sugar found in milk and other dairy products.

Sorbitol intolerance. A number of people are unable to digest this commonly used artificial sweetener.

Intestinal disorders. In some cases, diarrhea is caused by intestinal motility disorders like irritable bowel syndrome or colitis.

AT-HOME TREATMENT

Unless diarrhea persists, it's not a serious problem (very young, elderly, or seriously ill people are exceptions) and you can usually just wait it out. Within two to seven days, you should be good as new. These home remedies are aimed at relieving symptoms and preventing dehydration.

Drink, drink, drink. Dehydration is one of the most serious complications of diarrhea. You lose a lot of liquid and electrolytes, minerals like sodium and potassium that are essential for important bodily functions. Drink at least two quarts of fluid a day while the diarrhea lasts; three quarts if you also have a fever. Water, weak tea with a little sugar, and bouillon are all good choices. Some doctors recommend flat soda pop (non-diet), but be aware that anything with a high sugar content may increase diarrhea. Stay away from fruit juices, especially apple and prune, and caffeinated beverages, both of which can increase diarrhea.

You should also replace electrolytes with Gatorade or other replacement fluids. Special hydration formulas are available for infants. (Gatorade is not recommended for infants.) Since the sodium in these rehydration beverages can increase blood pressure, anyone with high blood pressure, heart disease, diabetes, glaucoma, or a history of stroke should consult with a physician before using electrolyte-replacement beverages or bouillon. For infants and children, use less-concentrated rehydration fluids like Pedialyte, Rehydralyte, and Ricelyte.

Sip, don't gulp. While it's important to drink plenty of fluids, don't gulp them. Gulping can overstimulate the gastrointestinal tract and cause cramping.

Keep it cool. Cool—not ice cold—drinks are best for an irritated gastrointestinal tract.

Try chicken broth. Warm (not hot) low-salt chicken broth or any kind of broth can be soothing and provide much-needed nutrients.

Keep eating. Too often, when people develop diarrhea they stop eating, believing that food is causing the problem. It's not. You need to eat to prevent dehydration and to get nourishment. Just keep it mild, not spicy.

Be a BRAT. Chances are good that you're not going to want a juicy steak for dinner. That's good. What your body needs are bland foods. Try the BRAT diet—Bananas, Rice, Apples, and dry Toast. Bananas help restore lost electrolytes. Soups and gelatins go down easily also. When you're feeling a little better, add other easily digested foods like crackers, noodles, cooked vegetables, and skinless fish. Do stay away from spicy or high-fat foods like pizza, burgers, ethnic dishes, and fried foods for a while.

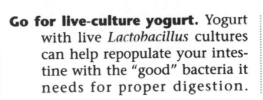

Go for live-culture yogurt. Yogurt with live *Lactobacillus* cultures can help repopulate your intestine with the "good" bacteria it needs for proper digestion.

12 Wᴀʏs ᴛᴏ Tʀᴇᴀᴛ Yᴏᴜʀ Dɪᴀʀʀʜᴇᴀ

- Drink plenty of fluids.
- Sip, don't gulp fluids.
- Drink cool beverages.
- Sip soup broths.
- Keep eating.
- Try the BRAT diet.
- Eat live-culture yogurt.
- Don't eat high-sugar foods.
- Use a heating pad on your belly.
- Avoid sorbitol.
- Try Pepto-Bismol, Kaopectate, or Imodium A-D as a last resort.
- Go for a bulk-forming laxative.

While there's little research to support yogurt as a diarrhea remedy, plenty of people have reported success with it.

Forget high-sugar foods. Now is not the time to eat your favorite chocolate or other high-sugar food. Fruit sugar may also increase diarrhea.

Try heat. A heating pad on your belly may relieve discomfort from intestinal cramps.

Read labels. You may be allergic to the artificial sweetener sorbitol. Try avoiding it and see what happens.

Get in the pink. Reaching for an over-the-counter diarrhea remedy like Pepto-Bismol isn't always the best idea. Diarrhea is often the body's way of ridding itself of troublesome bugs. But if you must have relief, Pepto-Bismol is a relatively safe, over-the-counter antidiarrheal medicine. Its mildly antibacterial effect can also help with traveler's diarrhea.

KO the problem. You're probably better off without them, but two other over-the-counter antidiarrheal medications can relieve symptoms. Kaopectate absorbs fluid and Imodium A-D slows the movement (motility) of the gut. Follow the instructions on the bottle. The elderly shouldn't take these medications because decreased motility can be dangerous in case of an infection and lead to even worse problems. Women who are pregnant or breast-feeding should consult with their physician before taking any drugs, including over-the-counter ones.

Try a bulk-forming laxative. Use a laxative for diarrhea? It may sound crazy, but over-the-counter bulk-forming laxatives like Metamucil (not chemical laxatives) contain fiber that absorbs water and adds mass to watery stools.

Pʀᴇᴠᴇɴᴛɪᴏɴ

If you are traveling, consult with your doctor about medications you can take to prevent traveler's diarrhea. In addition, there are some things you can do to help prevent the two to seven days of diarrhea, abdominal pain, cramps, gas, nausea, fatigue, loss of appetite, headache, vomiting, fever, and bloody stools of traveler's diarrhea, amebiasis, or giardia:

Never ice it. It doesn't matter how hot the temperature gets, forego ice cubes made from tap water when you're in a foreign country. That goes for ice in alcoholic drinks, too; alcohol does not kill the bacteria that causes traveler's diarrhea.

Go bottled. Drink only bottled mineral water or sodas. Don't drink water that is delivered to your table in a glass.

Thanks, I'll open it myself. Insist on opening your own bottles of soda, water, beer, and other beverages. Otherwise, you risk someone contaminating your bottle with dirty hands or a grimy dish towel. It's also the only way you can be sure someone didn't fill the bottle with water from the tap.

Nix lemonade and other fruit/ water blends. Often in tropical countries you'll find colorful glass jugs filled with lemonade, tamarind, or other juice/water drinks. Resist! You don't know the source of the water. Coffee, tea, or any water that has been boiled is safe.

Watch those dairy products. Stay away from milk or any other unpasteurized dairy product.

Pass on the raw. A foreign country isn't the place to indulge in raw oysters, ceviche (citrus-marinated raw fish), or sushi. Avoid raw vegetables, too, since these have probably been washed in tap water.

If you can't peel it, don't eat it. Eat only fruits you can wash with uncontaminated water and peel. The bacteria isn't *in* the food, it's *on* the food.

Pack your own. Whenever you're traveling in a foreign country, take along your own "emergency" kit full of granola bars, instant cocoa, tea, or similar items. When you make your own hot beverages, boil the water thoroughly.

Take along water purifiers. In some places, boiled water or bottled mineral water isn't available. Take along iodine drops or chlorine tablets to add to the water or pack a water purifier that has both a filter and iodine resin that can remove bacteria, viruses, and parasites. Pregnant women and

---

18 TIPS FOR PREVENTING DIARRHEA

To help avoid traveler's diarrhea, amebiasis, or giardiasis:
- Don't use ice.
- Drink bottled water.
- Open bottles of soda and other beverages yourself.
- Avoid lemonade and juice/water beverages.
- Avoid unpasteurized milk products.
- Forgo raw foods, including fish, shellfish, and vegetables.
- Peel all fruits yourself before eating.
- Pack your own treats.
- Use water purifiers.
- Don't buy from food and drink from street vendors.
- Never drink from lakes, streams, or rivers.

To prevent diarrhea from milk products:
- Avoid milk and other dairy products.
- Buy lactase-added products.
- Buy lactase supplements.
- Try soy-based milk substitutes.

To prevent infectious diarrhea in children:
- Have children wash their hands before eating and after going to the bathroom.
- Wash your own hands and the child's hands after changing diapers.
- Wash your hands before serving or preparing food.

people with thyroid disease or iodine allergy should not use iodine.

Don't buy off the street. Don't buy food from street vendors even if the food is hot.

Never drink from streams, lakes, or rivers. Boil water thoroughly or purify with iodine, chlorine, or water purifying filters.

If you have children, especially if they attend day care, try these tips to prevent infectious diarrhea:

Always wash hands before eating. Teach your children to wash their hands with soap and water before meals or snacks.

Always wash hands after going to the bathroom. This is an important hygiene step for your children to learn.

Wash your children's hands after changing their diapers. If there's an outbreak of diarrhea, be sure to wash your children's hands after changing their diapers.

Wash your own hands. Always wash your own hands after you change children's diapers or before preparing food.

If you think your diarrhea is caused by lactose intolerance, try these prevention tips:

Avoid milk and other dairy products. This includes products made from goat's milk, since goat's milk also contains lactose.

Buy milk and dairy products with added lactase. This enzyme allows people to digest milk sugars.

Buy lactase supplements. You can purchase lactase supplements (Lactaid) over the counter and add the caplets or drops to dairy products yourself.

Try milk substitutes. Plenty of soy and soy milk-based products are available.

Sources: **Peter A. Banks, M.D.,** Director, Clinical Gastroenterology Service, Brigham and Women's Hospital; Lecturer, Harvard Medical School, Boston, Massachusetts. **Richard Bennett, M.D.,** Assistant Professor of Medicine, Johns Hopkins School of Medicine, Baltimore, Maryland. **Harry S. Dweck, M.D.,** Director, Regional Neonatal Intensive Care Unit, Westchester Medical Center; Professor of Pediatrics, Associate Professor of Obstetrics and Gynecology, New York Medical College, Valhalla, New York. **Rosemarie L. Fisher, M.D.,** Professor of Medicine, Division of Digestive Diseases, Yale University School of Medicine, New Haven, Connecticut. **David A. Sack, M.D.,** Associate Professor, School of Public Health; Director, International Travel Clinic, Johns Hopkins University, Baltimore, Maryland. **Anne Simons, M.D.,** Coauthor, *Before You Call the Doctor*; Family Practitioner, San Francisco Department of Public Health; Family Practitioner and Assistant Clinical Professor, Family and Community Medicine, University of California San Francisco Medical Center, San Francisco, California.

Proven Tips to

Tame Your

Tresses

FEEL YOUR HAIR. IS IT DRY AND LIFELESS? Does it look like straw? Well, don't blame genetics for this one. Some people are born with hair that tends to be more dry, but most dry hair problems aren't due to health problems or family genes. If you've got dry hair, chances are good that you've been abusing your tresses.

CAUSES

Your hair may be dry due to exposure to harsh chemicals like hair dyes, bleaching agents, permanent-wave solutions, and chlorine in swimming pools and hot tubs. You may be shampooing too much or using harsh shampoos. Styling your hair with hot combs, hot rollers, and blow dryers may contribute to your dry locks. Even too much sun and wind can dry out your hair.

AT-HOME TREATMENT

With these simple, at-home remedies, your dry, fly-away hair can be helped.

Cut back on shampooing. Too much shampooing is one of the most common causes of dry hair. You don't have to shampoo every day. In fact, daily shampooing strips natural oils from your hair. Don't let your hair go too long without shampooing, either. Gentle shampooing can stimulate the oil glands in the scalp. Many hair-care experts recommend shampooing once every three days.

Take it easy. Dry hair is fragile and more subject to breakage. Shampoo gently without pulling or putting tension on the hair shafts. And don't scrub with your fingernails, since they can break dry hair and irritate the scalp. Use your fingertips, instead.

Go for gentle shampoos. As a rule, don't use a shampoo on your hair that you wouldn't put on your face. Dry hair needs a gentle, acidic cleanser with a pH between 4.5 and 6.7. While some people recommend baby shampoos, our experts say that the pH is too high for dry hair. Alkaline shampoos like baby shampoo just dry out the hair even more. Stick with the acidic shampoos.

10 WAYS TO MOISTURIZE YOUR LOCKS

- Cut back on shampooing.
- Treat your hair gently.
- Opt for gentle, acidic shampoos.
- Use a conditioner.
- Try hot oil treatments.
- Moisturize with mayonnaise or olive oil.
- Brush your hair gently.
- Choose boar-bristle or "vent" brushes.
- Massage your scalp.
- Try an egg shampoo.

Get into condition. Dry hair needs to be conditioned after every shampoo. Look for a conditioner that has little or no alcohol; alcohol tends to be drying. Also opt for fragrance-free products whenever possible, since they usually have less alcohol. If normal after-shampoo conditioning isn't effective, try using an overnight conditioner.

For hair that is severely dry and damaged, condition with Moisturel, a body lotion that contains petrolatum and glycerin. Apply it to damp hair, leave it on overnight under a shower cap, and rinse thoroughly in the morning.

Try hot oil. Over-the-counter hot oil treatments are great for restoring moisture to dry hair. Heat and place on the hair for five to twenty minutes (follow the package instructions). Wear a plastic shower cap while the oil is on and then wash your hair thoroughly with a gentle shampoo.

Pass the mayo, hold the mustard. It may sound a little crazy, but mayonnaise is one of the best hair moisturizers around. Use old-fashioned mayonnaise (not low cal or low cholesterol). First, shampoo your hair, then apply a tablespoon of mayonnaise. Wrap your hair in a plastic bag for 20 to 30 minutes before shampooing again and rinsing thoroughly. Olive oil is another effective moisturizer from your kitchen.

Go easy with the brush. Dry hair is fragile, and too much brushing can fracture the hair, causing it to fall. Brush gently and never when hair is wet.

Choose your brush with care. The type of hairbrush you use is important. Try a boar-bristle brush or "vent" brush, one with a rubberized tip, that doesn't pull the hair too much.

Try self-massage. Stimulate your scalp's oil glands by gently massaging it when you shampoo. With the tips of your fingers, gently massage all over the scalp.

Crack an egg. Here's a way to clean and shine your dry hair: Beat an egg in a cup, lather the egg into the hair, and then rinse. (Be careful to use tepid water, because hot water cooks the egg!) Don't bother shampooing afterward. Your "egg shampoo" will leave your hair beautiful and shiny.

Go easy on hair treatments. If you have dry hair, you don't necessarily have to abandon styling practices like dyeing or permanent waves, but space them out. Give your hair time to recover.

Be careful with heat. The combination of dry hair and hot combs, hot rollers, and blow dryers spells trouble—and more dry hair. Whenever you can, let your hair air dry. When you must use artificial heat, use a blow dryer on the low setting and avoid stretching or pulling on the hair while drying.

Sources: **Paul Contorer, M.D.,** Chief of Dermatology, Kaiser Permanente; Clinical Professor of Dermatology, Oregon Health Sciences University, Portland, Oregon. **Rose Dygart,** Cosmetologist; Barber; Hair-Care Instructor; Manicurist; Owner, Le Rose Salon of Beauty, Lake Oswego, Oregon. **Nelson Lee Novick, M.D.,** Author, *Super Skin: A Leading Dermatologist's Guide to the Latest Breakthroughs in Skin Care*; Associate Clinical Professor of Dermatology, Mt. Sinai School of Medicine, New York, New York. **Frank Parker, M.D.,** Professor and Chairman, Department of Dermatology, Oregon Health Sciences University, Portland, Oregon.

It's dry and flaky. It itches and feels rough to the touch. At its worst, it can become cracked and scaly and can develop chronic irritation. We're not talking about some exotic disease, but rather one of life's little trials—dry skin.

Everybody suffers from dry skin at one time or another. Dry skin not only feels itchy and rough; drying out the dermis makes it subject to wrinkling and can make us look older than our years.

The skin is made up of several layers. The outermost layer, the stratum corneum, becomes flaky, itchy, and unsightly when it doesn't contain enough water. Normally, this outer layer is kept moist by fluid from the sweat glands and underlying tissues. When the stratum corneum is allowed to dry out, dry, itchy, wrinkled skin results.

CAUSES

Some people have skin that is normally more dry. Their skin doesn't hold water very well. Other people have drier skin because they have less active sweat glands.

Plenty of other things can rob the skin of its natural moisture. Age, for example, can be a major factor in dry skin. As we age, the oil (sebaceous) glands produce less oil and the skin tends to dry out.

Dry air also makes for dry skin. The lower the water content or humidity of the air, the more water is taken from the skin. Dry skin is particularly a problem in areas such as the north central and southwestern parts of the United States where the winter months are cold and dry. If you add the drying effects of sun and/or high altitude, you've got a dry skin nightmare.

Another source of low humidity is heated or air-conditioned air in our homes and offices. When the humidity of indoor air drops below about 60 percent, the dry air sucks moisture from the skin.

The popularity of hot tubs in the last 10 or 15 years has contributed to the problem of dry skin. Paradoxically, water, especially hot water, can actually rob moisture from the skin. If you repeatedly wet and then dry the skin, over time the skin's outer layer changes and becomes less able to retain water.

External agents like detergents, chemicals, and harsh soaps can also be a factor in dry skin. This is especially true for people like nurses, dishwashers, cooks, bartenders, and anyone who has to frequently wash and dry their hands. These people often complain of red, dry, chapped, and cracked "dishpan hands." Harsh chemicals, solvents, soaps, and detergents can damage the outer layer of the skin, making it subject to drying and vulnerable to secondary infections.

AT-HOME TREATMENT

In general, dry skin can be effectively treated at home. In a few cases, dry skin (and dry mouth and dry eyes) can be caused by other medical problems. If your dry skin doesn't respond to the remedies suggested here, or if you develop a rash, blistering, or thick, scaly patches, see your doctor.

Bring on the moisturizer. Keep your skin protected with a moisturizing lotion or cream. After taking a bath or shower, apply the moisturizer while you're still damp. The cream or lotion will help seal in the water. Reapply moisturizers throughout the day whenever your skin feels dry.

Strike oil. There are a confusing number of moisturizers available. Which is best? Lotions are mostly water; thicker products like cold creams contain more oil and less water. Thicker, more oily moisturizers are better able to help the skin seal in moisture.

14 WAYS TO BE KIND YOUR DRY SKIN

- Moisturize.
- Choose thick, oily moisturizers.
- Try Vaseline "cream."
- Opt for unscented products.
- Take short, cool showers or baths.
- Use soap sparingly.
- Avoid scrubbing your skin.
- Add oil to your bathwater.
- Use a humidifier.
- Wear gloves to protect against drying chemicals.
- Don't use alcohol-based products and limit your alcohol intake.
- Use oil-based makeup.
- Turn down the heat.
- Avoid excessive sun exposure.

Try Vaseline. One of the oiliest products—and one of the best and least expensive skin moisturizers available—is Vaseline (petrolatum or petroleum jelly). Try mixing water with Vaseline to create a terrific moisture-protection cream.

Go scentless. Heavily scented products usually contain plenty of chemicals that dry your skin. Look for moisturizers that are scent-free.

Cool it. Opt for short, cool showers or baths. Bathe or shower only as often as necessary and never more than once a day. If you must have a long, hot bath, be sure to pat (not rub) yourself damp-dry with a soft towel, then apply a thick, oil-based moisturizer immediately.

Go easy on the soap. Too much washing with soap and water can damage and dry the skin. Oilated or superfatted soaps such as Dove, Basic, and Aveenobar are less drying.

If you suffer from chronically dry skin, take brief, cool showers or baths, and lather up only the groin, armpits, and bottoms of the feet. For extremely dry skin, use a soap substitute like Cetaphil.

Don't scrub. Many skin-care books recommend scrubbing your skin with various types of loofa sponges, buffing puffs, or grainy cleansers. Don't do it! It will dry out your skin even more.

Add oil. Adding a little oil to your bathwater can help seal in moisture. However, there's a secret to it: Add the oil after you've been in the tub and your skin is saturated with water. Or put the oil on your skin immediately after your bath. Mineral oil makes an effective and inexpensive bath oil. Even with an oil bath, limit your soak to no more than 20 minutes.

Try a humidifier. No one suffers from dry skin in the tropics, where the humidity hovers around 90 percent most of the time. When the humidity drops below 60 percent (the perfect "balance point" for skin and air), or the temperature drops below 50 degrees Fahrenheit, the skin begins to suffer.

If you live or work where the humidity drops below 60 percent, consider using an air humidifier. Even houseplants or a kettle of slowly boiling water can help increase indoor humidity.

Say no to alcohol. If you have dry skin, don't use alcohol-based wipes or astringents, which tend to dry the skin. Also avoid drinking too much alcohol (no more than two ounces per day), since alcohol lowers the water concentration of the blood and draws water from surrounding cells.

Go oil-based. Choose oil-based makeup rather than water-based makeup.

Keep it cool. Don't overheat your house or office. Keep the temperature a little cooler and your skin will be less dry.

Limit sun exposure. Sunlight is very drying to the skin. It also increases your risk of developing wrinkles, age spots, and skin cancer (melanoma). Cover up with hats and long sleeves or wear sunscreen when you're exposed to the sun. The fairer your skin, the higher sun protection factor (SPF) you should choose. Avoid sun exposure between 10:00 A.M. and 3:00 P.M., when the sun's rays are

most damaging to skin. After sun exposure, apply a cream-type moisturizer.

Protect your hands. Don't expose your skin to drying chemicals like cleansers, ammonia, turpentine, detergents, and window cleaners. Wear vinyl (not rubber) gloves and use less harsh alternatives whenever possible (for example, vinegar and water with a drop of liquid detergent for washing windows).

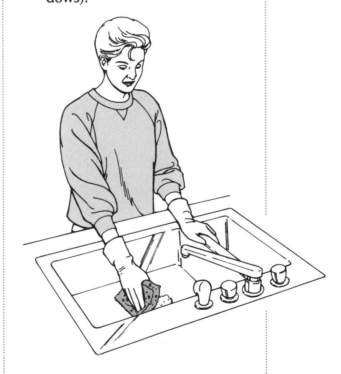

Sources: Frank Parker, M.D., Professor and Chairman, Department of Dermatology, Oregon Health Sciences University, Portland, Oregon. **Margaret Robertson, M.D.,** Staff Physician, St. Vincent Hospital and Medical Center, Portland, Oregon. **James Shaw, M.D.,** Chief, Division of Dermatology, Good Samaritan Hospital and Medical Center; Associate Professor of Medicine, Oregon Health Sciences University, Portland, Oregon.

•EAR DISCOMFORT

How to Ease

the Pain

YOU PROBABLY DON'T GIVE MUCH thought to your ears. Mostly, they're just there on the sides of your head—two outcroppings of cartilage and bone that serve as convenient hitching posts for an earring or two. But if throbbing pain, stuffiness, or a persistent ringing noise develops, you can bet that your ears will command most of your attention.

Despite its modest, innocuous exterior, the ear is a complex and delicate organ. It consists of three parts: the outer ear, the middle ear, and the inner ear. The outer ear consists of the pinna, or external ear, which captures sound waves and directs them inward, and the ear canal, which leads to the eardrum.

In the middle ear, sound waves vibrate through three tiny bones called the hammer, the anvil, and the stirrup. The vibrations continue into the inner ear, where a spiral structure called the cochlea transforms them into nerve impulses. These impulses are conveyed to the brain by the auditory nerve.

The eustachian tube in the middle ear connects the ear with the nasopharynx (the upper part of the throat). This tube allows the air pressure in the middle ear to equalize with the pressure outside of the body, thus helping to prevent rupture of the eardrum. However, the eustachian tube also provides a passageway for infecting microorganisms to enter the middle ear from the nose or throat.

The semicircular canals (also called the labyrinth) within the inner ear serve as the organ of balance. They detect the motion of the head and convey this information to the brain.

CAUSES AND SYMPTOMS

With so much going on inside our ears, it's no wonder things can go wrong. If untreated, some ear problems—especially ear infections—can be serious, causing permanent hearing loss. So don't play doctor at home: Any child showing symptoms of an ear infection should be taken to a doctor as soon as possible. Adults with persistent ear pain or hearing loss should also see a doctor.

The following is a list of the most common causes of ear discomfort, along with their corresponding symptoms. Sometimes, by playing detective and thinking about the circumstances associated with the discomfort, you'll be able to figure out what has caused your problem. Other times, the symptoms will be your only clue to what is going on inside your ear.

Middle-ear infection. These infections, also called otitis media, often follow a cold or an allergy. When mucus congestion is present, the eustachian tube swells and air is absorbed by the lining of the middle ear, creating a partial vacuum. The eardrum then gets pulled inward and fluid weeps from the lining of the middle ear. Bacteria or viruses from the nose and throat can travel up the eustachian tube and infect the stagnant, warm fluid in the middle ear, which provides a perfect environment for them to live in and multiply. When this happens, an infection is underway.

Some one-third of all children have more than three middle-ear infections during the first three years of life, resulting in 30 million doctor visits a year. While children

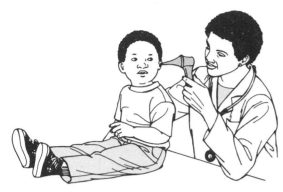

aren't the only ones who get ear infections, they are, by far, the most common victims. The reason is that their eustachian tubes are shorter and slope downhill toward the ear, which may make it easier for bacteria and viruses to penetrate. Children also get colds and sore throats more often than adults.

The most common symptoms of a middle-ear infection are severe, throbbing pain, stuffiness, and hearing loss. Infants who are suffering from ear infections may be unusually fussy, rub or pull at an ear, run a fever, or vomit. You may also notice that a baby or a toddler doesn't seem to hear you when you speak to him or her.

Swimmer's Ear. This is an infection of the outer ear canal that is usually caused by bacteria or, less commonly, by fungus.

Swimmer's ear gets its name from the fact that it is more likely to develop in the summer, when people are in the water a lot. Warm weather, coupled with water in the ear, provides just the right conditions for this type of infection to develop (bacteria thrive in warm, moist environments). In addition, exposure to large amounts of water tends to wash away the oily, waxy substance that normally lines and protects the ear canal from bacteria.

External ear infections don't occur only in swimmers or only in the summertime. They can develop at any time of year. Getting water in your ear from showering may cause an external ear infection. Sometimes you don't need to be around water at all. Cleaning the inside of the ear canal with cotton swabs, bobby pins, or other implements can cause outer-ear infections by scratching the very delicate skin in the ear canal and introducing bacteria.

Swimmer's ear may start out as an itching, tingling sensation inside the ear. Scratching, however, may compound the problem by injuring delicate ear tissue. The infection then starts to produce pain. Ear discharge and hearing loss may develop in severe cases.

One way to help you determine whether the infection is in the outer ear is to gently pull on your ear, wiggle it, and move it back and forth. If that hurts, it's likely to be an outer-ear infection, such as swimmer's ear.

Blocked eustachian tube. After middle-ear infection, the most common cause of an earache is a blocked eustachian tube. The eustachian tube, as mentioned above, is a thin, membrane-lined tube that connects the inside back portion of the nose with the middle ear. The air in the middle ear is constantly being absorbed by its membranous lining. The air is never depleted, however, as long as the eustachian tube remains open and able to resupply it during the process of swallowing. In this manner, the air pressure on both sides of the eardrum stays about equal. When the eustachian tube is blocked for one reason or another, the pressure in the middle ear can't be equalized. The air that is already inside the middle ear is absorbed and, without an incoming supply, a vacuum occurs in the middle ear, sucking the eardrum inward and stretching it painfully taut.

This type of earache is especially common in people who travel by air, particularly if they have a cold or a stuffy nose. As the plane takes off, the air pressure in the plane's cabin decreases; as the plane lands, the air pressure in the cabin increases. In each instance, the pressure change occurs very rapidly. While the air pressure in the middle ear normally manages to equalize on its own, if there is congestion in the upper respiratory tract, air may not be able to flow through the eustachian tube to reach the middle ear. (This type of earache can also result from pressure changes during an elevator ride in a tall building and during scuba diving.)

Referred pain. Sometimes, diseases and disorders in other parts of the head and neck can cause pain in the ear. The most common culprits in referred pain are the "five Ts:" tongue, tonsils, teeth, throat, and the temporomandibular joint (TMJ).

Tinnitus. Pronounced tin-EYE-tis, this sometimes tormenting condition is defined by its main symptom: a persistent ringing, hissing, clicking, buzzing, or crackling inside the ear. The noise may come and go, or it may be continuous.

Medical researchers have made substantial headway into discovering why tinnitus develops. When vibrations from the outside world pass through tiny movable bones behind the eardrum, they reach a fluid-filled chamber deep in the inner ear. Within the chamber, thousands of tiny hair cells pick up the vibrations and send electrical impulses through the auditory nerve—or hearing nerve—to the brain. The brain translates these signals into sound.

Sometimes, the hair cells can be damaged in such a way that they continuously send bursts of electricity to the auditory nerve, even when there are no outside noises causing vibrations. In short, these hair cells are permanently turned on, making the brain believe that sound vibrations are entering the ear nonstop. Among the many causes for hair-cell damage are excessive exposure to loud noise, earwax, middle-ear and inner-ear infection, a perforated eardrum, fluid accumulation, and stiffening of the middle-ear bones. Allergies, high or low blood pressure, a tumor, diabetes, thyroid problems, high levels of triglycerides in the blood, strokes, and injuries to the head and neck may all cause hair-cell damage. Tinnitus is also a prime symptom of Meniere's disease, an inner-ear disorder marked by loss of equilibrium, and an early symptom of acoustic neuroma, a tumor of the ear nerve, which controls hearing and balance. Degeneration of hair cells that occurs as a result of aging may also cause tinnitus in some people.

If there doesn't appear to be an obvious cause for your tinnitus, you would be wise to set up an appointment for a medical checkup to determine whether a more serious problem is causing the ringing. Unfortunately, however, treatment of an underlying medical condition may not cure the ringing in the ears.

Earwax. Normally, earwax is good for the skin in the outer ear canal. It acts as a trap for dust and other particles that might find their way into your ear and cause injury, irritation, or infection. It also contains enzymes to help fight bacteria. In addition, it "waterproofs" the skin of the ear canal, protecting it from water damage, which makes the skin susceptible to infections such as swimmer's ear. In fact, without wax, or with a diminished amount of it, the inside of your ears would become dry and itchy.

In rare cases, the ear canal can become almost completely blocked by wax, preventing the entry of air and sound and preventing the escape of trapped fluid. It should only be attended to when there is evidence of hearing loss or discomfort.

Perforated eardrum. If you feel a sudden, sharp pain in your ear following a trauma such as an explosion or a scuba-diving accident, you may have a perforated eardrum. While the pain may occur only at the time of the accident, the injury itself should be evaluated by a doctor to head off permanent disruption of the middle-ear mechanism. Most injury-related eardrum perforations are small and will heal spontaneously within a few weeks, as long as middle-ear infections are prevented or controlled (which is why you must see a doctor even for small perforations). Large perforations may require surgery.

AT-HOME TREATMENT

As we have said, serious ear pain or persistent discomfort should be checked out by a doctor. Once you've been diagnosed, however, there are several simple steps you can take at home to ease the symptoms of ear discomfort.

Blocked Eustachian Tube or Ear Infection. The following tips will help ease the pain caused by a blocked eustachian tube or an ear infection. Remember, these remedies will not cure an infection; they will just help relieve symptoms. Only an antibiotic prescribed by your physician can cure the infection.

Follow doctor's orders. The infection doesn't disappear when you leave the doctor's office. You must finish the course of medication that has been prescribed for you. Usually, the full time prescribed is ten to 14 days. You should read the label on the prescription bottle carefully and follow directions. Even if your symptoms are relieved, if you stop taking an antibiotic before the full time has elapsed, your ear infection may come back. When it does, the antibiotic may not work the second time around.

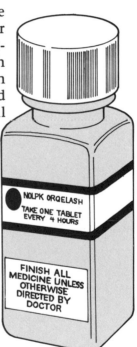

To help you with the symptoms of a cold or allergy, the doctor may also prescribe an antihistamine and/or a decongestant. Don't just guess at the proper use or administration of the medication. If you are unsure, call your doctor or pharmacist.

Keep your chin up. So that your eustachian tubes will drain properly into the back of your throat, keep your head slightly elevated. Try using an extra pillow at night.

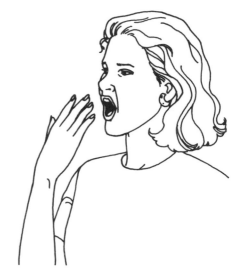

Warm the pain away. A heating pad placed on the affected ear may alleviate some of your discomfort. Don't set it too high, though; the pad should be warm, not hot.

Take a painkiller. Acetaminophen can help relieve the pain and fever associated with an ear infection.

Swallow it. When you swallow, the muscle that opens the eustachian tube is triggered. If you're on a plane, take your cue to start swallowing when the "fasten seat belt" sign goes on for landing. (If you plan to be napping, ask the flight attendant to wake you before landing.) Swallowing can also stave off the pain of an earache until you can see a doctor. You can also try chewing gum or sucking on hard candy to keep you swallowing. Pop some into your mouth just before the plane descends.

Yawn openly. Don't worry about giving offense. Yawning is the most effective way for you to unblock your eustachian tubes.

Pinch your nostrils together and blow. If your ears become uncomfortably blocked as a plane descends, try pinching your nostrils together with a thumb and forefinger. Block the external opening of the unaffected ear with your other hand, and close your mouth tightly. Try to blow through the pinched nostrils as if you were blowing your nose. Repeat, if necessary. You might feel a cracking sensation or hear a loud pop; that means it worked and you should feel some relief from the pain. If you have a sore throat or a fever, though, don't use this method; it might force the infection into your ears.

Stay clear. Decongestants or nasal sprays can shrink the ear's membranes, making it easier to keep the eustachian tube open. If you're flying, and especially if you suffer from allergies or sinusitis, take your medication at the beginning of the flight. Of course, if you are pregnant or nursing a baby, or if you suffer from a special medical con-

---

7 WAYS TO TREAT EAR PAIN

- Complete the entire course of any prescribed antibiotics.
- Keep your head elevated.
- Apply a warm heating pad to an aching ear.
- Take a painkiller, such as acetaminophen.
- Swallow hard or yawn to clear a blocked eustachian tube.
- To clear blocked ears on an airplane, pinch your nostrils together with a thumb and forefinger, block the external opening of the unaffected ear with the forefinger of your other hand, and blow through the pinched nostrils.
- Use a decongestant or a nasal spray, with your doctor's go-ahead.

dition, you should not take any medication without first consulting your physician.

Ringing in the Ears. Although tinnitus is not life-threatening, it affects nearly 36 million people in the United States. Seven million of them are so severely stricken that they cannot lead normal lives. Even at its worst, however, there are a number of measures you can take to make the situation more bearable.

Keep it down. As anyone who has been subjected to a blasting radio knows, the noise lingers on long after the melody ceases. If your ears continue to ring after listening to your stereo at top volume, you are probably developing tinnitus, as well as temporary or permanent hearing loss. Every additional exposure to loud noise damages the tiny hair cells in the inner ear even more, reducing the chance that damaged cells might heal or that the central nervous system might develop a tolerance level to block the noise out over time. People who attend loud rock concerts or who go hunting or target shooting may also be unwittingly damaging the tiny hair cells in their ears. To increase the chances that your ears might recover, turn the volume down—today.

Have a physical. Ringing sounds in the ears can often be traced to high blood pressure. The bad news is that if your blood pressure is high enough to cause ringing in your ears, it is probably causing other damage to your body, as well. High blood pressure is a primary risk factor in heart disease, a far more serious condition than ringing in the ears.

Put away the salt shaker. If an inner-ear disorder, such as Meniere's disease, is causing your tinnitus, you should cut the sodium from your diet. This has been found effective in helping reduce symptoms for many Meniere's disease patients. Limit salty snacks, cook with other seasonings in place of salt, and search out foods labeled "sodium-free," which means that the item has less than five milligrams of sodium per serving. Talk to your doctor to determine what your daily sodium intake should be.

Switch painkillers. In high doses, aspirin can cause reversible tinnitus for a day after it is taken. If it is taken on a regular basis—say, for arthritis or chronic pain—the hair cells may suffer permanent damage. Try to limit your intake of aspirin and see if your tinnitus improves. Also, be sure to check the labels on any over-the-counter medications you take, since many of them may contain aspirin. If you take aspirin for a chronic condition, talk to your doctor about alternative medications.

Avoid stimulants. Certain substances can prod the hair cells into unnecessary action. Try to limit your use of caffeine, which is found in coffee, tea, chocolate, and cola drinks. Also eliminate tobacco and other

> ## 9 TIPS TO QUIET RINGING EARS
>
> - Avoid loud noises.
> - Have your doctor check your blood pressure.
> - Cut sodium from your diet.
> - Don't take aspirin.
> - Cut down on caffeine and eliminate all uses of tobacco, marijuana, and cocaine.
> - Start a program of aerobic exercise.
> - Stay well rested.
> - Keep the problem in perspective.
> - Counter the noise in your ears with some quiet background music or "white noise."

addictive substances, such as marijuana or cocaine.

Get moving. If poor circulation is the cause of ringing in your ears, a little aerobic exercise can go a long way toward improving the situation. Start slowly and build up to a good, brisk walk once a day.

Sleep it off. Fatigue can lower your resistance to colds and flu, which can bring on swelling in the inner ear and tinnitus. Getting enough rest can help your body ward off illness.

Keep your cool. As annoying and frustrating as tinnitus is, it's important to keep the problem in perspective to preserve your quality of life. The condition is not life-threatening, but obsessively focusing on it can make your life a misery.

Give the noise some competition. Ringing in the ears can often be countered by a competing sound, such as low-volume background music or "white noise." These outside sounds may be more pleasant—or at least more bearable—than the internal ones.

If you have severe tinnitus, you might be able to mask the problem by wearing an electronic device that looks like a hearing aid and generates a competing but more pleasant sound. An audiologist can set the masking device to bring some measure of relief without interfering with conversational hearing. Unfortunately, maskers seem to help only a few people. Wearing the device can be bothersome, so many people choose to use it only at night to help them fall asleep.

Earwax. Under normal circumstances, earwax doesn't need to be removed; it's there naturally as a barrier against injury and infection. Usually, the wax accumulates a little bit at a time, gradually dries up, and comes rolling out of your ear on its own, carrying all the foreign matter along with it.

Leave it alone. The bottom line is that ears are self-cleaning. By inserting "cleaning" tools, you risk damaging your eardrum or the delicate lining in the ear canal, opening the door to infection. More importantly, inserting foreign objects into your ear pushes the wax farther into your ear canal, even up against your eardrum, possibly affecting your hearing. Never, under any circumstances, should you insert anything into your ear canal. That mandate includes cotton swabs, bobby pins, toothpicks, and so on. In fact, as the old saying goes, don't clean your ears with anything smaller than your elbow.

Try a little cotton. When the wax moves to the outside of the ear canal more slowly, simply wipe it off with a piece of moistened cotton once it becomes visible.

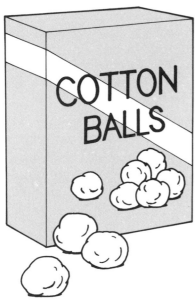

Don't play doctor. If you suspect that earwax is interfering with your hearing, you should seek medical attention. Some physicians recommend against rushing out for wax-softening drops until you know for sure what is causing your problem. (These drops can actually exacerbate certain ear problems.) You should not attempt to treat wax buildup that is causing symptoms; instead, go to the doctor. Likewise, if your ears are tender to the touch, reddened in an area that you can see, or draining fluid, see your doctor. Using any kind of eardrops or medication for these conditions before con-

sulting a doctor may only complicate the matter.

Swimmer's Ear. There are various home remedies for swimmer's ear. Try the following suggestions for relief from the irritation of a case of swimmer's ear.

Try eardrops. There are some over-the-counter antiseptic eardrops, such as Aqua Ear, Ear Magic, or Swim Ear, that may prevent or ease the symptoms of swimmer's ear. They are best used by people who already know what the symptoms of swimmer's ear feel like. As an alternative to store-bought drops, the Academy of Otolaryngology–Head & Neck Surgery says that a mixture of equal amounts of rubbing alcohol and white vinegar makes an effective at-home antiseptic, providing you have normal eardrums and your doctor says it's safe. White vinegar kills bacteria and fungus; alcohol absorbs water and may kill bacteria and fungus as well. Dropper bottles to apply the mixture are available at almost any pharmacy.

Call your doctor. If you keep your ears dry and use antiseptic eardrops, your swimmer's ear should abate in a few days.

3 WAYS TO DRY OUT A CASE OF SWIMMER'S EAR

- Try over-the-counter antiseptic eardrops.
- Use a homemade potion of equal parts of white vinegar and rubbing alcohol.
- Call your doctor if you have severe pain lasting more than an hour, or if there is discharge from the ear.

However, you should see your doctor if you have persistent pain that lasts more than an hour or if there's discharge from the ear. According to the Academy of Otolaryngology–Head & Neck Surgery, you should consult a doctor before swimming or administering any ear medication if you have ever had a perforated, punctured, ruptured, or otherwise injured eardrum or have had ear surgery.

PREVENTION

Of course, your best bet for avoiding ear discomfort is to keep your ears healthy. The following are some tips for preventing ear infections and swimmer's ear:

---

5 STRATEGIES FOR PREVENTING EAR INFECTIONS

- Keep up your resistance to colds and flu.
- Avoid people who have colds or other respiratory infections.
- Keep allergy symptoms under control.
- Blow your nose gently.
- Quit smoking.

Stay healthy. Middle-ear infections don't just appear out of thin air. They usually develop from a cold, an allergic reaction, or an infection of the tonsils or adenoids. If possible, steer clear of people who have colds or other respiratory infections and keep your allergies under control with antihistamines or decongestants (ask your doctor to recommend a medication that is right for you). You should also eat well, keep your stress level to a minimum, and get enough sleep, all of which may help boost your natural resistance to infections.

Go easy on your nose. When your nose is congested or runny, blow it softly, rather than with excessive force, which can drive infection into the ears. Also, never squeeze your nostrils shut in order to stifle a sneeze. The infection can be forced up the eustachian tubes and into your ears.

Kick the habit. Cigarette smoking can increase susceptibility to ear infections, especially in children subjected to secondhand smoke. Cigarette smoke can inflame the linings of the nasal passages and middle-ear cavity, and disrupt the eustachian tube's function. Secondhand smoke has the same effect, so ban smoking in your home, sit in the nonsmoking section in restaurants, and ensure that your place of employment has an isolated smoking area—away from your desk.

Avoid germs. Steer clear of pools, ponds, lakes, oceans, or any other body of water in which the water may not be clean. Dirty water means more bacteria, and more bacteria mean a greater chance of infection.

Stay dry. You can usually prevent a case of swimmer's ear by keeping the inside of your ears dry. Sometimes after swimming or bathing, you can feel water swishing around in your ear. Try shaking the water out of your ear. Simply tilt your head all the way over to the affected side and shake it vigorously toward the ground.

Cover your ears. Wearing a bathing cap can go a long way toward keeping the wet out of your ears. If you do choose to wear a cap, make sure that it fits tightly over your ears, across your forehead, and around the back of your neck.

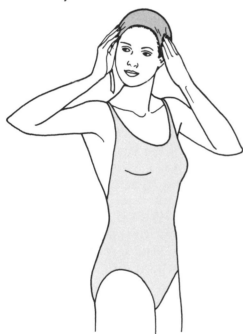

Leave your ears alone. The wax inside your ears is there for a reason. It provides a protective barrier against foreign organisms and excess moisture. Poking, swabbing, or scratching inside your ears only serves to break down this barrier, and it could turn a mild case of swimmer's ear into a more serious infection. Ears can function very well without the help of your fingers or other "cleaning" implements.

6 WAYS TO KEEP SWIMMER'S EAR AT BAY

- Avoid swimming in dirty bodies of water.
- Shake the water out of your ears after swimming, showering, or diving.
- Wear a bathing cap that tightly covers your ears.
- Never poke, prod, or scratch your ears.
- Don't insert any object smaller than your elbow—including fingers—into the ear canal.
- Don't clean your ears with cotton swabs.

Sources: Jay E. Caldwell, M.D., Director, Alaska Sports Medicine Clinic, Anchorage, Alaska. **John W. House, M.D.,** Associate Clinical Professor, Department of Otolaryngology, Head and Neck Surgery, University of Southern California at Los Angeles; President, House Ear Institute; Otologist-Neurotologist, House Ear Clinic, Los Angeles, California. **Donald B. Kamerer, M.D., F.A.C.S.,** Professor, Department of Otolaryngology, University of Pittsburgh School of Medicine; Staff Physician, Pittsburgh Eye and Ear Hospital, Pittsburgh, Pennsylvania. **Daniel Kuriloff, M.D.,** Associate Director, Department of Otolaryngology–Head and Neck Surgery, St. Luke's–Roosevelt Hospital Center; Associate Professor, Columbia University College of Physicians and Surgeons, New York, New York. **Alexander Schleuning, M.D.,** Professor and Chairman, Department of Otolaryngology/Head and Neck Surgery, Oregon Health Sciences University, Portland, Oregon. **James Stankiewicz, M.D.,** Professor and Vice-Chairman, Department of Otolaryngology–Head and Neck Surgery, Loyola University Medical School, Maywood, Illinois. **Jack J. Wazen, M.D.,** Associate Professor of Otolaryngology, Director, Department of Otology and Neurotology, Columbia University College of Physicians and Surgeons, New York, New York.

EXCESSIVE HAIR GROWTH

How to Get

Rid of It

A HAIRY CHEST AND A FIVE-O'-CLOCK shadow can make a man appear rugged and virile. But on a woman, well, that's another story. We spend plenty of our hard-earned cash—not to mention hours of our precious time—trying to keep up with the hair that grows where we expect it (our heads, underarms, and legs). But when dark, curling hairs start to appear on our faces, chests, backs, or breasts, in our culture, it may seem like a cosmetic liability. For some women, it even threatens their self-esteem.

There are two different words for such excessive hair growth: hirsutism and hypertrichosis. Just keep in mind that despite the serious sound of these terms, excessive hair growth certainly doesn't make you a freak. Some eight to ten percent of all adult women in the United States are suffering from the same problem right along with you.

SYMPTOMS

The main symptom of both hirsutism and hypertrichosis is an excess of hair in unwanted places—the face, chest, back, breasts, and so on. We are not talking about vellus hair, or "peach fuzz," that is present over most of the body. Hirsutism and hypertrichosis refer to an excess of terminal hair—the thick, pigmented hair that, before puberty, is present only on the scalp, eyebrows, and eyelashes.

The spectrum of abnormal hair growth in either of these conditions can range from scattered patches on the face and chest to a full beard.

CAUSES

Hirsutism is a result of increased amounts of or increased sensitivity to hormones called androgens. The causes can include menopause, pregnancy (rarely), an overactive adrenal gland, Cushing's disease, polycystic ovary syndrome, a pituitary tumor, an ovarian tumor, or the use of medications or herbs containing androgens. Hypertrichosis can also be caused by certain medications, physical factors such as chronic rubbing, and systemic (body-wide) disease.

Ethnic and geographic influences affect amount of hair. Among Caucasians, those of Mediterranean and Semitic descent tend to be hairier than Scandinavians and Anglo-Saxons. The least hairy peoples are Asians and American Indians.

If your mother and your mother's mother had excess facial hair, you probably don't have to be concerned that there is a medical problem underlying your excess hair growth. If, on the other hand, the people in your family tend to be sparsely whiskered, the sudden appearance of a crop of dark and/or coarse hair on your face, chest, back, arms, or legs should be reported to your doctor. Often, the excess hair will disappear once the underlying condition is corrected.

AT-HOME TREATMENT

Once you've ruled out any medical causes for excessive hair growth, you'll probably be eager to take care of the problem cosmetically. The following suggestions are ways to do just that.

Cover it up. Heavy makeup may be the answer for a mild case of excess facial hair. If your skin tends to be oily or is acne-prone, use water-based or non-comedogenic foundations and blushes.

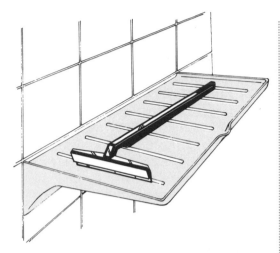

Shave it off. Shaving is an excellent way to get rid of the hair on your legs and under your arms. It is the easiest, cheapest way to go and, contrary to popular belief, it does not cause the hair to grow coarser or faster. However, for women, shaving is not usually the method of choice to eliminate unwanted facial hair. The reason is clear: the emergence of the five-o'-clock shadow when the hair begins to grow back.

Pluck away. If the overgrowth problem is mild and is confined to a small area, such as the chin, a pair of tweezers may be your tool of choice. The downside of tweezing is that it can be painful and may leave the area red and irritated temporarily. However, it can stave off regrowth for as long as four to thirteen weeks. And there is no medical basis for the old wives' tale that nine new hairs will grow in place of one that is plucked.

Go blonde. Bleaching is probably the most common home treatment for unwanted facial hair.

It doesn't eliminate the hair, but it does make it colorless and less noticeable. Most of the bleaches sold in drugstores involve mixing a powder and a cream together to activate the bleaching agent. Make sure the bleach is fresh; sitting on the shelf for several months can cause it to lose strength. If your facial hair is very dark, the bleaching process may not be 100 percent successful the first time, but a repeat bleaching should do the trick. Of course, it will have to be bleached again when the hair grows out.

Get waxed. Instead of plucking hairs one at a time, wax lets you pull many hairs out all at once. The wax is heated to a fluid state and spread on an area of skin. It hardens in a few seconds, and then it is stripped off, pulling hundreds of hairs out by the roots. This procedure can leave skin smooth and hair-free for up to six weeks.

Waxing is not without its drawbacks, however. It can be painful and time consuming, especially when you're covering large areas, like the legs. In addition, surface skin can sometimes be pulled off with the wax, causing long-lasting irritation and redness. In fact, irritation may occur even if the skin remains intact. Your best bet is to go to a salon that specializes in waxing. If you do try it at home, be sure to follow package instructions carefully.

Try cream. Depilatories are creams or lotions that chemically remove hair. Most drugstores offer a variety of inexpensive depilatories that are as easy to use as bleach. There are different depilatories for use on different parts of the body. Be sure you use the appropriate type of depilatory for the body area you will be applying it to. A depilatory may irritate sensitive skin; always test it on a small patch of skin before spreading it on a larger area.

After using depilatories, you may feel that the regrowth is unusually thick and stubbly. Don't worry—the same amount of hair grows back as was removed. It only feels like more because depilatories take off all the hair, including the light vellus hair, which then grows back all at once.

---

7 Hair-Removing Remedies

- Use heavy makeup to cover a mild case of excess facial hair.
- Shave the hair off your legs or underarms.
- Use tweezers to pluck scattered hairs from small areas.
- Try a hair bleach.
- Wax hair away.
- Use a depilatory cream.
- Try electrolysis.

Shock it into disappearing. Electrolysis is the only method of permanent hair removal, but this procedure requires a trained electrologist. A very fine probe is inserted into the hair follicle. Through the probe, a small electrical current is sent, destroying the hair root and rendering the follicle incapable of future growth. The procedure is most uncomfort-able when applied to the upper lip and the inner thigh; treatment on the forearms and chest area hurts least.

Improperly performed electrolysis can cause scarring and infection. However, when performed by a trained, skilled operator, there are generally few complications. To be safe, ask to see credentials—such as certification by the Society of Clinical and Medical Electrologists—before you get started.

A slight swelling or redness may appear along the treated area; this should subside within a matter of hours. Occasionally, slight scabbing may develop two to four days after treatment. If left alone, the scabs will fall off without causing any further problems.

Sources: Bruce R. Carr, M.D., Paul C. MacDonald Professor of Obstetrics and Gynecology, Director, Division of Reproductive Endocrinology, University of Texas Southwestern Medical Center, Dallas, Texas. Elizabeth Knobler, M.D., Assistant Clinical Professor of Dermatology, Columbia-Presbyterian Medical Center, New York, New York. Donald Rudikoff, M.D., Assistant Clinical Professor of Dermatology, Mount Sinai School of Medicine, New York, New York.

•EXCESSIVE PERSPIRATION

How to Keep

Your Cool in

Hot Situations

HAVE YOU EVER FELT LIKE A CHARACTER in an antiperspirant commercial? You're a half-hour late for a job interview and are about to raise your arm to flag down a bus, when you realize that your silk blouse is sporting a very large half-circle of sweat under each arm. Or perhaps you go to shake the hand of a prospective employer and realize that your palm is damp and clammy. Or your forehead drips profusely every time you eat spicy food.

Excessive perspiration is embarrassing because it always happens at just the wrong times—the times when we want to make our most confident, self-assured impressions.

What's going on here? Why does this happen? Is there a cure?

CAUSES

Sweat is the by-product of the body's temperature-control system. It is the body's way of cooling off. This internal thermostat sometimes responds to spicy foods, anxiety, and danger in the same way that it does to excessive heat. You may think that you would be more comfortable and self-confident without such sensitive reactions. But this is the price we pay for one of the systems that keeps us alive.

There's nothing complicated about the mechanics of sweat. The human body contains more than two million sweat glands (women may have more, according to some studies). These sweat glands come in two varieties: eccrine glands and apocrine glands. The eccrines are located almost everywhere on the body's surface—about 400 of them per square inch of skin, except in places like the palms of the hands, where as many as 3,000 may be concentrated. The eccrines are the smaller of the two types and originate deep within the skin, with narrow ducts threading to the skin's surface.

The task for the eccrine glands is primarily temperature control: When things get too hot, the sweat glands go into high gear, drawing fluid from the blood to produce sweat and transporting it through the pores to the skin surface. Once on the surface, sweat evaporates, cooling the skin. This, in turn, cools the blood, which has also been rushed to the surface in response to signals from the brain. The cooled blood then returns to the internal organs and muscles, cooling them down, too.

Apocrine glands are larger, fewer in number, and attached to hair follicles in the genital areas, the armpits, and the chest. The apocrines become active after puberty and are extremely sensitive to emotional stress, as well as sexual stimulation.

AT-HOME TREATMENT

Even the most inactive person sweats as much as a quart a day. Marathon runners may produce up to two gallons during the course of a race. Such extreme sweat production is still considered quite normal under the circumstances. You only start worrying about it when its presence becomes an embarrassment (see the profile on body odor). Some people perspire beyond this norm. Their bodies can bead with sweat even when they're sitting perfectly still in the shade. In medical terms, this condition is known as hyperhidrosis. If this sounds like you, here's what you can do:

145

Stay cool. Your body can quickly become overheated when the sun is at its highest and hottest, sending your heat-regulating mechanism into high gear. So, if you want to avoid excessive sweating, take the first, most logical step: Avoid the midday sun. Even worse is being outdoors on a warm day when the humidity is high. With high humidity, the air is already saturated with water, reducing its ability to evaporate the sweat from your skin. Not only will your sweat not evaporate, but you'll feel hot and sweaty.

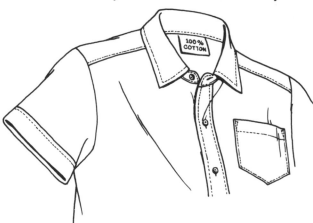

Go natural. Most synthetic materials appear to increase sweating because they do not absorb moisture. Natural fibers, on the other hand, allow skin to "breathe," keeping you cooler and more comfortable. Put away the polyester and reach for cotton in the summer months and wool during the winter.

Go on the wagon. Even before you feel its other effects, alcohol opens up blood vessels near the skin, increasing blood flow and stimulating perspiration. Non-alcoholic beverages are the better choice for staying dry on hot, humid days. In fact, cold water is perfect for quenching your thirst and replacing fluids that you may have sweated away.

Cool down your diet. Since eating hot, spicy foods can trigger perspiration, forgo them for milder fare when staying dry is a priority.

Lose the spare tire. Excess weight forces your heart to strain harder to pump blood throughout your body. This is true even when you are engaging in only moderate activity. Shedding a few of those extra pounds and maintaining the loss may help ease an excessive sweating problem.

Stay calm. Anxiety—even if it is temporary—can bring on excessive sweating. Most of us are familiar with this phenomenon (when we have to speak in front of many people, go on a job interview, and so on). If you are prone to having anxiety attacks, the smallest external or internal stresses can bring on a bout of anxiety, accompanied by excessive nervous sweating. To break this cycle, try to become conscious of when the anxiety is coming on, then divert the symptoms with physical activity, such as jogging, walking, or swimming, or with relaxation exercises, such as deep breathing. These activities may help you release stress and reach a more serene (and sweat-reduced) state.

Use an antiperspirant—all over.
For a little extra confidence, use an antiperspirant. In addition to your underarms, you can apply it to the palms of your hands and the soles of your feet. Antiperspirants inhibit eccrine perspiration, because they contain an aluminum salt that causes the area around the sweat gland ducts to swell, cutting off the outflow of perspiration. There are different aluminum salts in different products. Some acidic salts, such as aluminum chloride and aluminum sulfate, are more effective, but they can irritate your skin and stain clothing, especially linen and cotton. Aluminum chlorohydrate is the mildest of the aluminum salts and may be a better choice if the strong ones give you a problem.

The following are tips from the *FDA Consumer* that will help you get more protection and less irritation from your underarm antiperspirant:

• Repeat applications regularly. Antiperspirants work for only a certain length of time. The label will tell you how often you should apply your antiperspirant.

• Dry your underarms thoroughly before applying an antiperspirant. The active ingredient penetrates more effectively if your skin is dry.

• Don't apply an antiperspirant to freshly shaved skin, since this could cause irritation. (Try shaving at night, so you can wait until morning to apply your antiperspirant.) Also, never apply an antiperspirant to irritated or broken skin.

• If one product doesn't work, or if it irritates your skin, try another with a different active ingredient. Different antiperspirants work well for different people.

---

7 Tips to Help You Stay Dry

• Avoid getting overheated.
• Wear natural-fiber clothing.
• Avoid drinking alcoholic beverages.
• Avoid spicy foods.
• Maintain a healthy body weight.
• Try to stay calm and relaxed.
• Use an antiperspirant.

Sources: **Allan L. Lorincz, M.D.,** Professor of Dermatology, University of Chicago Medical Center, Chicago, Illinois. **Donald Rudikoff, M.D.,** Assistant Clinical Professor of Dermatology, Mount Sinai School of Medicine, New York, New York. **Alan R. Shalita, M.D.,** Chairman, Department of Dermatology, State University of New York Health Science Center at Brooklyn, Brooklyn, New York.

•Eye Redness

How to Get

Rid of that

"Morning-

After" Look

Watching a sentimental love story, having a new baby in the house, staying out a little too late, or an allergy attack can all leave your eyes looking weary and bloodshot. It's hardly the best way to make a good impression on the people you meet.

Luckily, you don't have to sport those ruby red eyes for long. Read on for tips on how to perk up your peepers.

Causes

Eye redness is usually caused by simple dryness or irritation. However, it can be a symptom of a more serious condition, such as chronic or acute glaucoma, inflammation of the eye, blood diseases, gout, thyroid diseases, tumors, or conjunctivitis. But before you start worrying, you should know that with many of these medical problems, there are other symptoms present as well. For example, in the case of acute glaucoma, eye redness will be accompanied by dilated pupils, blurring of vision, and pain. With iritis, an inflammatory disease that usually develops inside the eye, there is often discomfort and increased pressure within the eye.

Because the medical problems associated with eye redness can be serious if left untreated, experts recommend that you have your eyes checked if you notice any of the following:
- Redness that persists for more than a couple days
- Pain
- A change in vision
- Sensitivity to light
- Redness or blood over the pupil (the dark center of the eye)
- Discharge from one or both eyes

At-Home Treatment

If you're sure that your eye redness was caused by an everyday irritant—long hours in contact lenses, allergies, fatigue, air pollution, or dry air—there are some things you can do to help get rid of the red and relieve irritation.

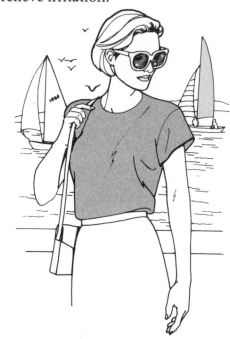

Keep 'em covered. A good-quality pair of sunglasses can protect your already sore eyes from further irritation. You really should wear them if you're skiing, boating, or sunbathing on a bright day. Unprotected eyes can fall prey to painful snow blindness and ultraviolet burns. Also, skiing without protective eyewear can cause your eyes to become extremely dry. Sunglasses may also provide welcome camouflage for red eyes until the redness clears up.

Just add moisture. Sometimes all your dry eyes need to feel better is lubricating eyedrops, such as Visine. However, eyedrops should not be used for more than a few consecutive days, since continual use can worsen the problem.

Some over-the-counter drops have preservatives in them, which can further irritate sensitive eyes. Others contain a decongestant that may cause a rebound effect (the same problem occurs with nasal spray). The decongestant contracts the eye's arteries, making the eye look whiter. However, over time, the arteries can become dependent on the chemical in order to stay contracted. When the chemical wears off, the arteries dilate again and make the eye appear red.

Eyedrops and artificial tears can be especially helpful for older people, who don't produce as many tears as they once did.

When you do choose to use eyedrops, be sure to read the label for instructions. If the redness still doesn't clear up in a few days, a call to the doctor is probably warranted.

Try a soothing compress. A warm or cold compress can temporarily relieve dryness and itching. The temperature of the compress depends on what feels best to you. Simply soak a washcloth in water and place it over your eye. Cupping cool water in your hand and holding it under the eye may have the same effect.

Take an allergy pill. If an allergy, such as hay fever, is behind your red, itchy eyes, then treat

---

8 WAYS TO CLEAR UP THE REDNESS

- Use over-the-counter eyedrops, but only for two or three days in a row.
- Use a warm or cold compress.
- Rinse your eyes with cool water.
- Take an antihistamine, if allergies are the culprit.
- Get a good night's sleep.
- Wear sunglasses on bright days.
- Wear goggles when skiing or swimming in chlorinated pools.
- Use lubricating eyedrops when traveling by plane.

---

the allergy with an over-the-counter antihistamine, and your eyes will feel better, too. Of course, if you are pregnant, nursing a baby, or have a special medical condition, you should not take any medications without first consulting your doctor.

Sleep it off. If too little sleep is the problem, a good night's rest may be all your eyes need to feel better and clear up.

Protect your eyes from chlorine. Wearing a pair of well-fitting goggles in the swimming pool can prevent the irritation and redness caused by chlorine.

Lubricate "airplane eyes." The cabin of an airplane has notoriously dry air that can be extremely irritating to the eyes. Over-the-counter lubricating drops will help keep sensitive eyes from drying out.

Sources: Jon H. Bosland, M.D., General Ophthalmologist, Bellevue, Washington. Charles Boylan, M.D., Specialist in Pediatric Ophthalmology, A Children's Eye Clinic, Seattle, Washington. Carol Ziel, M.D., Ophthalmologist, Wausau, Wisconsin.

●Eyestrain

How to

Rejuvenate

Overworked

Eyes

It's been a long week. You've been staring at the computer screen, working on an important report. It's almost over, but you feel as though you can't read another word. Your head is aching and your eyes are tired, dry, and sore. You're suffering from eyestrain.

Causes

Eyestrain has numerous causes, from stress to astigmatism (a defect in vision caused by an abnormal curvature of the cornea or lens, both of which help the eye focus an image) to jaw disorders. Tension in the neck and back muscles can also cause the eyes to tire.

Many diseases may show themselves as eyestrain. Glaucoma, a condition in which pressure within the eye increases, is one such condition. Even some conditions that are not directly related to the eye, such as temporomandibular joint syndrome, which causes facial pain (see the profile on TMJ), may show up as eyestrain.

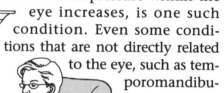

One of the reasons eyestrain is so common is that the eye's lens gradually loses some of its ability to change shape—and thus focus an image clearly—as we age. This condition, referred to as presbyopia, becomes most pronounced after age 40. It affects the eye's ability to focus on an image up close, which is why older individuals often need to hold reading material at arm's length.

At-Home Treatment

Because there are so many causes of eyestrain, it's best to consult an eye-care professional for a complete diagnosis if you've been suffering from eyestrain for a month or more, or if it seems to have become more frequent or bothersome. Even if your eyestrain isn't persistent, you should always get an eye examination once a year, especially if you are over 35 years of age or if you have a family history of glaucoma or diabetes.

In the meantime, here are some ways to ease the strain on your eyes:

Keep it well-lit. Reading in dim or harsh light doesn't actually harm the eyes, but it may make their job more strenuous. Too much light can cause glare, so don't overdo it.

Use an indirect approach. Indirect lighting makes for more comfort, as far as the eyes are concerned. Try facing light fixtures upward, allowing their light to bounce off a ceiling or wall.

Give your eyes some extra help. Reading glasses can assist your eyes by magnifying close work. Particularly if you're over 40, you may find that these glasses ease your eyestrain. You can purchase a pair without a prescription at a drugstore or pharmacy. Simply try on several pairs until you find one that has the right degree of magnification.

Cut through the glare. Particularly if you do a great deal of computer work, you may want to get your prescription lenses made with polarized ultraviolet

(UV) filters. These lenses cut glare by filtering out some wavelengths of light and can make life much easier on your eyes.

Relax your peepers. If you're doing visually demanding work, such as sewing, reading, or working at a computer terminal, take a break for a few minutes each hour. Get up and switch to a project that does not require so much of your eyes. In fact, taking a break is far more effective than doing any of the eye exercises that used to be so popular (these exercises are now generally regarded as ineffective). Walking away from your work for a few minutes will also give your neck and shoulders a rest; tension in these areas can aggravate eyestrain.

Try an eye bath. Here's a saltwater soak for tired eyes: Stir half a teaspoon of salt into a quart of warm water. Then, moisten cotton balls in the water, and place them on your closed eyelids for about ten minutes. If you don't have ten minutes, splashing your face with cool water or laying a cool, damp towel across your eyes can be soothing.

Close your eyes. Sometimes when you're concentrating on a computer screen or on printed material, you forget to blink. Infrequent blinking leaves the eyes with insufficient lubrication. In these situations, consciously make yourself blink often to prevent your eyes from becoming too dry.

Don't overmedicate. Some eyedrops decrease redness by constricting the blood vessels in the eyes. These drops are not designed to relieve eyestrain; in fact, repeated use will actually have a rebound effect, irritating your eyes and making them redder in the long run. However, the occasional use of an over-the-counter eye lubricant, sometimes called artificial tears, may help you find relief.

Humidify. Dry eyes are sometimes the result of dry air. Increasing the humidity in your home or office may help. If you don't have a humidifier, a pot of water set on a radiator may do the trick. Potted plants also add moisture to the air, and they are more attractive and less expensive than humidifiers.

Don't smoke. Your sore, irritated eyes may be a result of all that cigarette smoke. Give your eyes—not to mention the rest of your body—a break and quit smoking.

Make sure your computer is eye-friendly. Staring at a computer screen for hours every day can definitely put a strain on the eyes. Try the following suggestions for lightening their load:
• Create the right amount of ambient light. Ideally, the light in the room should be the same brightness as the computer screen.
• Invest in an antiglare screen. The glass ones are more effective than the mesh type.
• Make your computer's background light and the letters on its screen as dark as possible.

12 WAYS TO EASE YOUR STRAINED PEEPERS

- Make sure the light where you work is neither too bright nor too dim.
- Use indirect lighting instead of direct, glaring illumination.
- Invest in a pair of nonprescription reading glasses.
- Try prescription lenses made with polarized ultraviolet (UV) filters for computer use.
- Take a break for a few minutes every hour.
- Soak your eyes with cotton balls moistened with a saltwater solution.
- Take care to blink frequently.
- Don't use eyedrops that are meant for red eyes.
- Try lubricating drops, sometimes called artificial tears.
- Keep your environment from getting too dry.
- Quit smoking.
- Take steps to make working at a computer easier on your eyes.

Black-on-white contrast is the easiest on the eyes.

• Place your terminal at an angle that is 15 degrees lower than the top of your head. This angle is more comfortable for the eyes than staring straight ahead at the screen.

• Use a document holder. Getting your work off a flat surface and putting it in the same line of sight as your computer screen will help ease eyestrain.

• Keep the light low. Offices are often overlit, since their lighting was originally designed for people looking down at the work on the surface of their desks. However, more work is now done on computer screens, meaning that people spend more time with their eyes looking straight ahead, and getting too much light in their eyes. Try turning off every other fluorescent ceiling fixture or at least removing a few of the bulbs from each fixture above your desk. If this is not an option, perhaps you can rotate the position of your desk to get the too-bright lighting out of your line of sight or wear a visor to help block overhead light.

• Have your prescription glasses modified for computer use. The different sections of bifocals and trifocals are often not positioned properly for focusing comfortably on a computer screen. Ask your optometrist about lenses made for computer use.

Sources: Andrew S. Farber, M.D., F.A.C.S., Ophthalmologist, Terre Haute, Indiana. Henry D. Perry, M.D., Clinical Associate Professor of Ophthalmology, Cornell Medical College, New York, New York. Arnold Prywes, M.D., Head, Glaucoma Clinic, Long Island Jewish Medical Center, New Hyde Park, New York; Assistant Clinical Professor of Ophthalmology, Albert Einstein Medical College New York, New York; Chief of Ophthalmology, Mid-Island Hospital, Bethpage, New York. James E. Sheedy, O.D., Ph.D., Associate Clinical Professor, School of Optometry, University of California at Berkeley, Berkeley, California.

What to Do

When Your

Temperature

Rises

BY THE TIME YOUR FEVER IS HIGH enough for you to take notice, you probably already feel pretty terrible. You may be swelteringly hot and drenched in sweat, or shivering as though you were wandering naked through an Arctic village. Your head may be pounding and the familiar pressure behind your eyes is probably growing worse and worse. There's nothing like a fever to really put you out of commission.

The first thing you should know about fevers is that there is quite a range in what is considered a "normal" body temperature. The body's natural temperature-control system, located in a tiny structure at the base of the brain called the hypothalamus, is usually set somewhere around 98.6 degrees Fahrenheit. A normal temperature—measured orally—ranges from 96.7 to 99.0 degrees Fahrenheit (taken rectally, it measures one degree Fahrenheit higher; under the arm, one degree Fahrenheit lower). Your own normal temperature probably varies by more than two degrees during the course of a day, with the lowest reading usually occurring in the early morning and the highest in the evening.

CAUSES

Fever is not a disease in itself but a symptom of some other condition— usually an infection caused by bacteria, fungi, viruses, parasites, or even an allergic reaction. When the body is invaded by one of these, white blood cells (the immune system's first line of defense) are triggered to attack, releasing a protein called endogenous pyrogen. This protein causes the brain to tell the hypothalamus to increase the body's

temperature. If that temperature is over 100 degrees Fahrenheit, you have a fever.

The fact is that fever may actually do the body some good. An untreated fever tends to be self-limiting (meaning that it will usually drop on its own) and—contrary to popular belief—is not likely to escalate to the point that it causes harm. Nor does lowering fever mean that you are lessening the severity of the illness; indeed, fever may be not only a by-product of the immune response, but a way of enhancing it.

This heightened immune response is brought about by pyrogen, the same protein that causes the hypothalamus to increase your body temperature. Pyrogen also has the ability to withhold iron from the blood, which may help keep infectious organisms from flourishing. The bottom line is that by leaving a fever untreated, you may be going along with Mother Nature's way of dealing with infection.

Letting a fever run its course is not the best idea for everyone. While a fever of 102 to 103 degrees Fahrenheit is not usually dangerous in an otherwise healthy adult, it can be risky for infants and very young children, who can develop seizures. A high fever can also be dangerous for very elderly individuals, in whom fever can aggravate an underlying illness, such as a heart arrhythmia or a respiratory ailment. A continually escalating fever in either group should be monitored carefully by a physician. In otherwise healthy adults, if a high fever (above 102 degrees Fahrenheit) or shaking and chills last for more than a day, a doctor should be called. Any fever that doesn't have an apparent cause should be reported to your doctor.

AT-HOME TREATMENT

So, you've got a low fever and have decided to let it run its course, on the assumption that it may be your body's way of healing itself. But you still feel as though you've been repeatedly run over by a very large truck. What should you do?

Let your body tell you what to wear. If you are chilly, bundle up. If you feel uncomfortably warm, however, shed some clothing. When your skin is exposed, the sweat glands can release moisture that will evaporate and cool you down. In fact, the less clothing you wear, the faster the fever will go down.

Don't sweat it. Unless you are cold, burying yourself under a pile of blankets or quilts and letting yourself bake won't help; you can't sweat a fever away. The blankets will only make you more uncomfortable. Simply let your body be your guide. If a light sheet makes you feel comfortable, consider that your body's dictum and obey.

Give yourself a sponge bath. Another way to cool yourself down is to take a sponge bath. You can even sit in a tub of shallow water and splash yourself. Don't fill the tub; the water evaporating off your skin into the air is what cools you

down. And use tepid water; don't try to freeze the fever away by making the water ice cold—the shivering that will result may make the fever rise again.

Keep drinking. Fever, particularly if it is accompanied by vomiting or diarrhea, can cause dehydration and electrolyte imbalance. (Electrolytes, which include calcium, sodium, and potassium, are compounds in the blood that are necessary for metabolism.) Keep your fluid levels up by drinking plenty of cool water or fruit juice.

Take your body's cue when it comes to food. There's no need to force yourself to eat if a fever has stolen your appetite. With food, as with feelings of being hot or cold, your body will tell you what it needs. As long as you keep drinking, your body will be able to get by without too much food.

As your fever breaks and you start feeling better, your appetite will improve. You may even feel ravenously hungry for a while. To restock on nutrients, try eating a variety of foods, including fruits, vegetables, whole grains, low-fat dairy products, low-fat meats, fish, and poultry. The more variety in your diet, the more likely it is that you will provide your body with all the nutrients it needs.

You may think you could eat a horse, but keep one thing in mind: If you haven't eaten much for a few days, your digestive system may need to be reacclimated, too. Go ahead and eat, but start slowly with easy-to-digest foods.

Take an analgesic. Antipyretics are drugs that seek out the trouble-making pyrogen and put it out of commission. Aspirin and acetaminophen both fall into this category. Of course, if you are pregnant, nursing a baby, or suffer from a special medical condition, you should consult a physician before taking any medications. Also, never give aspirin to a child who has a fever coupled with any signs of chicken pox, flu, or even a cold. The drug may trigger a potentially fatal condition known as Reye's syndrome.

Monitor your temperature. It's important to take your temperature periodically with a fever thermometer to make sure that your fever is not continually rising, and so you know when it has broken.

There are two basic types of glass fever thermometers—oral and rectal. The only difference between the two is the shape of the bulb: thin and long on the oral and short and stubby on the rectal. Rectal temperatures are the most accurate; oral temperatures can be thrown off by breathing through the mouth, smoking, or having just had a drink of something hot or cold. Rectal readings are, in general, one Fahrenheit degree higher than oral temperatures. (If neither of these methods is convenient, temperature can also be taken by placing an oral ther-

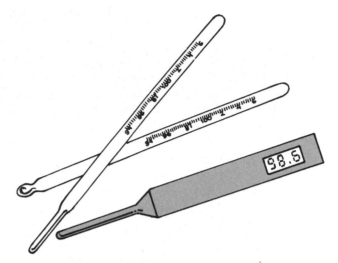

mometer under the armpit for at least two minutes, which will give a reading about one Fahrenheit degree lower than an oral temperature.)

Glass thermometers have several disadvantages: They may break in handling or even in the mouth. If a thermometer breaks in your mouth, don't worry—there is only a tiny amount of mercury in the tube. Just be sure to remove any slivers of glass from your mouth. Glass thermometers also need to be shaken down to 96 degrees Fahrenheit in order to allow the body's true temperature to register. On the other hand, glass thermometers have a big advantage: They are cheap, with most selling for about three dollars at your local pharmacy.

More convenient—and somewhat more expensive (costing about seven to ten dollars)—are the newer digital thermometers, which register temperature accurately to within a tenth of a degree. These thermometers are also fast. It takes less than a minute for the thermometer to register an oral or rectal temper-

8 WAYS TO STOP A FEVER FROM GETTING YOU DOWN

- Bundle up if you're chilled; shed clothing when you feel too hot.
- Don't try to "sweat it out."
- Sponge yourself down with tepid water or sit in a shallow, tepid bath and splash yourself with water.
- Make sure to keep up your fluid intake.
- Eat if you have an appetite, but don't force food down if you don't.
- Take aspirin or acetaminophen if you have no medical conditions prohibiting it.
- Take periodic temperature readings to monitor your fever's progress.
- Give your body a chance to heal.

ature, as compared to three minutes with glass thermometers. (Axillary temperatures—those taken in the armpit—can take up to four minutes.) Most digital thermometers run on a "button," or hearing-aid, type battery that boasts a two- to three-year life with normal use. A newer method of measuring temperature is a heat-sensitive strip you hold against your forehead. The color change in the strip tells you your approximate temperature. Pharmacies generally carry a selection of thermometers.

Get some rest. Common sense tells us that minor illnesses, such as the common cold, can hit us hardest when we are stressed out, run down, and generally not taking very good care of ourselves. Is your present illness a message from your body telling you to "chill out"? Only you know for sure if you've been burning the candle at both ends. You know what Mom's advice would be: Take a day off, stay in bed, rest up. Give your body the opportunity to put its energy into fighting off disease, instead of moving mountains. If you're like most 90s women, you deserve a break. Take it.

Sources: Pascal James Imperato, M.D., Professor and Chairman, Department of Preventive Medicine and Community Health, State University of New York Health Science Center, Brooklyn, New York. Matthew J. Kluger, Ph.D., Professor of Physiology, University of Michigan Medical School, Ann Arbor, Michigan. Harold Neu, M.D., Professor of Medicine and Pharmacology, Columbia University College of Physicians and Surgeons, New York, New York.

•FINGERNAIL PROBLEMS

How to Grow

Nails that Are

Strong and

Healthy

YOUR FINGERNAILS ARE AMONG THE most-used parts of your body. Although you may take their utility for granted while you're scratching an itch, peeling an orange, or opening a soda can, you probably curse them when they don't look long and beautiful, even after all that abuse. However, while less-than-beautiful nails may be slightly annoying, more serious fingernail problems, such as fungal infections and deformities, can be truly disconcerting. Nails are made up of keratin, the same type of protein that hair is made of. Each nail actually consists of several parts, all of which play an important role in its health and growth:

- Nail plate: This is what you see as the fingernail.
- Nail bed: This lies beneath the nail plate and is attached to it. The capillaries in the nail bed nourish the nail and give it its pinkish color.
- Nail matrix: You don't see most of the nail matrix. It is located below the cuticle at the base of the nail. Cells in the matrix produce the fingernail. If the matrix is damaged, your nail will be distorted or may stop growing completely.
- Lunula: This is the moon-shaped portion at the bottom of your nail. It's the part of the matrix that you can see.
- Cuticle: This fold of skin is made of dead cells. It keeps foreign substances, like infection-causing bacteria, out.
- Nail fold: The ridge of skin around the nail.

SYMPTOMS AND CAUSES

Plenty of things can go wrong with fingernails. One of the most common complaints dermatologists hear is that fingernails are brittle—either soft and brittle or hard and brittle.

Hard, dry, brittle nails can be compared to dry skin, since the two have many of the same causes: indoor heat, exposure to detergents, and too-frequent use of chemicals, such as nail-polish removers. Such nails are often shingling; they split like roof shingles at the end of the nail.

Nails that are soft and brittle, on the other hand, need to be kept dry. This condition can be caused by using too much lotion or by constantly having your hands in water.

Trauma, the medical profession's term for injury, is another major problem for fingernails. For example, you might have slammed your fingernail with a hammer, causing a blackish-purple bruise to form under the nail. (A bruise like this is a good reason to contact a physician.)

Injuries can also open the door to infections, especially fungal infections. Although these generally plague toenails more often than fingernails (because of athlete's foot), fungal infections can strike the nails on the hands—with some unpleasant consequences.

With an infection, the nail plate may look chalky-white, yellowish, brownish, or even green. The nail may separate from the bed, or the nail fold may be red and irritated-looking.

The problem you most want to avoid is separation of the nail plate from the nail bed, a condition called onycholysis. It can be caused by an injury, infection, allergy to nail cosmetics, exposure to chemicals, or diseases like psoriasis. If the nail appears white, it may have separated. In this case, you should see your doctor, and you'll want to be careful not to aggravate the problem further. Unfortunately, once the nail separates, it won't reattach until a new nail has grown out.

You should also take good care of the nail matrix. If this is damaged, it will start producing a deformed nail or, even worse, no nail at all.

Some fingernail problems might provide a peek into your health. The symptoms listed here may possibly signal the health problems listed. However, they do not provide definite diagnoses. If you notice any of these, call your physician.

- Pale or bluish nails: This may indicate anemia.
- Pink color slow in returning when nail is squeezed: This may indicate decreased or slowed blood circulation.
- White spots: These occur as the result of an injury to the nail; they're not due to zinc deficiency as some people believe.
- Beau's lines: These horizontal depressions occur after a traumatic event, such as a high fever. Medical experts can actually date the event by measuring the nail and figuring in the growth rate.
- White lines parallel to the lunula: These indicate some sort of systemic (bodywide) illness.
- Clubbed nails: These nails are shaped like the backside of a spoon and may indicate cardiopulmonary disease or asthma.
- Spoon nails: These dip inward and could mean certain types of anemia or injury.
- Pitted nails: These punched-out looking spots might indicate psoriasis.

- Anything resembling a wart around the nail: This could be a skin cancer and should be examined by a doctor.
- Dark spot: This could be melanoma, the most dangerous type of skin cancer. If the spot "bleeds" into the cuticle or nail folds or if you're fair-skinned, this is a warning sign that requires immediate medical attention.

AT-HOME TREATMENT

Here's what the experts recommend you do to keep your nails as healthy and attractive as possible:

Protect them from harsh substances. Janitors are exposed to strong cleaning fluids, bartenders to citrus fruits, anyone who cleans house to detergents and cleansers, and so on. If you must come in contact with these substances, wear gloves. Without a barrier to protect your hands, your nails can become brittle, separated, or infected, which could lead to deformity or nail loss.

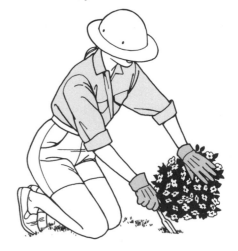

Cover them up. You should wear vinyl gloves—not latex or rubber gloves—for wet work. Latex or rubber will make hands sweat, which may cause further problems. If your hands still perspire when you wear vinyl on them, try wearing cotton gloves underneath. Cotton gloves can also be worn for dry work, such as gardening. These will help protect your nails from damage or possible injury.

Stay well manicured. In the case of fingernail problems, well manicured means short. (Try giving that advice to actress/singer Barbra Streisand or Olympic star Florence Griffith Joyner.) Shorter nails are less vulnerable to damage.

Treat them with respect. Your nails are not screwdrivers, and they were not designed to stand up to the force of a hammer. Mistreatment can lead to injury, which can mean infection, impaired nail growth, or damaging bruises. If your nail turns black and blue, go to your doctor or the emergency room. A medical professional will have to relieve the pressure on the injured blood vessel underneath the nail.

Try a conditioning nail treatment. Soak your dry, brittle nails in tepid water, then massage in a moisturizer. The moisturizer will help hold in the water, since there are no naturally occurring fats in your nails to do the trick. You can also try a humectant; this is a product that contains phospholipids, urea, or lactic acid. All humectants will hold in water. Some products that contain humectants are Complex 15, Aqua-

derm, and Moisturil. You can also use a white petroleum jelly.

Dry out an infection. If your nail becomes infected, especially with a yeast organism, keep it as dry as possible. Consult your physician for other treatment advice.

---

12 TIPS TO IMPROVE YOUR NAILS' HEALTH

- Avoid harsh chemicals that may dry out the fingernails.
- Don vinyl gloves when doing wet work, cotton gloves when doing dry work.
- Keep your nails short.
- Avoid injury to your nails—don't use them as tools.
- Soak your hands in tepid water, then massage in a moisturizer.
- Keep an infected nail away from moisture.
- Gently push back cuticles with a moist towel. Never clip or cut them.
- Clip the dry part of a hangnail with fine scissors and apply an over-the-counter antibiotic ointment.
- Avoid sculptured and artificial nails, as well as nail wraps.
- Don't use any nail product that contains formaldehyde.
- Don't use nail-polish remover more than once a week.
- Don't try to force-feed yourself gelatin or calcium. Neither will help your nails grow or make them stronger.

Leave your cuticles intact. Never use mechanical instruments to cut your cuticles, the finger's barrier to bacteria and moisture. When you clip them you break this barrier and invite infection. You may soak your cuticles in warm water, then push them back with a moist towel. Orange sticks are not recommended, since they, too, may damage the cuticle.

Carefully cut a hangnail. Picking or tearing at a hangnail can make you vulnerable to infection. Any break in the skin is a potential entrance for bacteria. Instead, use fine scissors to clip the dry part of the hangnail, and apply an over-the-counter antibiotic ointment. Moisturize your hands, nails, and cuticles to prevent future hangnails.

Choose health over vanity. Artificial, sculptured nails can hold in more moisture than is healthy, paving the way for fungal and yeast infections. The reactions caused by the glues used in nail wraps can cause permanent damage to the nail bed and root. The most serious problem that can occur is separation of the nail from the bed. To cut down the risk of any of these problems, forgo the artificial nails and learn to love the short look. If you notice any pain or tenderness, you should seek medical attention.

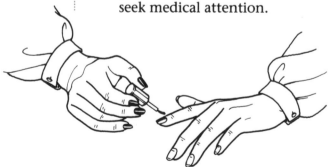

Take some time between manicures. You should apply and remove nail polish no more than once a week, since the acetone present in many polish removers can dehydrate the nails. Even the milder, nonacetone polish removers may leave sensitive nails dry and brittle.

Avoid formaldehyde. These days, most fingernail polishes and nail hardeners do not contain formaldehyde. But some still do. If you're using such a product, you may suffer from an allergic reaction or irritation, causing nail separation.

Don't pin your hopes on Jell-O. Unfortunately, gelatin just doesn't build strong nails, so don't feel like you have to force it down. The same goes for calcium, which has very little, if anything, to do with the hardness of your nails. In fact, with the exception of extreme cases (crash diets or malabsorption problems), your diet does not much affect your nails.

Sources: C. **Ralph Daniel III, M.D.**, Clinical Professor of Medicine (Dermatology), University of Mississippi Medical Center, Jackson, Mississippi. **Lawrence A. Norton, M.D.**, Clinical Professor of Dermatology, Boston University School of Medicine, Boston, Massachusetts. **Richard K. Scher, M.D.**, Professor of Clinical Dermatology, Columbia University School of Medicine, New York, New York.

What to

Do About

an

Invisible

Demon

OK, SO IT'S NOT SOMETHING THAT makes for polite cocktail-party conversation. But it's happened to all of us—usually at the worst possible times: on a first date; at a job interview; in school, as we stood at the blackboard delivering an oral report. We do our best to stifle the sound, but the smell is unmistakable.

CAUSES

Everyone passes a certain amount of flatus—or "breaks wind," as we delicately describe it. Most of the time, this happens unnoticeably, without any undue sound or smell. In fact, the average person expels from 400 to 2,000 milliliters of oxygen, nitrogen, carbon dioxide, hydrogen, and methane each day from the anus. But under some circumstances and in some people, the process does not go so smoothly. Undigested food products pass from the small intestine into the large intestine and colon, where the mass is fermented by large amounts of bacteria that are normally present there. These benign bugs pitch into whatever comes their way. It is this bacterially produced gas that gives flatus its characteristic odor when expelled.

Certain foods are more likely to be passed through the small intestine undigested than others. These, of course, are the foods that are most likely to cause gas.

The worst offenders are beans, dark beer, bran, broccoli, Brussels sprouts, cabbage, carbonated beverages, cauliflower, onions, and milk (for those who are lactose intolerant). Foods that cause problems for some people include raw apples, apricots, bananas, bread and other products containing wheat, carrots, celery, citrus fruits, coffee, cucumbers, eggplant, lettuce, potatoes, pretzels, prunes, radishes, raisins, soybeans, and spinach.

AT-HOME TREATMENT

There are some things you can do to prevent or relieve flatulence:

Avoid the culprits. If a food is causing your problem (see the list of the most common flatulogenics, or gas-producing foods, above), then the logical thing to do is to avoid it. If you're not sure what's causing the problem, try cutting out as many of the common offenders as possible. When you feel better, start adding back the foods one by one. If the small quantities don't bother you, gradually increase your intake.

Cut out dairy products. Many people, especially those of Jewish and Asian ancestry, do not readily digest milk and milk products. The troublemaker is lactose, the milk sugar contained in these foods. The body uses an enzyme called lactase to digest lactose. But people who are lactose intolerant don't produce enough lactase in their intestines to digest the milk sugar. And switching to low- or nonfat dairy products won't help; the lactose is in the nonfat part of the milk. There is less lactose in

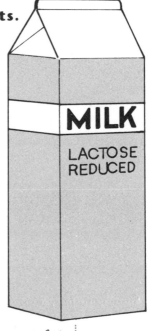

cultured buttermilk, but not everyone likes the taste. Try cutting down on or eliminating milk products for a few days. If the flatulence seems to die down, then you may be lactose intolerant. This is not a definitive test. Only your doctor can say for sure if you're lactose intolerant.

10 WAYS TO DEFEAT YOUR GAS PROBLEM

- Avoid the foods that cause you gas.
- If you are lactose intolerant, either cut out dairy or consume only lactose-reduced milk products. Use over-the-counter drops to reduce lactose in milk or take lactase tablets when you eat regular dairy foods.
- Try a gas-free method of preparing beans.
- Take Beano when you eat gassy foods.
- Try to stay calm—minimize the stress in your life.
- Try mild aerobic exercise.
- Apply pressure to the abdomen, rock back on forth on the floor with your knees drawn up to your chest and your arms wrapped around your legs, or use a heating pad on your tummy.
- Don't wear clothing that constricts the abdomen.
- Try activated charcoal tablets.
- Take an anti-gas medication.

If you do discover that you are lactose intolerant, you don't have to banish dairy forever. There are several brands of lactose-reduced milk on the market that may be easier for you to digest. You can also buy lactase drops to add to your carton of regular milk. Lastly, you can buy lactase tablets at your supermarket or pharmacy. Taking these tablets with your first bite of a dairy product should prevent gas.

De-gas your beans. Beans are almost the perfect food—a great, low-fat source of fiber and protein. However, for many people, eating beans has one big drawback—gas. Rather than give up this vegetarians' delight, however, you can try adjusting the way you prepare it. Here is a tried-and-true method for cooking gas-free dried beans: Soak the beans overnight, then dump the water out. Cook the beans in new water for about half an hour, and then, drain that water out. Again, put in new water, and cook for another 30 minutes. Drain the water out one last time, put new water in, and finish cooking.

Head gas off at the pass. Beano is an over-the-counter food modifier that has an enzyme to break down some gas-producing sugars. Beans, cabbage, broccoli, carrots, oats, and other vegetables and legumes may be more agreeable if you use Beano.

Relax. Anxiety, anger, and depression can have a significant effect on your gastrointestinal tract. Emotional stress can make an existing flatulence problem worse. When you are under stress, muscles in the abdomen tighten, causing potentially painful spasms. Eating under stress can cause you to swallow air, which can also worsen the problem. (See the profile on stress for ways to help you release tension and invite calm back into your life.)

Work it out. Sometimes, flatulence is due to a faulty digestive process rather than diet. The passage of food through the digestive tract should be smooth and unhindered. Mild aerobic exercise, such as brisk walking, may help ease food's journey. You can also try the age-old technique used by parents to calm a fussy, gassy baby: Apply pressure to your abdomen. You can do this by pressing down on the painful area or by lying facedown on the floor with a pillow bunched up under your abdomen. Try rocking back and forth on the floor with your knees drawn up to your chest and your arms wrapped around your legs. A heating pad placed on your abdomen may also help.

Forgo tight clothing. If flatulence is a problem for you, you'd be well advised to avoid wearing clothing that constricts your abdominal area, such as a girdle. The tight fit can compress the abdomen and cause pain. This advice goes double if you expect to be sitting for a long time, on an airplane or in a car, for example.

Swallow charcoal. No, not the kind that you use in your barbecue grill—activated charcoal tablets, which are available without a prescription at drugstores. These tablets absorb excess gas, which may, in turn, calm your flatulence. Because activated charcoal absorbs and neutralizes some chemicals, be sure to ask your pharmacist whether it will interfere with any prescription medications you might be taking.

Try an anti-gas medicine. When all else fails, try taking one of the variety of non-prescription preparations containing simethicone (such as Mylanta, Maalox, or Phazyme). These medications may help ease gassiness and the symptoms that go along with it.

Sources: **Sharon Fleming, Ph.D.**, Associate Professor of Food Science, Department of Nutritional Sciences, University of California at Berkeley, Berkeley, California. **Lawrence S. Friedman, M.D.**, Associate Professor of Medicine, Jefferson Medical College, Thomas Jefferson University, Philadelphia, Pennsylvania. **Mindy Hermann, R.D.**, Spokesperson for the American Dietetic Association. **Norton Rosensweig, M.D.**, Associate Clinical Professor of Medicine, Columbia University College of Physicians and Surgeons, New York, New York.

●Flu

What to Do

When You've

Been Bitten by

the Bug

THE FLU: IT'S THE SCOURGE OF WINTER, the working woman's nemesis, that inconvenient, debilitating pirate of fun. Who hasn't felt its icy-cold hand close around her throat, leaving her a shivering mass of feverish chills and achy exhaustion? Perhaps you're feeling it now. Take heart—millions of other women are probably suffering right along with you (misery loves company, right?). Another (small) consolation: It probably won't kill you.

So where did this awful flu come from? Well, it probably started with the children in your community. According to public-health experts, most flu outbreaks begin with an increasing level of absenteeism in the schools and an increasing number of children hospitalized for some sort of respiratory illness. Adults are usually the next ones hit.

Again, a bout of influenza isn't usually fatal. There are some serious complications that can develop, however. The most common ones involve parts of the respiratory system—for example, pneumonia (inflammation of the lungs), which affects both adults and children, and croup (infection of the larynx), which affects young children.

Despite evidence to the contrary, a few myths about the flu continue to prevail. One myth has to do with what people often refer to as the "24-hour flu." This is an illness characterized by the sudden onset of vomiting and diarrhea, accompanied by a general feeling of malaise. It can be quite intense in the first few hours, but tends to subside completely after 24 hours. While this illness is, indeed, caused by a viral agent, it is not caused by the influenza virus, and so is not a form of the flu at all. The correct term for this type of upset is "gastroenteritis," which simply means an infection of the gastrointestinal tract.

Another myth is the belief that using medicine to keep the fever down helps fight the illness. Experimental studies on flu in animals show that more of the virus is excreted over a longer period of time when the body temperature is lowered with medication. So while such treatments may make you feel better, they don't necessarily help you get over the virus. (See the profile on fever for more on how a fever can actually help the body fight infection.)

SYMPTOMS

Influenza symptoms tend to be similar, regardless of the type or strain of the virus. They include a high fever, a sore throat, a dry cough, severe muscle aches and pains, fatigue, and loss of appetite. Some people also experience pain and stiffness in the joints. Usually, the aches, pains, and fever last only three to five days, while the fatigue and cough can continue for several weeks.

Signs that it's time to see your doctor include a high fever that lasts more than three days, a cough that persists or gets worse (especially if it is associated with severe chest pain or shortness of breath), or a general inability to recover. Other problem signs are extreme difficulty in breathing, blood in coughed-up mucus, bluish skin, or a barklike cough. These symptoms could indicate a secondary infection.

If you have an underlying lung or heart disease, you should consult your physician at the first sign of the flu.

CAUSES

People tend to use the term "flu" to describe any viral upper-respiratory-tract infection. But, strictly speaking, influenza is a very distinct viral agent.

There are two types of viruses that cause influenza—type A and type B. Each type encompasses several different strains, named for the place where they were first identified (the Hong Kong flu, the Russian flu, and so on).

The unusual characteristic of the flu viruses is that once a strain has spread throughout a population, it changes in structure, becoming capable of causing a new form of influenza. The antibodies that were produced by the body to combat the virus the first year are no longer effective, because the virus has taken on different qualities.

Scientists are generally able to predict what type of virus to expect each year, but about every ten years, an entirely different strain of the flu pops up. The new strain is often associated with a much higher rate of infection and death. The last new strain reported in the United States was in 1977.

Because influenza is thought to be transmitted by airborne particles from an infected person's respiratory tract, large numbers of people in a community, or even in a country, can easily contract the disease in a relatively short period of time. Overcrowded living conditions also promote the transmission of the virus.

To dispel a common misconception: Being cold or chilled does not make you more susceptible to geting the flu (or to the common cold, for that matter). Scientific studies on humans have shown that those exposed to severe temperatures for several hours are no more likely to become ill than those who are kept warm and dry. The myth probably originated because one of the first symptoms of the flu is severe chills. People feel that they "caught a chill," leading to the illness. Another factor contributing to the misunderstanding is that since the flu spreads most easily when temperatures and humidity are low, most cases occur during the coldest times of the year.

AT-HOME TREATMENT

Even if you don't manage to evade this relentless bug, you can do a few things to ease some of the symptoms and give your body a chance to fight back.

Hit the sheets. Getting some quality rest time is important, especially if you have a high fever. This shouldn't be hard to do, considering that you probably feel as though you have been run over by an 18-wheeler. Use this time to take a needed break from the daily stresses of life. If you absolutely have to go to work, at least go to bed earlier than usual and be a little late in morning.

Stay hydrated. Drink plenty of nonalcoholic, decaffeinated beverages. Keeping yourself hydrated is very important, and the liquids also keep mucous secretions fluid. Caffeine, being a diuretic, actually increases your fluid loss and should be avoided. Some good choices are clear broth and juice.

Use a humidifier. Influenza viruses survive better in low humidity. Hence, humidifying your home during the drier winter months actually helps prevent the spread of the flu virus, at least inside your house. It also makes you feel better once you have contracted the virus. A warm- or cool-mist humidifier can do the trick. If you don't have a humidifier, try placing a pot of water on a warm radiator.

Take a cough suppressant. A dry, hacking cough can keep you from getting your much need- ed rest. There is over-the- counter relief. Cough remedies containing dextromethorphan are best for a dry cough. Of course, if you are pregnant, nursing a baby, or suffer from a special medical condition, you should always consult a physi- cian before taking any medica- tion.

A cough that brings up mucus, on the other hand, is considered "productive." Do not try to suppress it with cough medicines. Drink fluids to help bring up the mucus of a productive cough. Fluids will help ease it a little, too. You can also try an over-the- counter expectorant, keeping in mind the same warnings that apply to cough suppres- sants.

When all else fails, take an anal- gesic. Since a high temperature may actually help your body fight off the infection, you may want to try to let the fever run its course. However, if you're suf- fering from a terrible headache, taking aspirin, acetaminophen, or ibuprofen may give you some needed relief. Lowering your temperature will also help you feel a bit better by prevent- ing dehydration and cutting down on the severe, shaking chills associated with fever.

Aspirin and ibuprofen tend to work better against aches and pains, whereas aceta- minophen works best on the fever. Be aware of the precau- tions: Aspirin and ibuprofen can irritate the stomach, and people with a history of gas- trointestinal problems and/or ulcer disease may have their conditions complicated by these drugs. Also, in young people (aged 21 and under) the combination of aspirin and the flu has been associated with Reye's syndrome, an often fatal illness characterized by sudden, severe deterioration of brain and liver function. It is best not to administer aspirin to mem- bers of this age group during flu season. Again, consult your doctor about any medications if you are pregnant, nursing a baby, or have a special medical condition.

PREVENTION

Flu vaccines are about 80 percent effective when received before the flu season begins (ideally in September or October). So if you really can't afford to get sick, a flu shot may not be a bad idea for you. A flu shot is a priority if you fall into one of the high-risk groups that are listed below:

- Individuals with chronic heart and lung disease. The flu virus can aggravate these conditions to the point of causing serious complications and even death.
- People over the age of 65, especially if they are living in a nursing home or chronic-care facility. (Viruses can spread like wildfire in such environments.) What's more, the flu virus attacks the already weakened immune systems of elderly people. This can lead to pneumonia and even death.
- Individuals with other chronic diseases, including asthma, diabetes, kidney disease, or cancer. When the body is already fighting a disease, contracting another illness can cause serious problems.
- Individuals under the age of 21 who take aspirin regularly for problems such as chronic arthritis. Reye's syndrome may be triggered by the flu virus in children and young adults who are on aspirin therapy.
- Health-care providers. Catching the flu may not seriously endanger these individuals, but it can be spread to the patients they treat.
- Pregnant women who fall into any of the high-risk groups mentioned. In this instance, the vaccine must be given after the first trimester of the pregnancy to prevent the possibility of harming the fetus.

Sources: Evan T. Bell, M.D., Specialist in Infectious Diseases, Lenox Hill Hospital, New York, New York. W. Paul Glezen, M.D., Pediatrician, Influenza Research Center, Professor of Microbiology and Immunology, Professor of Pediatrics, Chief Epidemiologist, Baylor College of Medicine, Houston, Texas. Marcia Kielhofner, M.D., Clinical Assistant Professor of Medicine, Baylor College of Medicine, Houston, Texas.

5 WAYS TO BEAT THE FLU-BUG BLUES

- Get some rest.
- Drink plenty of fluid.
- Keep your home humid in cold weather.
- Suppress a dry cough with an over-the-counter cough suppressant; encourage a "productive" cough with plenty of fluids or an expectorant.
- As a last resort, take an analgesic.

•FLUID RETENTION

How to Get

Rid of Excess

Water Weight

and Swelling

THERE'S PROBABLY NOT A WOMAN IN the world who hasn't experienced a bout of excess fluid retention—before a menstrual period, during pregnancy, after a salty meal, during hot weather, after standing up for long periods of time, and so on. Some people, because of a deeper problem, such as a heart, blood-vessel, or kidney disorder, experience the problem more frequently.

Water retention usually causes nothing more serious than a bloated, uncomfortable feeling. Sometimes, however, retaining too much fluid can be harmful. During pregnancy, it is associated with preeclampsia, a dangerous condition characterized by excessively high blood pressure.

SYMPTOMS

How do you know when you are retaining water? One telltale symptom is an overnight weight gain of a few pounds or more. The large initial weight loss that occurs at the beginning of a diet is also due to excess water weight. Other signs include not being able to zip your favorite jeans, your rings or shoes feeling tight, and visible swelling of the ankles, legs, or fingers.

Here's an old midwives' trick for gauging the degree of water retained: Pick a spot where you seem to be experiencing swelling (the ankle, for instance). Press one finger into the skin for a second or two. When you stop pressing, if a dimple or indentation remains for more than a few seconds, you are probably retaining fluid.

CAUSES

For women, one of the most frequent causes of water retention is the hormonal changes that accom-

pany menstruation and pregnancy. These changes influence the levels of salts retained in the body (sodium and potassium salts control fluid regulation). Other causes include a high dietary sodium intake (from eating salty foods), potassium deficiency, or problems with circulation, kidneys, or the urinary system.

AT-HOME TREATMENT

Excessive fluid retention during pregnancy should always be monitored by a physician, since it may be a warning sign of preeclampsia. It is normal to retain some water during pregnancy, which usually shows up as a swelling of the fingers, feet, and ankles. However, if it's becoming difficult to distinguish between the top of your ankles and the bottom of your calves, you should probably point it out to your obstetrician. If you suffer from any kidney disorder, heart disease, or blood-vessel disorder, excess water retention may also be a warning sign that should be checked out by a doctor.

However, if it's just a simple case of the I-can't-zip-my-skirt blues, try the following tips:

Drink, drink, drink. Many people suffer from the misconception that drinking more fluids will result in more water-weight gain. This is, in fact, the opposite of what really happens. The best cure for water retention is to up your fluid intake to eight to ten eight-ounce glasses every day. The best choices are water, fruit juice (some say that cranberry is good for fighting fluid retention), and decaffeinated coffee and tea. Caffeine does act as a diuretic but excessive amounts can cause nervousness, heart palpitations, and insomnia. Also, during the premenstrual period, coffee and tea may aggravate headaches and irritability. Alcohol also acts as a diuretic, but, as we know, has a number of undesirable effects that preclude drinking it during the course of a normal day.

Go bananas. Eat a banana or a handful of raisins—both of which contain high amounts of potassium. Potassium helps eliminate fluid retention. If you don't think a banana is enough, you can also ask your doctor for a recommendation about taking a potassium supplement.

Shift your weight. If you must stand for long periods of time, shift your weight from one foot to the other or rock back and forth from your heels to your toes to exercise your leg muscles. This will help force blood back up into your legs and reduce swelling.

Skip the water pills. Over-the-counter diuretics can be dangerous and habit-forming. In the long run, they may make your body dependent on ever-increasing amounts of them to eliminate water. Then, when you stop taking the pills, you may start to retain more fluid than you did before. If you really feel that you need a diuretic, talk to your doctor and ask for a recommendation. Also ask your doctor how long you should continue taking the diuretics, in order to avoid the rebound effect.

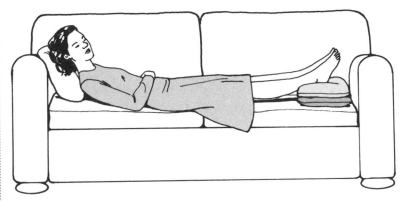

Put your feet up. You enlist the aid of gravity in draining fluid from a swollen limb when you elevate the limb. It's even more beneficial to raise the extremity above the level of your heart. If your hand is swollen, sit up with your hand propped up so that your thumb is about even with your nose. Support your arm or leg on some pillows or on the back of a couch.

Get some support. If being on your feet all day causes minor swelling, try over-the-counter support hose for relief. A doctor can also prescribe stockings that are specially made to apply more pressure to the lower leg in order to help keep fluids from collecting. These are available in various lengths and degrees of compression. Prescription stockings can be especially helpful to pregnant women who suffer from excess water retention. (They may also help prevent or minimize the development of varicose veins.)

Exercise. If your legs are swollen, it's important to keep them moving. Get up periodically and stretch your legs. If you're at your desk, take a stroll around it; if you're on a plane, promenade up and down the plane's aisle occasionally to

18 WAYS TO BEAT THE BLOAT

- Drink eight to ten eight-ounce glasses of water or fruit juice every day.
- Avoid alcohol.
- Eat high-potassium foods like bananas or raisins.
- While standing for long periods of time, shift your weight from foot to foot or rock back and forth from heel to toe.
- Don't take over-the-counter diuretics.
- Elevate a swollen limb above the level of the heart, if possible.
- Wear over-the-counter or prescription support hose.
- Start a program of walking every day.
- If you can't exercise, stretch and flex your leg muscles often.
- Don't sit with your legs crossed.
- Find out if your medication could be to blame.
- Don't wear clothing that is too tight.
- Maintain a healthy body weight.
- Cut down on high-sodium foods.
- Learn to relax.
- Don't wear tight shoes or socks.
- Wear shoes made from natural materials and socks that let your feet breathe.
- During pregnancy, sleep on your left side with pillows between your knees.

loosen them up and stimulate blood flow. Even better, take advantage of a lunch break or layover at the airport to take a longer walk. The movement helps your leg muscles push blood and other fluids back toward the heart. In general, this kind of aerobic activity builds up the strength and efficiency of your heart and leg muscles. If your hands swell during exercise, wear a pair of stretch gloves during your workout.

For people who are limited in their activity (people with arthritis, for example) flexing is the next best thing to walking. While sitting, flex your knee and ankle joints up and down. Doing a tighten-and-release routine on the thigh and calf muscles can also help. During pregnancy, however, flexing calf muscles may result in a painful leg cramp.

Give up feminine sitting positions. Don't sit with your legs crossed. This position can limit blood flow through the veins in the thighs, aggravating the swelling in the lower legs.

Consult your doctor. Certain prescription drugs, including some blood-pressure medications (such as reserpine and nifedipine) and hormonal regulators (such as birth-control pills), can cause fluid retention. Ask your physician if your medication could be causing the problem.

Loosen up. Avoid tight garments that can apply too much pressure on the upper thighs and waist. By restricting the removal of fluids in the lower legs, this pressure can cause swelling. Common culprits are belts, garters, and girdles. Wristwatches, rings, and bracelets (for the wrist or ankle) can also aggravate or cause swelling if they are worn too tightly.

Shed a few pounds. Being overweight is associated with higher levels of water retention and may make you more susceptible to the inflammatory effects of heat and humidity. Along with numerous other benefits, maintaining a healthy weight can help combat water retention problems.

Go the low-sodium route. Sodium makes the body retain fluid. Cutting out table salt isn't the only way to reduce your sodium intake. Avoid salty snacks; choose no-salt potato chips, pretzels, and popcorn instead. Check the labels of any processed foods that you eat, because they can be very high in sodium. Fresh and frozen fruits and vegetables, whether eaten raw or steamed, are practically salt-free. If you cook them, don't add salt. Try to stay below 2,500 or 3,000 milligrams of sodium per day.

Chill out. Even though water retention is not directly affected by stress, some doctors see an indirect link. Stress can make you feel lethargic and sedentary. The inactivity these feelings produce can aggravate swelling.

Buy well-fitting footwear. Tight footwear and hosiery can cause, or aggravate, swelling. Here are some tips to make sure that you get the right size:

• Buy shoes in the late afternoon. Your feet can swell by as much as half a shoe size as the day goes on. Shoes that are too tight can cause swelling or make it more pronounced.

• Stand up to measure your foot. The most accurate measurements of the length and width of your foot can be obtained while you are on your feet.

• Choose lace-up shoes. When your feet swell, your footwear has to give. Slip-on styles are not very forgiving, but lace-up shoes can always be loosened to allow your feet more room.

• Stick with a flat or low heel. Walking in flat or low-heeled shoes is a more natural movement for your foot, with the sole flexing from heel to toe. Higher heels restrict this movement. Because the lower circulatory system relies on the movement of the leg muscles to keep fluids moving, the confinement of high-heeled shoes can contribute to swelling by limiting your proper stride.

• Wear a style that fits your feet. Some shoe styles suit some shapes better than others. For example, shoes with shallow toe boxes are no good for you if you have thicker toes. People with broad feet will not be comfortable in pointy-toed shoes.

• Take a walk on a hard floor. Because your feet spread more on hard surfaces than they do on soft carpeting, walking on a hard surface will better help you determine if a pair of shoes is too tight.

• Let your feet breathe. Socks made of certain acrylic fibers may tend to pull moisture away from the feet. However, some doctors still feel that the traditional natural fibers, cotton and wool, are best for keeping the feet cool and dry. Try a pair of each, and see which one works best for you. You will probably want to avoid nylon altogether, since it tends to generate heat and absorb moisture like a sponge. If your feet sweat heavily regardless of the type of socks you wear, try changing your socks two or three times a day.

• Don't assume that a pair of socks will fit. No matter what the package says, one size does not fit all. Sock size is based on shoe size, but what about people who have thicker ankles or calves? If a pair of socks makes you feel like your legs are clamped into a vise, don't wear them. Elastic banding that is too tight can lead to or aggravate swelling by restricting circulation.

Stay well-ventilated. Shoes made from leather and canvas are porous and will keep your feet cool and dry by allowing them to "breathe." Rubber and vinyl are nonporous and will trap moisture, resulting in excessive heat and humidity, which can aggravate swelling.

Sleep on your left side. During pregnancy, lying on your back causes the growing uterus to put pressure on certain blood vessels that are important to circulation. Lying on your left side with pillows between your knees can restore circulation and reduce water retention.

Sources: **Missy Donnell, O.T.R., C.H.T.,** Occupational Therapist, The Hand Clinic, Austin, Texas. **Glenn B. Gastwirth, D.P.M.,** Deputy Executive Director, American Podiatric Medical Association, Bethesda, Maryland. **Claudia Holland, M.D.,** Assistant Clinical Professor of Obstetrics and Gynecology, Columbia-Presbyterian Medical Center, New York, New York. **Pamela Kirby, O.T.R./L., C.H.T.,** Occupational Therapist, Certified Hand Therapist, The Hand Center, Greensboro, North Carolina. **Allan D. Marks, M.D.,** Associate Professor of Medicine, Director, Hypertension Clinic, Temple University Health Sciences Center, Philadelphia, Pennsylvania. **William F. Ruschhaupt, M.D.,** Staff Physician, Department of Vascular Medicine, Cleveland Clinic Foundation, Cleveland, Ohio. **Robert C. Schlant, M.D.,** Professor of Medicine (Cardiology), Emory University School of Medicine, Atlanta, Georgia.

Relief for

Tender Tootsies

THERE'S AN OLD SAYING, "WHEN YOUR feet hurt, everything hurts." If you've suffered from painful feet—and four out of five of us have—you know just how true it is. As women, we have fives times the risk of developing serious foot problems than men do.

When you think of the abuse we put our feet through, it's no wonder they often hurt. If your feet are like most, they'll carry you 70,000 miles in your lifetime, or three times around the world! In a single day, they'll absorb 1,000 pounds of force. And many of us ask our feet to accomplish all this while crammed into pointed, high-heeled shoes with little or no support.

Little engineering wonders, the feet are usually able to respond to our demands. Each foot has 26 bones. Together the feet have nearly one-quarter of all the bones in the body. They have 33 joints for flexibility and 19 muscles that control the movement of various parts. Tendons stretch tautly between muscles and bones, moving parts of the feet as the muscles contract. Two arches in the midfoot and forefoot, constructed like small bridges, support each foot and provide a springy, elastic structure to absorb 1,000 pounds of force every day. Nerve endings in the feet make them sensitive and sometimes ticklish. Holding the whole structure together are more than 100 strong, fibrous ligaments.

CAUSES

Most foot pain results from two major causes: ill-fitting shoes and inherited structural weaknesses. The majority of women's foot problems are caused by so-called "fashionable shoes." In fact, shoe-related foot problems are ten times more common in women than in men. Take a look at most women's shoes, even flat ones, and you'll see that they offer little or no arch support and feature pointed toe boxes that pinch the toes. If you add a heel higher than an inch, it causes a woman's weight to rock onto the ball of the foot, the Achilles tendon to shorten, and the pelvis to shift forward.

The result of such poorly fitting shoes is problems such as corns, bunions, blisters, toe deformities, and over time, even tendinitis, back problems, and joint irritation and dysfunction. A common problem foot doctors (podiatrists) see in women is "forefoot shock": pain, fatigue, and a wobbly gait caused by the body's weight being centered on the ball of the foot. Lower back muscles strain to cope with the imbalance, which can result in chronic back pain.

Structural problems that can cause pain involve weaknesses in the foot's construction. Some feet, for example, are apt to "overpronate," or roll excessively inward with each step. Pronation is a normal mechanism that "unlocks" the foot and gets it ready to push up. Problems come when the foot overpronates, which in turn, overworks the tendon and causes pain.

Sometimes foot pain is caused by injuries or medical conditions. Too often, women who begin a new exercise routine or overdo an old one, for example, suffer plantar fasciitis. Caused by an inflammation of the heel tendons, plantar fasciitis is characterized by severe pain in the heel, especially when getting up in the morning.

Medical conditions can cause foot problems or make them worse. Diabetes, for example, reduces blood circulation to the feet and can make them susceptible to infections, some serious enough to warrant amputation.

AT-HOME TREATMENT

If you do develop foot pain, try these tips to get you walking comfortably again:

Change shoes. Often people wear their shoes long after they've worn out and can no longer properly support their feet. It's especially important that you replace your exercise shoes regularly. A good pair of running shoes should be replaced after 400 to 600 miles; walking shoes after 600 miles. Aerobics shoes should last at least six months; tennis shoes about 50 hours. Any time your feet ache, legs feel tired, knees are sore, or hips hurt, replace your shoes.

Take a load off. Much foot pain is due to fatigued muscles. Take frequent breaks, especially if you have to stand for long periods of time. Whenever you can, elevate your feet at a 45-degree angle to your body and relax for 10 to 15 minutes. Elevating the feet reduces swelling.

Try massage. A foot massage can make you feel relaxed all over. With massage oil, baby oil, or moisturizing lotion, use medium to light strokes with your thumbs and fingers to loosen up the muscles. Then starting with the ball of the foot and working across and down the entire foot, massage gently with your thumbs in small, circular motions. Making long, deep strokes with your thumbs, rub the along arch all the way to the toes. Gently squeeze, rotate, and pull each toe. Finally, cupping the foot between both hands, gently squeeze up and down the whole length of the foot.

Cool your heels. Many people suffer from swollen feet at the end of the day. Refresh your feet by applying a washcloth filled with ice.

Stay in good trim. Ingrown toenails are inherited, but improper nail trimming can make them worse. Trim the nails straight across, and then trim the sides to keep the nails from cutting the skin and causing infections.

9 WAYS TO TREAT YOUR SORE TOOTSIES

- Replace worn-out shoes.
- Put your feet up.
- Try a foot massage.
- Ice your feet.
- Trim your toenails correctly.
- Don't perform bathroom surgery.
- Learn about your foot type.
- Consider orthotics.
- Don't ignore foot pain.

Avoid bathroom surgery. For problems like corns and calluses, the temptation is to get out a straight-edged razor blade and play surgeon. Resist the urge! Instead, soak your feet and file down the excess skin with a pumice stone. If you have corns between your toes ("kissing corns"), use cushions between the toes to prevent further corn buildup.

Get to know your feet. Not all kinds of shoes are meant for all feet. The rigidity of high-arched feet calls for shoes that provide good cushioning and shock absorption. Flat feet are quite flexible and need shoes that control excess motion.

To determine your foot type, wet your bare feet and stand on a concrete floor or a piece of paper. Does your foot outline appear narrow and curved like a half-moon? If so, you have high arches. Does your foot outline look like a slab? If so, you have flat feet. You may need the help of a professional if you have flat feet.

Consider orthotics. If you're bothered by painful feet despite wearing supportive, well-fitting shoes, your problem may be structural, and the solution may be orthotics, or shoe inserts. You can find over-the-counter orthotics in the foot-care section of your pharmacy. Or you can have some custom-fit by a health professional for your foot's particular problem.

Pay attention to pain. Your feet cannot talk to you except through pain signals. Don't ignore pain. Early warning signs that something may be wrong include burning, numbness, cramping, swelling, and redness. If self-care doesn't help, see a foot doctor.

PREVENTION

Most common foot problems can be prevented before they become a problem. Try these tips:

---

6 WAYS TO PROTECT YOUR DOGS

- Wear shoes that fit.
- Buy activity-specific shoes.
- Keep your feet dry and clean.
- Stretch and warm up before exercising. Don't overdo your exercise routine.
- Exercise your feet.
- Maintain your ideal weight.

Get fit. When you shop for shoes, find a salesperson who can properly measure and fit your feet. Buy shoes in the afternoon when your feet are slightly swollen. Look for shoes that:

• Have room for your toes. Avoid overly pointed shoes that pinch the toes and can cause corns, calluses, and toe deformities.

• Have enough width. Too often, shoes squeeze the forefoot and result in painful bunions (inflammation and swelling of the big toe joint).

• Don't move independently of your foot. When you lift your heel, the shoe should come with it and not slip.

• Have cushion. You can often prevent problems by wearing shoes with plenty of cushion in the forefoot and heel areas.

• Offer arch support. Look for shoes that support the arch or buy shoes large enough so that you can put in an arch support.

• Fit when you buy them. Don't plan to "break in" shoes that aren't comfortable. If they don't fit in the store, don't take them.

Buy the right shoe. Every activity, like walking, running, aerobics, or tennis, involves its own set of repetitive movements needing specific support and cushioning. That's why they make specific shoes for specific sports. Don't wear your old sneakers to your aerobics class. Instead, invest the money in the right, activity-specific shoes. In the long run, it'll save you money and pain.

Bring along your walking shoes. Fashion and custom dictate that women can't always wear "sensible" shoes to work or social occasions. Minimize the amount of time you have to wear high-heeled shoes by bringing walking shoes and wearing them to and from work and during breaks.

Keep your feet clean and dry. Problems like toenail fungus and athlete's foot multiply when feet aren't kept clean and dry. Wash your feet daily (the feet have 250,000 sweat glands that produce about a cup of moisture a day). Dry your feet thoroughly, especially between the toes. Dust them with talcum (not cornstarch), and wear cotton or wool socks. Wear different shoes each day to allow each pair to dry out. In public showers, wear sandals.

Stretch first. Often foot injuries occur because people don't stretch or warm up before exercising. Stretch, warm up, and slowly build up the amount of exercise you do.

Exercise your feet. Feet are healthiest when they are strong and flexible. Exercise your feet by walking in shoes that provide good support and cushioning.

Specific exercises can get your feet in shape, too. Try the golf-ball roll: Rest your shoeless foot on top of a golf ball, and roll it against the floor using only the weight of the foot—don't stand on the ball. You can also scatter beans on the floor and practice picking them up with your toes.

Try the circle/stretch: Sit in a chair with your feet out in front of you and make four or five small circles in both directions with your feet. Then stretch out your toes as far as you can, and flex them up towards you. Repeat six times.

Maintain your ideal weight. Being overweight puts excess strain on your feet. Keep your weight within normal limits.

Sources: **Hugh Fraser, D.P.M.**, St. Vincent Hospital and Medical Center, Portland, Oregon. **Kathleen Galligan, Ds.C.**, President, Oregon Chiropractic Association; Chiropractor, Shontay Chiropractic, Lake Oswego, Oregon. **Michael Martindale, L.P.T.**, Physical Therapist, Portland Adventist Medical Center, Portland, Oregon. **Andrew Schink, M.D.**, Past President, Oregon Podiatric Association, Eugene, Oregon. **Martyn Shorten, Ph.D.**, Former Director, NIKE's Sport Research Laboratory. **David Wisdom, M.D.**, Orthopedic Surgeon, St. Vincent Hospital and Medical Center, Portland, Oregon.

Say Hello to

Healthier

Gums

If you brush your teeth and your gums bleed, even just a little, you may have gingivitis, the first stage of gum disease. While it's not life threatening, it could spell bad news for your teeth. According to the American Dental Association (ADA), gum disease, not cavities (dental caries), is the leading cause of tooth loss among adults.

Gingivitis (pronounced "jin-ja-VI-tus"), is inflammation, swelling, and bleeding of the gum tissue. It's caused by the bacteria that naturally coat your teeth. The bacteria form a sticky, whitish film on the teeth called plaque. When you forget to brush or don't brush your teeth thoroughly enough, the bacteria in the plaque form toxins that irritate your gums and make them red, swollen, and likely to bleed easily.

Almost everyone has a certain amount of gingivitis. When gingivitis is left untreated, however, it can become a big problem. Over time, the toxins in the bacteria can destroy gum tissue, causing it to separate from the teeth and form pockets. These pockets hold even more bacteria and cause the teeth to detach further from the gums. At this point, gingivitis has progressed to periodontitis, an irreversible form of gum disease that can destroy the bone and soft tissue that support the teeth.

CAUSES

Take a moment to look at your gums. Are they red? Do they look slightly puffy and swollen? You're not alone. Gingivitis is very common. In fact, the ADA says that three out of four adults have gingivitis. Most gingivitis is caused by not brushing and flossing correctly or often enough and not having teeth professionally cleaned on a regular basis.

However, other factors can increase your risk of developing gingivitis. Women often experience increased gingivitis during pregnancy or menstruation, times of hormonal fluctuation. If you're under a lot of stress, you may also find your gums more swollen, inflamed, and subject to bleeding easily.

Some diseases can increase your risk of gingivitis. Diseases like diabetes and drugs like Dilantin (phenytoin) can cause gingivitis to flare up. Even bad habits like breathing though the mouth, which tends to dry out the gums and cause an overgrowth of tissue, can increase your gingivitis risk.

AT-HOME TREATMENT

A sage once said, "In the cause is the solution." This is certainly true of gingivitis. The major cause of gingivitis is poor oral hygiene; the solution is good oral hygiene. If you catch gingivitis before it has progressed to the periodontitis stage, it is entirely reversible and the damage can be repaired with these home remedies.

Go dry. To relieve the boredom of brushing and make it easier for you to do it longer, brush your teeth without toothpaste while you're watching television or doing some other activity.

Try three on three. Whenever you can, brush your teeth three times a day for at least three minutes. Most people spend

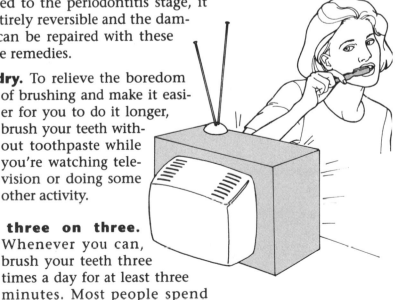

less than one minute a day brushing their teeth. That's not enough to clean out the bacteria that cause plaque.

Get regular. Find an oral hygiene routine that works for you and stick with it. Start at one spot and work around the entire mouth. It will help keep you from missing areas.

Don't brush too hard. Have you ever drunk something cold or hot and felt a "stinging" or sensitive sensation? Although sometimes dental sensitivity is evidence of something more serious, often it's a sign that dentin, the tissue just below the gums, has been exposed by brushing too hard.

Try this: Apply the bristles of the toothbrush to the back of your hand. Press with the brush as hard as you normally would when you brush your teeth and try to move the brush around. Then apply only a tiny amount of pressure and move the brush. It becomes obvious that the hard pressure doesn't allow the brush's bristles to move easily. So, when you brush, lighten up.

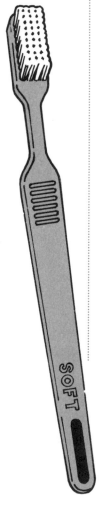

Don't travel. Avoid brushing up and down, moving quickly over several teeth. Instead, brush only a couple of teeth at a time, holding the brush in one place.

Soften up. Toothbrushes come in "hard," "medium," and "soft." Choose a soft brush that is less likely to damage your gums. With softer bristles, you don't have to worry so much about your brushing technique.

Careful around hormonal fluxes. Fluctuating hormones can make women more susceptible to oral bacteria and plaque. Be especially careful in your brushing and flossing during pregnancy and menstruation.

Brush everything! Don't forget to brush your tongue and the roof of your mouth (palate). This will increase circulation in your mouth and cut the number of bacteria.

Go electric. Hate to brush? Try an electric toothbrush. The new "rotary" electric brushes are even better. Since not all electric toothbrushes are equal, ask your dentist for a recommendation about the type that's best for you.

Hello, flossy? It doesn't matter how well or how long you brush, you can't get the bristles between your teeth. That's why flossing is so important. Use either the unwaxed or waxed variety (waxed is easier to slide between teeth) and try to floss at least twice a day. A good idea is to carry floss in your car or keep some in your desk at work. After a meal, call on flossy.

Have patience. If you haven't been brushing and flossing as often or as well as you should and now you have gingivitis, an increased oral hygiene program will likely stimulate even more gum bleeding at first. Don't panic. It may take a couple of weeks to eliminate the oral bacteria and allow your gums to heal. If bleeding continues for more than three weeks despite good oral hygiene, see your dentist.

Try water. Anything that removes food debris and bacteria from your teeth can help fight gingivitis. Water irrigation devices like Waterpik can help clean debris and massage your gums. (Sorry, but they don't take the place of proper brushing and flossing.)

Control that tartar. "Tartar-control toothpastes"—you've seen them advertised on television. Don't all toothpastes control tartar? Well, yes and no. Toothpastes that claim to have tartar-control formulas contain special chemicals that help slow some of the hardening (mineralization) of plaque. Brands that display the American Dental Association Seal of Acceptance or Recognition have been put through a rigorous testing process to ensure that their advertising claims are true.

Arm and Hammer it. One of the least expensive and most effective agents to keep your teeth and gums healthy is baking soda. It's a good abrasive—removes foods, neutralizes bacteria, and even polishes off stains—and doesn't damage tooth enamel. Brush your teeth once or twice a week with a baking soda paste (baking soda and a little water). Brush thoroughly, especially around the gum line.

Go for the rinse. No mouthwash will take the place of brushing or flossing, but one brand,

---

21 WAYS TO BE KIND TO YOUR GUMS

- Brush three times a day for three minutes.
- Try dry brushing.
- Brush in a consistent pattern.
- Don't brush too hard.
- Avoid a "traveling" brush stroke.
- Use a toothbrush with soft bristles.
- Brush especially carefully if you're pregnant or menstruating.
- Brush your tongue and palate.
- Try an electric toothbrush.
- Floss regularly.
- Have patience with gingivitis symptoms.
- Try a water irrigation device.
- Use a tartar-control toothpaste.
- Brush with a baking soda paste.
- Rinse after eating.
- Try a saltwater rinse.
- Use the gum stimulator at the end of your toothbrush.
- Eat a balanced diet.
- Manage your stress.
- Have your teeth professionally cleaned regularly.
- Pay attention to warning signals.

Listerine, has been proven by the ADA's Council on Dental Therapeutics to reduce plaque. Ask your dentist if he or she thinks adding Listerine to your oral hygiene routine might help.

Try a dash of salt. Rinsing your mouth for 30 seconds with a warm saltwater solution (half a teaspoon of salt to four ounces of warm water) can soothe inflamed tissue. And remember, be sure to spit (don't swallow) the salt water.

Rinse out. You can't always grab a toothbrush or dental floss right after you eat. So, after eating, at least rinse your mouth thoroughly with plain water. It will flush out some debris and help reduce your risk of gingivitis.

Stimulate those gums. You've seen those rubber tips on the ends of toothbrushes. Wonder what they are for? They're gum stimulators to clean between the teeth, massage the gums, and increase gum circulation. Here's how to use them: Place the rubber tip between two teeth. Turn the tip toward the teeth's biting surface until it's at a 45 degree angle to the gumline. Then make circular motions with the stimulator for 10 seconds. When you finish, move on to the next tooth.

Watch your diet. Researchers say that gingivitis in people who have poor diets progresses more rapidly than in those who eat a balanced diet. Eat a wide variety of foods that includes plenty of fresh fruits and vegetables, whole grains, legumes, low-fat dairy products, and protein sources like lean meats.

Manage your stress. Dental experts know that people under stress are at greater risk for gingivitis. Reduce your risk by effectively managing your stress.

Get a regular cleaning. No matter how thoroughly you clean your own teeth and gums, it's important to have your teeth professionally cleaned and checked to prevent gum disease. A professional cleaning will also clean below the gum line. Most dentists suggest twice a year as a good schedule for cleaning and checkups. If you already have gum disease, you may need to see your dentist more often. Talk with your dentist about the best cleaning and checkup schedule for you.

Watch for warnings. Call your dentist immediately if you notice any of these warning symptoms (don't wait for your regularly scheduled checkup):
• You have persistent bad breath.
• Pus appears between the teeth and gums.
• The way your teeth fit together (the "bite") feels off.
• Your teeth are loose or are separating.
• Your gums bleed consistently.
• At the gumline, your gums appear "rolled" instead of flat.
• Your partial dentures fit differently than they used to.
• You feel pain or sensitivity to hot and/or cold.

Sometimes bleeding gums are a sign of a systemic bleeding disorder. Call your doctor if, in addition to bleeding gums, you have these symptoms: easy bruising, prolonged bleeding from minor cuts, and nosebleeds without trauma.

Sources: Jack Clinton, D.M.D., Associate Dean of Patient Services, Oregon Health Sciences University School of Dentistry, Portland, Oregon. Sandra Hazard, D.M.D., Managing Dentist, Willamette Dental Group, Inc., Portland, Oregon. Ken Waddell, D.M.D., Dentist, Tigard, Oregon. Ronald Wismer, D.M.D., Past President, Washington County Dental Society; Dentist, Beaverton, Oregon.

Ways to Keep

from Losing

Your Locks

YOU'RE STANDING IN THE SHOWER shampooing your hair when you notice a clump of hair in the drain. Or you notice more hair than usual on your pillow or in your hairbrush. You're a woman. You can't be going bald. Or maybe you can.

If your scalp is like most, it holds about 100,000 hairs. You lose 50 to 100 of those hairs every day. It's part of the hair's normal growth and replacement cycle. But sometimes, that hair loss is altered or accelerated by any number of factors including drugs, radiation, disease, aging, and stress.

CAUSES

The most common cause of hair loss in women (and men) is pattern balding. Normal "terminal" hair shafts are replaced by shorter, "peach-fuzz" vellus hair. This nonpigmented vellus hair gives the bald or thin appearance to the hair.

Both men and women suffer from pattern balding. In men, it tends to be hereditary and involves the metabolism of male hormones (androgens) in the hair. Male hair loss can begin at age 20 or earlier. In women, pattern balding is also related to a hormonal mechanism, but usually doesn't begin until after menopause. In men, hair loss begins at the forehead on either side of the front and continues to the top of the head. In contrast, pattern balding in women is more diffuse, usually less extensive, and starts on the back of the crown. Some women experience hair loss at times of hormonal fluctuation such as during pregnancy, menstruation, or during postmenopausal hormone therapy.

Hair loss may also be related to taking a wide range of medications or herbs with heavy metals in them. Chemotherapy drugs, of course, are notorious for causing hair to fall out, but more common drugs like some cholesterol-lowering drugs (clofibrate, gemfibrozil), most arthritis medications, beta-blocking drugs for high blood pressure, and some ulcer drugs can also cause distressing hair loss.

In some cases, hair loss is a reaction to extreme psychological stress, surgery, or severe influenza with fever. It may also be a symptom of a more serious health problem such as thyroid disease or systemic lupus erythematosus.

AT-HOME TREATMENT

There's no cure for pattern baldness in women or men. But you can control other causes of hair loss and have a healthful lifestyle that promotes healthy hair.

Don't get sick. It's not always easy, but you can increase your chances of staying healthy and therefore keeping your mane intact. Live a healthful lifestyle: Exercise regularly. Manage your stress (stress lowers the immune system). Eat a balanced, low-fat diet. Protect yourself with safe-sex practices (syphilis can cause hair loss).

6 WAYS TO MAINTAIN YOUR CROWNING GLORY

- Stay healthy.
- Check out your medications.
- Eat a balanced diet.
- Don't overuse supplements.
- Manage your stress.
- Eliminate or space out hair-stressing styling treatments.

Look to your medications. If you're losing your hair and you take medications, you should suspect a possible correlation. Hundreds of different medications—from exotic ones like chemotherapy to common ones like steroids and aspirin, when used chronically—can cause hair loss. Some people can take a drug and not experience hair loss as a side effect; others will have their hair fall out by the handful. It just depends on your sensitivity. Talk with your doctor to see if your hair loss is associated with medications or herbs. Don't stop taking your medication without talking with your doctor first.

Check out your diet. What you eat—or don't eat—may be the hair-loss culprit if your diet is deficient in iron or protein. Dietary iron and iron metabolism are especially important in a woman's hair cycle. Often women who crash diet or who have eating disorders like bulimia or anorexia nervosa suffer from hair loss.

Go easy on the hair treatments. Too much of a good thing can be bad for your hair. Corn-rowing, tight braiding, bleaching, teasing, straightening, and using hot rollers to make your hair look beautiful can also cause the hair shafts to break. Forget the 100 brush strokes at night, too. The less you do to your scalp and hair, the better.

If you can't give up those styling treatments, at least try to space them out to reduce the trauma.

Don't overdo supplements. Too much of some vitamins or minerals can also cause hair loss. Don't go on a megavitamin regimen. Too much vitamin A or D or selenium can cause hair loss. Also, don't take herbal products that may contain heavy metals. If you experience hair loss and you're taking supplements, discontinue them and see if your hair fall decreases. You may also want to see your doctor to ensure that the supplement has not caused other complications.

Manage your stress. Everyone has heard stories of people experiencing a traumatic event and losing their hair. But even moderate or chronic low-grade stress can cause gradual hair loss or thinning. Try meditation, regular exercise, music appreciation, progressive relaxation, or any other stress management techniques that might work for you.

Sources: **Douglas Altchek, M.D.,** Assistant Clinical Professor of Dermatology, Mt. Sinai School of Medicine, New York, New York. **Marty Sawaya, M.D., Ph.D.,** Assistant Professor of Dermatology and Biochemistry, State University of New York at Brooklyn, Brooklyn, New York. **Alvin Solomon, M.D.,** Associate Professor of Dermatology and Pathology, Emory University School of Medicine, Atlanta, Georgia.

How to Calm a

Throbbing

Ache

"**I** HAVE A HEADACHE." IT SEEMS LIKE the most common, benign complaint in the world. Take an aspirin or another analgesic, and it'll probably be gone within an hour. Fair enough, but what if the throbbing pain makes the hour seem like an eternity? Worse, what if the pill doesn't stop the pain?

A headache is a symptom, not a disease. And it is usually not a symptom of a serious illness. However, the pain can be severe or frequent enough to wear down your patience and seriously affect the quality of your life.

CAUSES AND SYMPTOMS

The following is a breakdown of the causes and symptoms of the three basic types of headaches: vascular, muscle-contraction, and inflammatory headaches.

Vascular headaches. The most common kind of vascular headache is the migraine. One theory about migraine headaches is that they occur when the blood vessels in the head expand and press on the nerves, causing pain. Another theory is that they result when the blood vessels react to outside stimuli by blocking blood flow to parts of the brain; this may cause the visual impairment and numbness that often accompany or precede a migraine headache. The blood vessels then become full of blood and press on surrounding nerves, causing pain.

Women are more prone to migraines than are men, and a certain personality type—compulsive, perfectionist, excessively neat, and very success-oriented—seems to be the most susceptible to this type of headache. Migraines may be trig-

gered by a sudden, sharp reduction in caffeine intake or by allergies to certain foods or food additives. Emotional stress can also cause migraine headaches, as can drinking alcohol, smoking, or an interruption in routine eating and sleeping habits. Cyclical, seasonal, and emotional factors all may play a part. The tendency to have migraines may be inherited.

The main symptoms of a migraine are sharp, pulsating, incapacitating pain on one or both sides of the head, pallor, sweating, nausea, and sensitivity to light. A warning sensation (called an aura) may indicate that a migraine is coming. Before the pain begins, some people may see flashing lights or "shooting stars," hear noises, smell fragrances or odors, or feel a tingling sensation in the arms or legs.

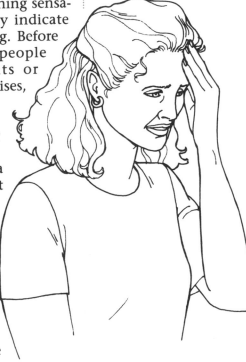

Cluster headaches, a form of migraine most commonly experienced by men, occur in groups of up to six a day, lasting for weeks or months. Their chief symptom is intense pain on one side of the head, accompanied by tearing of the eye and a runny nose on the same side.

Muscle-contraction headaches. These headaches occur when the muscles of the face, neck, or scalp contract and tighten. A tension headache is a good example.

A muscle-contraction headache usually occurs as a result of a clenched jaw, aching neck, or tightened head and face muscles. These headaches can also be brought about by abnormalities in the eyes, neck, teeth, or jaws, or by poor posture, especially by holding the head at an awkward angle—while watching television, for example.

The major symptom of muscle-contraction headaches is a tight squeezing pain in the forehead or jaws or around the back of the head or neck. This constant, dull pain usually occurs on both sides of the head.

Inflammatory headaches. These headaches are the result of pressure within the head. The causes range from relatively minor conditions, such as sinusitis, to more serious problems, such as brain tumors (don't panic; these are rare).

Clogged sinuses and sinus infections are probably the chief cause of this type of headache. The sinuses are the cavities, lined with mucous membranes, within the facial bones. When mucus, which normally flows freely down the sinuses or out the nose, cannot drain properly, it collects in the sinuses and causes excess pressure on the surrounding tissues, leading to a headache.

Another cause of inflammatory headaches is aneurysm (a bulge in a blood vessel) in the head. Aneurysms may not cause pain until they rupture or enlarge rapidly. For this reason, sudden severe pain in the head is a reason to seek medical help as quickly as possible.

Since brain tumors are usually associated with swelling in the surrounding tissues—which causes increased pressure within the skull—they usually cause dull, constant headaches and a sensation of pressing. High blood pressure, which causes blood to rush through the vessels with too great a force; infections, which inflame sensitive tissue; and fever, which may enlarge the blood vessels, including those in the head, can also cause inflammatory headaches.

The symptoms of an inflammatory headache are a dull, aching pain, often occurring early in the day, and a feeling of pressure in the head. The pain is heightened by sneezing, coughing, bending over, or doing anything that increases the amount of blood in the head.

If you suffer from frequent, severe headaches that put you out of commission several times a month, you need to seek medical attention. Likewise, if your headaches are associated with physical exertion, changes in vision, or weakness, numbness, or paralysis of the limbs, call your doctor. A headache specialist or a headache clinic may be a good idea if you're already seeing a physician and aren't getting any relief.

AT-HOME TREATMENT

The following tips can help relieve the pain of a headache in progress. In most cases, they can be used in conjunction with your doctor's treatment. They are also very effective for your run-of-the-mill tension headache. So if a headache's got you down, try these suggestions.

Use drugs prudently. Over-the-counter analgesics may give you a few hours of relief from a headache, but using them too frequently can actually worsen the pain. As a rule, if your headaches cause you to take more than two doses a day, you should see a doctor.

Take a load off. One of the most effective ways to treat a bad headache may be to just lie down and close your eyes for half an hour or more. For migraines, it seems that sleep is the only way to find relief from the pain. If you suffer from severe headaches, you should know that the sooner you get to bed, the sooner you will feel better.

Out go the lights. When you sit or lie down to rest, make sure the room is darkened. Light can exacerbate your headaches, especially if your symptoms resemble those of a migraine. Bright light or light from a computer screen can also cause headaches. Tinted glasses may head off a headache in the works.

Cool it. Dip a washcloth in ice-cold water and place it over your eyes or place an ice pack on the site of the headache. Both are good ways of relieving the ache. Along these lines, there are some products available that make it easier to put your headache on ice. The "headache hat," is an ice pack that surrounds the head, and the ice pillow is a frozen gel pack that is inserted into a special pillow. If you can't find these products at your local drugstore, ask your pharmacist about ordering them. For most people, ice will bring relief within 20 minutes, if it is applied early.

Heat it up. Some people cannot tolerate the discomfort of ice, or it just doesn't help ease their headache. If you're one of these people, try using warmth instead. A warm washcloth over your eyes or on the site of the pain for half an hour can be very soothing. Rewarm the cloth as necessary.

Police your stress level. Every now and then, stop what you are doing and check your tension level. Notice whether your jaws are set tightly, your forehead is scrunched, or your fists are clenched. When you stop at a red light, check to see if your hands have the wheel in a death grip. If you find that you are clenching your muscles, stop, relax, and take a deep breath.

You can also try doing a relaxation exercise, such as the following, which can be memorized or recorded on a cassette tape. The exercise relaxes the facial area, neck, shoulders, and upper back, and takes about five minutes. Before you begin, make sure you won't be disturbed—close the door and take the phone off the hook.

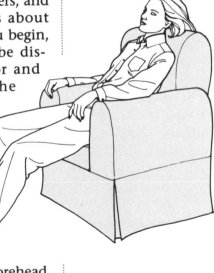

1) Settle back quietly and comfortably into a favorite chair or sofa. Allow your muscles to become loose and heavy.

2) Wrinkle up your forehead, hold it, then smooth it out. Picture your entire forehead becoming smoother as the relaxation increases.

3) Frown, creasing your eyebrows tightly, feeling the ten-

sion. Let go of the tension, smoothing out your forehead once more.

4) Close your eyes more and more tightly. Feel the tension as you hold them shut. Relax your eyes until they are closed gently and comfortably.

5) Clench your jaws and teeth together. Feel the tension build, then let go and relax, letting your lips part slightly. Allow yourself to feel relief in the relaxation.

6) Press your tongue hard against the roof of your mouth. Again, feel the tension, then relax.

---

9 WAYS TO RELIEVE THE PAIN

- Don't overdo the over-the-counter analgesics.
- Lie down and close your eyes for half an hour or more.
- Turn off the bright lights.
- Use a cool compress or an ice pack.
- Try a warm compress.
- Periodically check your stress level. Use relaxation exercises to help you keep tension in check.
- Avoid cigarettes, alcohol, and caffeine.
- Start a program of regular aerobic exercise.
- Wait until your nausea is relieved before taking pain medications.

---

7) Purse your lips together more and more tightly, then relax. Notice the contrast between tension and relaxation. Feel the relaxation all over your face, forehead and scalp, eyes, jaws, lips, and tongue.

8) Press your head back against your chair, concentrating on the tension in your neck. Roll your head to the right and feel the tension shift.

Repeat to the left. Straighten your head and bring it forward, pressing chin to chest. Finally, allow your head to return to a comfortable position.

9) Shrug your shoulders up to your ears, holding the tension, then drop. Repeat the shrug, then move the shoulders forward and backward, feeling the tension in your shoulders and upper back. Drop your shoulders and relax.

10) Allow the relaxation to spread deep into your shoulders and back. Relax your neck and throat. Relax your jaws and face. Allow the relaxation to take over and grow deeper and deeper. When you are ready, slowly open your eyes.

Just say "no" to cigarettes, booze, and coffee. Tension may make some people reach for a cigarette, but smoking won't help. In fact, smoking may bring on or worsen a headache, especially if you suffer from cluster headaches. Alcohol can also bring on migraines and cluster headaches, not to mention the morning-after doozy. Alcoholic beverages contain tyramine, an amino acid that may actually stimulate headaches.

The stimulant effects of caffeine can create all kinds of headache problems. They can raise your anxiety level, make your muscles tense up, and give you trouble sleeping—all of which can cause headaches. Another problem is caffeine-withdrawal headaches. If you drink several cups of coffee a day during the work week, but cut your consumption on weekends, you may get headaches on the weekends from the lack of caffeine. If this sounds like your problem, try slowly decreasing your caffeine intake by one-half cup per week until you are drinking the equivalent of one cup of coffee per day. A five-ounce cup of drip coffee contains about 150 milligrams of caffeine. A five-ounce cup of tea brewed for three to five minutes may contain 20 to 50 milligrams of caffeine. And cola drinks contain about 35 to 45 milligrams of caffeine per 12-ounce serving. Also, check the caffeine content of any over-the-counter drugs in your medicine cabinet.

Get moving. Regular aerobic exercise can help you in two ways. The release of energy helps you work out physical and emotional tension, and the activity stimulates your body's production of endorphins (natural pain-relieving substances).

Take care of your tummy first. If there's one thing worse than a bad headache, it's a bad headache accompanied by nausea. Stomach upset may also produce gastric juices that hinder the absorption of certain over-the-counter and prescription analgesics, making these drugs less effective at relieving your headache pain. The headache will be much easier to treat after the nausea is taken care of. You may find some relief by drinking peach juice, apricot nectar, or flat cola. Over-the-counter anti-

nauseants such as Emetrol and Dramamine may also be useful.

AT THE DOCTOR'S

If you do decide to visit a doctor for your headaches, here's what to expect:

Vascular headaches. These are diagnosed by a careful review of the circumstances surrounding the headaches, as well as by a physical examination to rule out any other disorder that might be causing them. Elimination tests may be done to identify the exact cause of migraines suffered by people who seem to react to certain foods or changes in eating and sleeping habits. In an elimination test, all the substances that are suspected of causing the trouble are eliminated and then reintroduced one at a time.

A doctor's treatment for a migraine already in progress usually consists of a drug therapy program chosen from a variety of painkillers, sedatives, and special migraine drugs. For the occasional migraine sufferer, tranquilizers and sedatives may relieve some of the symptoms.

One commonly prescribed drug, called ergotamine, constricts the blood vessels and thus prevents the swelling that causes pressure on the surrounding nerves. This drug is usually taken to stop an approaching migraine. Antidepressant drugs, taken in small doses, may prevent migraines in a patient who experiences them regularly. Recently, physicians have begun to use drugs called beta-blockers to prevent migraines. These drugs work in the body to block what are called the beta effects, one of which is the dilation, or enlargement, of the blood vessels. Other drugs called calcium-channel blockers are also effective in preventing migraine headaches, probably because they prevent the initial dilation of blood vessels.

Muscle-contraction headaches. A doctor can diagnose muscle-contraction headaches, but can do very little to treat them, aside from treating any underlying physical problems or prescribing painkillers, muscle relaxants, or tranquilizers. Tension headaches are good candidates for at-home treatment (see above).

Inflammatory headaches. With inflammatory headaches, a physician will try to determine whether sinuses are causing the problem. If not, the doctor may order an electroencephalogram (EEG), which is a visual record of electrical activity in the brain; X-ray studies; a computed tomographic (CT) scan, which provides a cross-sectional picture of the brain; or a magnetic resonance (MR) imaging study, which yields images comparable to those obtained with CT, but without the use of X rays. These tests may reveal the presence of a tumor, an aneurysm, or another abnormality.

Inflammatory headaches are treated according to their cause. Those triggered by a sinus infection can be treated with painkillers, antibiotics, or antihistamines and decongestants, which dry out and help drain the sinuses. Treatment of inflammatory headaches resulting from more serious disorders may include surgery.

PREVENTION

The following tips may help prevent headaches before they occur:

Keep regular hours. Try to make your sleeping schedule consistent. Go to bed and get up at

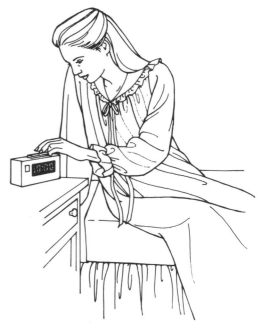

the same time every day. Oversleeping causes changes in body chemistry that can precipitate headache pain.

Eat to beat your headaches. At Diamond Headache Clinic in Chicago, patients are advised to eat a diet low in tyramine, an amino acid that is known to promote headaches, nausea, and high blood pressure in certain individuals. The following diet keeps tyramine levels to a minimum.

Beverages

Foods allowed: Decaffeinated coffee, fruit juices, club soda, non-cola sodas. Caffeine sources to be limited to two cups per day.

Foods to avoid: Caffeine (does not contain tyramine, but aggravates headache symptoms), coffee, tea, colas in excess of two cups per day. Hot cocoa, all alcoholic beverages.

Meat, Fish, Poultry

Foods allowed: Fresh or frozen turkey, chicken, fish,

beef, lamb, veal, pork, eggs (limit three per week), tuna fish.

Foods to avoid: Aged, canned, cured, or processed meats; canned or aged ham; pickled herring; salted, dried fish; chicken liver; aged game; hot dogs; fermented sausages (no nitrates or nitrites allowed) including bologna, salami, pepperoni, summer sausage; any meat prepared with meat tenderizer, soy sauce, or yeast extracts (it's not the yeast itself that's a problem, but yeast contains an enzyme that alters an amino acid to become tyramine).

Dairy

Foods allowed: Milk: homogenized, low-fat, or skim. Cheese: American, cottage, farmer, ricotta, cream cheese. Yogurt: limit to one-half cup per day.

Foods to avoid: Cultured dairy, such as buttermilk, sour cream, chocolate milk. Cheese: blue, Boursault, brick, Brie types, camembert types, cheddar, Swiss, gouda, Roquefort, Stilton, mozzarella, parmesan, provolone, Romano, Emmentaler.

Breads and Cereals

Foods allowed: Commercial breads: white, whole wheat, rye, French, Italian, English muffins, melba toast, crackers, bagels. All hot and dry cereals: cream of wheat, oatmeal, cornflakes, puffed wheat, rice, bran, etc.

Foods to avoid: Hot, fresh, homemade yeast breads; breads and crackers containing cheese; fresh yeast coffee cake, doughnuts, sourdough breads; any breads or cereals containing chocolate or nuts.

Starches

Foods allowed: Potatoes, sweet potatoes, rice, macaroni, spaghetti, noodles.

Vegetables, Legumes, and Seeds

Foods allowed: Asparagus, string beans, beets, carrots, spinach, pumpkin, tomatoes, squash, corn, zucchini, broccoli, green lettuce. All except those listed in the next paragraph.

Foods to avoid: Pole, broad, lima, or Italian beans; lentils; snow peas; fava, navy, or pinto beans; pea pods; sauerkraut; garbanzo beans; onions (except as a condiment); olives; pickles; peanuts; sunflower, sesame, or pumpkin seeds.

Fruit

Foods allowed: Apricots, prunes, apples, cherries, peaches, pears. Citrus fruits and juices: Limit to half cup per day of orange, grapefruit, tangerine, pineapple, lemon, or lime.

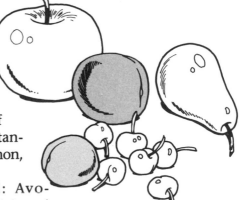

Foods to avoid: Avocados, bananas, raisins, (one-half cup allowed per day), figs, papaya, passion fruit, red plums.

Soups

Foods allowed: Cream soups made from list of allowed foods on these pages, homemade broths.

Foods to avoid: Canned soups, bouillon cubes, soup bases containing autolyzed

yeast or monosodium glutamate (MSG)—read labels.

Desserts

Foods allowed: Fruits listed
above, sherbets, ice cream,
cakes and cookies made without chocolate or yeast, gelatin.

Foods to avoid: Chocolate-
flavored ice cream, pudding,
cookies, or cakes; mincemeat
pies.

Sweets

Foods allowed: Sugar, jelly,
jam, honey, hard candy.

Foods to avoid: Chocolate
candies, chocolate syrup, carob.

4 Steps to a Headache-Free Life

- Rise and retire at the same time every day.
- Eat a diet free of tyramine, a chemical that may cause headaches.
- Keep a headache journal.
- Get information and support from a headache association.

Miscellaneous

Foods allowed: Salt (in moderation), lemon juices, butter
or margarine, cooking oils,
whipped cream, white vinegar
and commercial salad dressing
in small amounts.

Foods to avoid: Pizza, cheese
sauce, soy sauce, monosodium
glutamate (MSG) in excessive
amounts, yeast, yeast extracts,
brewer's yeast, meat tenderiz-
ers, seasoning salt, macaroni
and cheese, beef stroganoff,
cheese blintzes, lasagna, frozen
dinners, any pickled, preserved,
or marinated foods.

Be a headache detective. If you
get frequent headaches, keep a
headache diary. This will help
you figure out what factors
seem to cause your headaches.
Record each headache and rate
it on a zero-to-three scale of
intensity: no headache, mild
headache, moderate-to-severe
headache, incapacitating headache. Be conscious of what
foods you eat and track your
period, as well as any hormone-
replacement medications or
oral contraceptives you may be
taking. Try to pick out patterns.

Get support. The following associations provide support and
information for headache sufferers:

The American Council for
Headache Education (ACHE).
ACHE provides patient information and referrals to
headache specialists. The organization also sends out free
informational pamphlets about
headache treatment. In the
future, ACHE plans to set up
patient-support groups around
the country. You can contact
ACHE at 1-800-255-ACHE.

The National Headache
Foundation. This organization
sends out free headache information to patients and publish-
es a headache newsletter. You
can contact the Foundation at
1-800-843-2256.

Sources: **Sabiha Ali, M.D.**, Neurologist,
Houston Headache Clinic, Houston, Texas.
James R. Couch, Jr., M.D., Ph.D., Professor and
Chairman, Department of Neurology,
University of Oklahoma Health Sciences Center,
Oklahoma City, Oklahoma. **Seymour
Diamond, M.D.**, Founder, Diamond Headache
Clinic, Chicago, Illinois. **Fred D. Sheftell, M.D.**,
Director and Founder, The New England Center
for Headache, Stamford, Connecticut.

Strategies to

Banish the

Burn

You've just eaten a big, delicious meal. But now you feel uncomfortable. You begin to belch and your chest and throat start burning like fire. Is this the end? Are you having a heart attack? Not likely. You're experiencing heartburn, one of Americans' most common and most misunderstood ailments.

Heartburn has nothing to do with the heart. It often has to do with overindulging at the table and eating more than your stomach can comfortably hold. When you eat too much or too quickly, some of the acidic stomach contents can slip back up and burn the tender esophagus, the tube that carries food and drink from your mouth to your stomach.

Symptoms

If you suffer from this acid reflux, you're not alone. An estimated 10 to 20 percent of all Americans—or 25 to 50 million people—suffer regularly from the burning, belching, and regurgitation of bitter stomach acids known as heartburn. The discomfort occurs between the stomach and the neck. Most people feel it right below the breastbone. Some have pain so severe they're convinced they're having a heart attack.

Causes

When you eat, food travels down the esophagus. A valve at the lower end of the esophagus, called the lower esophageal sphincter (LES) opens, allowing food to enter the stomach. Normally, the LES then closes to keep food and industrial-strength stomach acids from splashing ("refluxing") back into the esophagus and throat.

Sometimes, however, the muscles around the LES lose their tone, and the valve can't close completely. Then strong digestive stomach acids can slip back up the esophagus and into the throat, causing the severe burning we call heartburn.

People often experience heartburn right after eating because that's when stomach acids reflux up the esophagus. When the stomach is full (or overly full), the pressure inside the stomach builds. The weakened LES can't close against the pressure, and the burning acids are pushed into the esophagus and throat.

Pregnant women often complain of heartburn. That's because the presence of the growing fetus competes with the stomach for space and interferes with digestion. The changing hormones also tend to relax the LES.

At-Home Treatment

If you overindulge and end up with a case of heartburn, here are some tips to ease the burn.

Try an OTC antacid. Over-the-counter antacids (tablets, granules, or liquid) can help ease the burning sensation. Alka-Seltzer and Bromo-Seltzer work well, but because of their sodium content shouldn't be used by people who have high blood pressure, heart disease, diabetes, glaucoma, or a history of stroke. Maalox, Mylanta, and Di-gel are all effective in neutralizing acid, but be sure to follow package instructions, as these products can cause diarrhea. Tums or Rolaids tablets work too, but because they contain large amounts of calci-

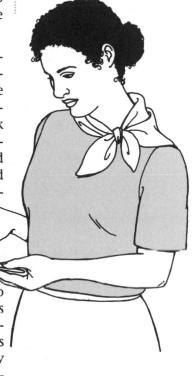

um, they shouldn't be used if you suffer from kidney disease. Women who are pregnant or breastfeeding should consult a physician before taking any antacid product.

Take antacid before bed. When you lie down, acid reflux increases, and the esophagus can be bathed in acids. Leave a bottle of antacid by your bed and take a dose before you go to sleep to ease the burn.

Prop up. Elevate the head of your bed about six inches with bricks or wooden blocks so that you're sleeping on a gentle slope. This uses the force of gravity to help keep stomach acids where they belong.

13 WAYS TO TREAT THE BURN

- Try over-the-counter antacids.
- Take antacids before bed.
- Elevate the head of your bed.
- Give up the waterbed.
- Try drinking milk.
- Don't eat before retiring.
- Avoid overeating.
- Exercise regularly.
- Cut down on fats and fried foods.
- Avoid spicy foods.
- Eliminate coffee from your diet.
- Cut out red and black pepper.
- Ease off the alcohol.

Give up the float. Sure, waterbeds feel cozy and comfortable, but they can wreak havoc on heartburn sufferers. Unfortunately, you can't properly elevate your head and chest while lying on a water-filled mattress. Opt for the more standard bed.

Pass the milk. Some people find that a glass of milk soothes the burn.

Give up the P.M. snacks. When nighttime heartburn attacks are a problem, don't eat within a few (two to three) hours of retiring. If you do eat at night, stay upright until all the stomach contents are digested.

Skip seconds. The stomach is like a balloon—the more food you stuff into it, the more pressure develops and the greater the risk you'll reflux stomach contents into the esophagus.

Exercise regularly. People who exercise regularly suffer less heartburn than couch potatoes. For one thing, exercise helps moderate weight. It also makes your digestion more efficient. Caution: Don't work out strenuously right after eating. Wait a few hours.

Phooey on fat and fried. Take an honest look at your diet. Does it contain too much fat and fried foods? A high-carbohydrate, low-fat diet is the best for heartburn.

Check the spices at the door. Sometimes hot, spicy foods like chilies and curries contribute to heartburn.

Pass on coffee. Caffeine may not be the component of coffee that causes your heartburn. You may discover that even decaffeinated coffee gives your esophagus fits. That's because the oils in coffee can affect the LES. Pass on the coffee and see if your heartburn improves.

Ease off pepper. For some people with heartburn, sprinkling or grinding red or black pepper onto their food isn't such a hot idea.

Cut down on booze. Alcohol relaxes the esophageal sphincter and irritates your tender stomach.

Don't sip soda. Carbonated beverages like soda pop create gas and cause the stomach to distend. That, in turn, can cause the acids to roll back up into the esophagus.

Be wary of the bends. Squatting, bending, or heavy lifting, especially if you've just eaten, can bring on heartburn.

Opt for gum/hard candies. Acid from the stomach can make your esophagus and throat sore and irritated. Try chewing gum or sucking on hard candies, both of which stimulate saliva and can soothe irritated tissues.

Check your drugs. A number of drugs such as aspirin, sedatives, tetracycline, asthma medications, calcium-channel blockers, vitamin C, and others, can contribute to heartburn. If you're taking aspirin, try a less-irritating painkiller like acetaminophen. Talk with your pharmacist or physician about other drug substitutions.

Watch for warning signals. Some heartburn symptoms are actually warnings of other, more serious health problems such as hernia, ulcers, or even (rarely) cancer. Chronic heartburn can actually burn holes in the esophagus (esophageal ulcers).

If symptoms persist for more than two weeks and aren't responsive to home remedies, call your physician.

If you're pregnant and suffer from persistent heartburn that isn't responsive to the remedies mentioned here, call your doctor. Do not take any medication without talking with your doctor first.

Some heart attacks may feel like heartburn. Call for emergency medical help immediately if you experience:
• pain that radiates to the jaw or out to an arm or shoulder
• sweating
• nausea
• shortness of breath
• dizziness
• feelings of "impending doom."

PREVENTION
You can usually prevent heartburn before it starts.

Everything in moderation. Avoid eating too much. Eat smaller portions. Instead of one big meal, try several smaller meals. By not filling your stomach so full, you can avoid the pressure that disables the esophageal valve.

Slow down. It takes about 20 minutes after you begin eating for your brain to catch up with your stomach and register "full." By eating more slowly, you'll give yourself time to feel full before you overeat.

Chew it up. Chew your food thoroughly. It will contribute to good digestion.

12 Strategies to Prevent the Burn

- Avoid eating too much.
- Eat more slowly.
- Chew your food thoroughly.
- Don't smoke.
- Cut caffeine from your diet.
- Wear loose clothing.
- Be careful not to swallow air while you eat.
- Maintain a healthful weight.
- Manage your stress.
- Avoid mint.
- Don't drink liquids with meals.
- Keep a food/heartburn diary.

Quit smoking. Smoking cigarettes irritates the LES, the esophagus, and the stomach lining and can contribute to heartburn.

Nix caffeine. Foods and beverages containing caffeine like tea, coffee, and chocolate all interfere with the proper functioning of the LES. Cut out or cut way back on these food items.

Loosen up. Anything that constricts the stomach increases pressure and may contribute to heartburn. Give up those tight pants and belts.

Watch your air. Swallowing air while you eat is a habit that can contribute to heartburn. Talking while eating and drinking carbonated beverages both contribute to swallowing air.

Don't eat and sleep. Lying down immediately after eating encourages reflux.

Drop the excess weight. People who are overweight often suffer from heartburn. That's because all the extra pounds stress the LES. If you're overweight, lose excess baggage by eating a low-fat diet and getting regular exercise.

Relax. Emotional stress increases stomach acid, interferes with digestion, and can contribute to heartburn. Learn to manage your stress with meditation, biofeedback, progressive relaxation, or other techniques.

Say no to mint. Often when you have a stomach upset, mint tea or an after-dinner mint is an effective home remedy. But not with acid reflux. Mint helps to relax the LES, which increases heartburn.

Drink between—not with—meals. Drinking liquids with meals dilutes the stomach contents, making them more liable to reflux.

Keep track. Eating some foods may precipitate heartburn. To discover what makes your heartburn worse or better, keep a food/heartburn diary to see if you can correlate specific foods with the onset of heartburn.

Sources: **Nalin M. Patel, M.D.,** Author, *The Doctor's Guide to Your Digestive System*; Clinical Instructor, University of Illinois at Urbana-Champaign, Champaign, Illinois. **Anne Simons, M.D.,** Coauthor, *Before You Call the Doctor*; Family Practitioner, San Francisco Department of Public Health; Family Practitioner and Assistant Clinical Professor, Family and Community Medicine, University of California San Francisco Medical Center, San Francisco, California. **David M. Taylor, M.D.,** Author, *Gut Reactions: How to Handle Stress and Your Stomach*; Assistant Professor of Medicine, Emory University, Atlanta, Georgia; Assistant Professor of Medicine, Medical College of Georgia, Augusta, Georgia. **Douglas C. Walta, M.D.,** Gastroenterologist, Portland, Oregon.

IT'S A PROBLEM SO PERSONAL, WE'D rather not discuss it even with a doctor, unless we're forced to do so. The anal pain, burning, itching, and bleeding of rectal hemorrhoids may not be the stuff of party conversations, but it's so common that up to three out of four of us have them and every year we spend $150 million trying to ease our misery.

Hemorrhoids (also called "piles") are essentially varicose veins of the anus. Three veins line the anal canal and lower rectum and drain blood away from the anal area. When these veins become swollen and stretched out, they're called hemorrhoids.

These enlarged veins may be found inside or just outside the anal canal. When they protrude out through the anal opening, they occur under the surface of the skin and they are called "prolapsed." Regardless of whether hemorrhoids are inside or outside the anal canal, they can hurt, burn, itch, and irritate the anal area, and sometimes bleed.

CAUSES

Lots of things contribute to the development of hemorrhoids—gravity, for one. Because human beings stand upright, the pull of gravity exerts its downward force on all the body's veins.

Hemorrhoids appear to run in families. If one parent had hemorrhoids, it's likely you'll develop them; if both your parents had them, it's almost certain you will, too. It may be that some people inherit more fragile veins than others. Or it may simply be that family members tend to have similar dietary and personal habits. However, the prevention strategies offered here can help you beat the genetic odds.

Your dietary and bowel habits are big factors in determining whether or not you'll develop hemorrhoids. People who eat foods with little fiber ("roughage"), tend to become constipated. During a bowel movement, the veins expand or dilate and then return to normal size afterward. However, straining during bowel movements because of constipation or hard stools can interfere with the veins' normal functioning. The once-efficient veins may drain poorly and remain permanently swollen. These swollen veins pressure nerves in the area and produce itching, burning, and pain. Defecation, especially hard stools, can rupture the delicate, swollen vessels and cause bleeding.

If you're overweight, you're more likely to suffer from hemorrhoids. The extra pounds put added pressure on the anal veins. Also, people who are overweight often eat low-fiber foods and are sedentary, both factors in constipation.

Some people use laxatives for constipation. Unfortunately, laxatives are likely to compound hemorrhoid problems. Improper use of laxatives is a major cause of hemorrhoids.

How often you defecate can have an impact on hemorrhoids, too. People who "hold it" rather than going when they feel the urge tend to increase the pressure in the bowel area, leading to undesirable straining during elimination.

Women often complain of developing painful hemorrhoids during pregnancy. As the uterus grows larger with the developing fetus, it puts pressure on the veins of the lower abdomen. In addition, prolonged pressure from pushing during labor and delivery can cause hemorrhoids. Fortunately, pregnancy-related hemorrhoids usually retract after the baby is born (unless hemorrhoids were present prior to pregnancy).

Sexual practices may contribute to the development of hemorrhoids. Anal sex puts undue pressure on the veins in the anal area.

Women who work at jobs where they must sit or stand for long periods of time often develop hemorrhoids. In prolonged sitting, the heart muscle has to work harder to return the blood to the heart. In standing for long periods, the pull of gravity is allowed to continuously drag on the anal veins.

Sometimes hemorrhoids are a symptom of a more serious health problem. For example, hemorrhoids may be due to pressure on the veins caused by diseases of the liver or heart, or by a tumor.

AT-HOME TREATMENT

If you develop hemorrhoids, there's plenty you can do to ease your discomfort and prevent more hemorrhoids from developing. Try the following tips:

Stay soft. A diet high in fiber will help to keep your stools soft and bulky and avoid excess strain on your painful hemorrhoids. Most nutrition experts recommend adding fiber to your diet gradually, particularly if you've been used to eating processed foods. Adding too much fiber to your diet too quickly can cause gas, cramping, and diarrhea. Even the gradual addition of fiber may cause you to have more gas. Don't worry. This side effect should subside within a couple of weeks as the bacteria in your gut becomes accustomed to your new diet.

To increase the fiber in your diet, eat more fresh fruits and vegetables (see the list below), and make your recipes more fiber-rich by adding bran, chick peas, cooked brown rice, and other whole grains to casseroles, meatloafs, soups, salads, and other dishes.

These foods are particularly rich in fiber:

Vegetables
Carrots
Brussels sprouts
Eggplant
Cabbage
Corn
Green beans
Lettuce (dark, leafy varieties)

Grains
Whole wheat
Whole rye
Brown rice
Milled corn
Unprocessed oatmeal
Rolled oats
Unprocessed bran

Fruits
Apples
Oranges
Pears
Figs
Prunes
Apricots
Raisins

Legumes
Lima beans
Soy beans
Kidney beans
Lentils
Chickpeas

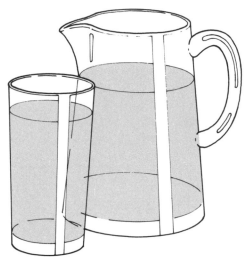

Drink more water. People who are constipated often don't drink enough fluids. It's especially important to drink plenty of water when you're eating more fiber. Water helps keep the digestive process moving along and helps soften your stools. Drink at least eight eight-ounce glasses of water every day.

Try a stool softener. For most people, adding fiber and water to their diets adequately softens stools so that elimination is less painful to their hemorrhoids. However, if hard stools are still a problem for you, ask your physician to recommend a stool softener-type laxative such as Colace or Correctol or one that contains bulking agents such as Metamucil or Effer-Syllium. Keep in mind that laxatives are a short-term rather than a long-term solution to constipation. Adding fiber to your diet, drinking plenty of water, and regular exercise are more effective, long-term solutions.

Do not use laxatives that act on the muscles of the rectum. Prolonged use of these types of laxatives can irritate the anal area and cause permanent rectum malfunction.

Go for a walk. Regular exercise, especially brisk walking, will help keep your digestive and elimination processes working in tip-top shape.

Clean up. When you have hemorrhoids, it's vitally important to keep the rectal area clean. Feces can irritate the delicate tissues around the anal opening. Rinse the area gently with warm water while sitting on the toilet. Then pat (don't rub) the area dry and dust with a non-perfumed, nontalc powder.

Go for the witch hazel. Some people like to use over-the-counter, pre-moistened wipes (Tucks) that contain 50 percent witch hazel and are designed for use in the anal area. They can be used to clean the anus after elimination or just to cool and soothe inflamed tissues. How-

15 WAYS TO END THE TORMENT
- Eat more fiber.
- Drink plenty of water.
- Try stool-softening laxatives.
- Move around more.
- Keep the anal area clean.
- Try witch hazel astringent.
- Rinse the anal area well.
- Use soft, unscented toilet paper.
- Avoid scratching.
- If you're pregnant, take breaks and lie down often.
- Sit on a "doughnut" cushion.
- Take a sitz bath.
- Soothe the area with a warm washcloth.
- Use an ice pack.
- Check with your doctor for proper diagnosis.

ever, some people find witch hazel irritating. You might want to try these wipes and see if they work for you.

Rinse well. Soap can irritate delicate anal tissues. Always rinse your anal area completely after showering or bathing.

Change your toilet paper. It's important not to irritate anal tissues. Look for toilet paper that is soft and unscented.

Don't scratch it. Vigorously rubbing with dry toilet paper or a towel can irritate the skin and can cause it to bleed.

Lie down. Pregnant women who suffer from hemorrhoids should avoid prolonged sitting or standing. Whenever possible, take a break and lie down.

Try a doughnut. If you have to sit a great deal, you can get some relief by sitting on a doughnut-shaped cushion made especially for hemorrhoid sufferers. They're inexpensive, inflatable rings of vinyl that are generally available over the counter in pharmacies or from mail-order health supply catalogs.

Have a sitz. Sitting for 20 to 30 minutes or so, three or four times a day, in a sitz bath (four to six inches of warm water) can help. Sit on a towel or on a doughnut cushion. The warm water will soothe inflamed tissues and relax muscle spasms.

Try a warm washcloth. When you can't take a sitz bath, use a warm washcloth. Moisten the cloth with warm water and apply to irritated tissues.

Ice it. You can soothe swollen and inflamed hemorrhoids with an ice pack. Wrap a couple of ice cubes in a plastic bag and put it in a clean cloth. Apply the ice pack for 20 minutes to hemorrhoids; then remove it for 10 minutes before reapplying. Don't place ice directly on the skin, as this can cause frostbite.

Have your hemorrhoids diagnosed. Simple hemorrhoids are usually responsive to the home remedies discussed in this chapter. However, sometimes hemorrhoid-type symptoms may be masking another, more serious problem. For example, anal itching may be caused by poor anal hygiene. Or the problem could be perianal warts, intestinal worms, allergies to medications, psoriasis or other forms of dermatitis, or a local infection. Pain in the anal area may be caused by fissures, small cracks in the skin around the anus.

Anal bleeding may not be due to hemorrhoids. It can be a symptom of colorectal cancer, a serious disease that claims 60,000 lives annually. Any rectal bleeding should be examined by a doctor.

Don't self-diagnose your hemorrhoids. Check with your physician first to rule out more serious health problems.

PREVENTION

These tips will help decrease your risk of getting hemorrhoids.

Stay regular. Constipation is one of the major causes of hemorrhoids. The best ways to prevent constipation and hard stools are the natural ones.

Eat a diet rich in fiber (whole grains, legumes, fresh fruits and vegetables). Fiber is able to pass through the digestive tract without being broken down by digestive enzymes. As it moves along, it absorbs large volumes of water. By the time the fiber reaches the colon and combines with digestive wastes, it produces bulky, heavy, soft stools that are easy to eliminate.

Drink plenty of fluids (nonalcoholic). Try to drink at least eight eight-ounce glasses of water every day. Fresh fruit can contribute fluids, too.

Exercise regularly. A program of regular exercise, such as brisk walking, helps the digestive tract work more efficiently.

Stay lean. Excess weight contributes to hemorrhoids. If you're overweight, shed the excess pounds by eating a low-fat, high-carbohydrate diet with plenty of fiber and participate in some form of moderate exercise.

Move around. If your job requires you to sit or stand for prolonged periods of time, try to schedule frequent breaks. Instead of sitting while on your break, take a brisk walk.

---

7 STRATEGIES FOR DODGING HEMORRHOIDS

- Stay regular.
- Exercise regularly.
- Stay lean.
- Take frequent breaks from prolonged sitting or standing.
- Don't strain.
- Avoid overly long toilet sessions.
- Squat, don't sit, on the toilet.

Go with the urge. When you feel like you need to go to the bathroom, go. Don't hold it.

Don't bear down. When you sit on the toilet, relax. Don't bear down or strain. Take the time you need.

Don't dally. Don't sit around on the toilet any longer than necessary. Even when you don't strain, toilet sitting places undue strain on the veins.

Squat rather than sit. It's more natural to squat rather than sit to move your bowels, but our toilets aren't designed for squatting. Try putting your feet on a small step stool to raise your knees closer to your chest.

Sources: Gayle Randall, M.D., Assistant Professor of Medicine, Department of Medicine, University of California, Los Angeles, School of Medicine, Los Angeles, California. Norton Rosensweig, M.D., Associate Clinical Professor of Medicine, Columbia University College of Physicians and Surgeons, New York, New York. Anne Simons, M.D., Coauthor, *Before You Call the Doctor*; Family Practitioner, San Francisco Department of Public Health; Family Practitioner and Assistant Clinical Professor, Family and Community Medicine, University of California San Francisco Medical Center, San Francisco, California. Thomas J. Stahl, M.D., Assistant Professor of General Surgery, Georgetown University Medical Center, Washington, D.C.

•HICCUPS

Put an End to

the Jerk

YOU'RE HAVING LUNCH WITH YOUR boss, and everything has gone perfectly. You've been at your best, and the boss has reacted well to all your carefully thought-out suggestions. Now you've reached dessert and you're wondering if you'll get that promotion you've been angling for. Suddenly, HICCUP! So much for the great impression you've been making.

A hiccup is a jerky or spasmodic inhalation of air. Most medical experts say that hiccups occur when the vagus nerve or one of its branches becomes irritated and stimulates the phrenic nerve. The phrenic nerve then sends a signal to the diaphragm, the abdominal muscle that controls breathing, to contract. At the same time, the flap of tissue called the glottis that acts as a gateway to the lungs closes suddenly, stopping the air from being drawn into the lungs, and causing the hiccup sound.

CAUSES

Why do we hiccup? No one really knows. Experts say hiccups are a common reaction to digestive disturbances. However, hiccups can occur for no apparent reason.

Doctors know that almost everyone, even infants, experiences bouts of hiccups an average of three to five times a year. Hiccups are rhythmic and come about every 30 seconds. Doctors also say hiccups are more of a nuisance than anything else and that they go away by themselves after a brief period, usually one or two minutes to an hour. However, for a few unlucky folks, hiccups can become chronic and last months or even years. If your hiccups last more than 12 hours, see a doctor.

AT-HOME TREATMENT

Most hiccup home remedies work on one of two principles: overstimulating the vagus nerve or increasing the amount of carbon dioxide in the blood. The first method fools the vagus nerve with a number of sensations like taste and temperature, causing it to send messages to the brain that tell it to respond to these new sensations. The brain turns its attention to the sensations and turns off the hiccup response. The second type of remedy brings more carbon dioxide into the blood, which makes the brain more concerned about eliminating the carbon dioxide than continuing to hiccup.

Stick your fingers in your ears. Putting your fingers in your ears creates pressure and stimulates the vagus nerve branches. Of course, doctors warn you not to put anything smaller than your elbow into your ear canals. So don't stick your fingers in too far.

Get spooked. Having someone surprise you can overwhelm the vagus nerve.

Tempt them with sugar. Try placing a teaspoonful of sugar on the back of your tongue, where "sour" is usually tasted. The nerve endings in the mouth become overwhelmed and the hiccups disappear.

Drink up. Swallowing water can help quiet nerves and stop the hiccup reflex. Some people have success gargling with water.

SUGAR

Pull it. Stick out your tongue and gently pull on it with your thumb and forefinger. This can stimulate the gag reflex, which stops the hiccups.

Give 'em the tickle. If you're ticklish, try having someone tickle you. Or tickle the soft palate of the roof of your mouth with a cotton swab.

Suck in and hold. Holding your breath with your mouth and nose closed can help increase the carbon dioxide in your blood and stop hiccups.

Bag it. You can also increase the carbon dioxide by breathing into a paper bag.

Cut the acid. Decrease digestive irritation and quiet the nerves with one or two antacid tablets, particularly brands that contain magnesium. Pregnant and breast-feeding women should talk with a physician before taking any medications, even over-the-counter ones.

Suck lemons. Overwhelm the vagus nerve with a sour sensation by sucking on a lemon wedge.

Ice it. Cold sensations can fool the vagus nerve, too. Cool the hiccups by sucking on an ice cube.

PREVENTION

If you'd like to avoid embarrassing hiccups, there are several strategies you can use.

Push away from the table. Too much food in the stomach can cause hiccups. Don't eat too much at one time.

Slow down. Eating too fast doesn't allow for adequate chewing. Air

---

10 TIPS TO GET RID OF HICCUPS

- Stick your fingers in your ears.
- Have someone scare you.
- Drink or gargle water.
- Try a spoonful of sugar.
- Pull on your tongue.
- Have someone tickle you.
- Hold your breath.
- Take an antacid.
- Suck on a lemon wedge.
- Eat ice cubes.

---

becomes trapped in pieces of food and stimulates a hiccup attack. Eat slower, chew your food thoroughly, and take smaller sips of beverages.

Stay away from spicy foods. Some spices irritate the lining of the food tube. They can also cause "acid reflux," in which stomach acids slip back up the esophagus. The extra acid can stimulate hiccups.

Skip the drinking games. In some circles, going to parties and drinking alcoholic beverages quickly is popular. The gulping causes the esophagus to expand quickly and brings on hiccups.

Sources: **Allan Burke**, M.D., Assistant Professor of Clinical Neurology, Northwestern University School of Medicine, Chicago, Illinois. **Howard Goldin**, M.D., Clinical Professor of Medicine, The New York Hospital—Cornell Medical Center, New York, New York. **Anne Simons**, M.D., Coauthor, *Before You Call the Doctor*; Family Practitioner, San Francisco Department of Public Health; Family Practitioner and Assistant Clinical Professor, Family and Community Medicine, University of California San Francisco Medical Center, San Francisco, California. **George Triadafilopoulos**, M.D., Associate Professor of Medicine, University of California Davis; Staff Physician, VA Northern California Systems of Clinics, Venicia, California.

•HIGH BLOOD CHOLESTEROL

How to Lower

Your Risk of

Heart Disease

IF YOU'VE BEEN TOLD THAT YOU HAVE A high level of cholesterol in your blood, you need to take steps to lower it—today. High cholesterol is a leading cause of heart disease, which can result in heart attacks and death. Lowering your cholesterol level may add several years to your life and keep you healthier, happier, and more active.

Heart disease is a leading cause of death in the United States. This year, about one-and-a-half million people in this country are expected to have a heart attack; 300,000 of them will die before they can get to a hospital. An additional 200,000 will die later on. Almost half those fatalities will be women.

What causes a heart attack? In most cases, an attack occurs when the blood supply to part of the heart muscle is severely reduced or stopped. This stoppage is caused when one of the arteries that supply blood to the heart is obstructed, usually by atherosclerosis. (Atherosclerosis is the deposition of fatty plaques on the walls of arteries. These plaques can block the flow of blood to the heart and cause a heart attack.)

Although it's not clear where the plaques come from in each individual case, the most common causes are a blood-cholesterol level that's too high, a hereditary tendency to develop atherosclerosis, and increasing age (55 percent of all heart attack victims are 65 or older, and only 5 percent are under 40). Other factors that contribute to the likelihood that heart disease will develop are cigarette smoking and high blood pressure. Men and post-menopausal women are also at higher risk.

According to the American Heart Association (AHA), total levels of blood cholesterol under 200 milligrams per deciliter represent a low risk of coronary heart disease. Levels between 200 and 240 are considered to be a "borderline" risk, and over 240 is considered a dangerously high risk. More than 27 percent of the U.S. population falls into a high-risk category.

While total levels of blood cholesterol are considered important, other factors come into play, as well. For example, if someone has a borderline-high total cholesterol level, but has very low levels of high-density lipoprotein (HDL), the "good" cholesterol believed to prevent heart disease, he or she may still have a high risk of heart disease. In general, doctors worry about the ratio of low-density lipoprotein (LDL—the "bad" cholesterol usually implicated in atherosclerosis) to HDL.

A desirable HDL level is over 50. For LDL, a level below 130 is desirable, a level of 130 to 160 is considered borderline-high, and over 160 represents a high risk of heart disease. Although these numbers aren't absolute (for example, levels of triglycerides, another fatty acid, also enter into the big picture), they do represent a fairly good predictor of heart-disease risk.

On average, for every one-percent increase in total blood cholesterol, there is a two-to-three percent increase in heart disease rates. This means that for a person with a total cholesterol level of 220, the risk of heart disease is 10 percent higher than for a person with a total cholesterol level of 200. A person with a level of 250 has a 50 percent higher risk than the person with 200.

High blood cholesterol is one of several potential causes of heart disease. If you've also been diagnosed with high blood pressure, read the chapter on high blood pressure for suggestions on controlling that problem as well.

SYMPTOMS

High blood cholesterol itself causes no symptoms. However, the conditions that it may lead to—angina (chest pain caused by inadequate blood flow to the heart), heart attacks, and strokes—do cause severe symptoms, including crushing chest pain, loss of consciousness, dizziness, and loss of motor control, memory, or speech. Ultimately, these conditions can result in death.

CAUSES

Cholesterol is a soft, fatlike substance found in all the body's cells. It is used to form cell membranes, certain hormones, and other necessary substances. Some cholesterol in the blood is produced by the liver. The rest comes from the foods that we eat.

Many people mistakenly believe that their high blood-cholesterol level is caused by eating too many foods that contain cholesterol. This is not exactly true. Eating too much saturated fat is the biggest cause of high blood-cholesterol levels. Saturated fat is the kind of fat found in full-fat dairy products and animal fat (it just so happens that many foods that are high in saturated fat are also high in cholesterol). Another culprit is partially hydrogenated vegetable oil, which contains trans-fatty acids. These acids increase the cholesterol-raising properties of a fat.

20 WAYS TO LOWER YOUR BLOOD CHOLESTEROL

- **Make a lifetime commitment to lowering your risk factors.**
- **Take action today.**
- **Don't be taken in by "magic-bullet" solutions.**
- **Substitute saturated fats with polyunsaturated and monounsaturated fats.**
- **Stick with low-fat varieties of meat.**
- **Count fat grams.**
- **Cut your fat intake to a very low percentage of your total daily calories.**
- **Stay away from animal fats.**
- **Learn fat-free ways of preparing food.**
- **Do not eat poultry skin.**
- **Avoid the fat hidden inside pastries.**
- **Increase your fish intake while cutting down on higher-fat meats and poultry.**
- **Avoid egg yolks.**
- **Keep meat serving sizes down to three ounces.**
- **Avoid organ meats.**
- **Take a one-teaspoon dose of a soluble-fiber product, such as Metamucil or Citrucil, every day.**
- **Stop smoking.**
- **Start a program of mild aerobic exercise.**
- **Know that it's never too late to improve your health.**
- **Follow the American Heart Association's dietary guidelines.**

AT-HOME TREATMENT

You can't change certain risk factors for heart disease, such as your age or your genes. However, you can change unhealthy habits that boost your risk. The following tips are designed to help you do just that.

Start a new life. Make a commitment to lowering your blood cholesterol and improving your heart's health. That means changing your way of thinking, not just a temporary effort. Set your mind to developing lifetime good habits, instead of jumping on and off of the wagon as you see fit. This is especially important with weight-loss efforts, since yo-yo dieting has been shown to cause cholesterol levels to rise.

Don't wait until you're in a high-risk group. It's true that much attention is paid to people with a total blood-cholesterol level over 240, but the numbers can be misleading. In fact, most heart attacks occur in people whose total cholesterol level is between 150 and 250. People whose cholesterol levels are above 240 account for only about 20 percent of the heart attacks. So even if you're not in a high-risk group, you still should make a point of maintaining healthful habits.

Avoid the culprit. The cardinal rule of cholesterol-lowering is to stay away from saturated fats. How do you know which are saturated? If it comes from an animal, in the form of a dairy product (except for the skim and fat-free varieties), meat, poultry, or seafood, it definitely contains saturated fat. Skinless, white-meat poultry contains less saturated fat than most beef, lamb, and pork; seafood (except for certain oily varieties of fish) contains the least. With straight fats, it can be hard to tell which spread is better. As a rule, those that are most liquid at room temperature have less saturated fat. For example, pick the most liquid kinds of margarine, such as the tubs or squeeze bottles.

Don't look for an easy out. Rice bran, garlic, oat bran, fish oil, and others have been touted as the magic-bullet solution to your cholesterol problem. Of course, it's tempting to look for a shortcut, but when you're dealing with your health, realize that there's just no such thing. If your cholesterol is high, it is most likely because you eat too much saturated fat and cholesterol. You need to address the source of the problem and concentrate on replacing fatty foods in your diet with whole grains and vegetables, instead of seeking the one magical substance that will make high cholesterol disappear.

Read the label. Pay attention to the small orange labels stuck to packages of meat at the grocery store. They're not advertisements, they're grades of meat. "Prime," "Choice," and "Select" are the official U.S. Department of Agriculture ways of saying, "fatty," "less fatty," and "lean."

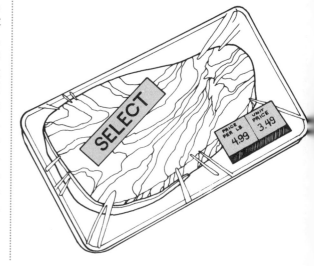

Prime means that the meat is about 40 to 45 percent fat by weight. Choice is from 30 to 40 percent fat, and Select (or diet lean) is from 15 to 20 percent fat. Choose Select meats, whenever possible.

Keep tabs on fat grams. The American Heart Association's dietary guidelines specify the percentage of your daily calories that should come from fat. However, most package labels show grams of fat, not percentages. This makes it difficult to tell whether you're getting too much fat. Here's how to figure out how many grams of fat, and how many grams of saturated fat, you can have each day. Multiply your total number of daily calories per day by .30, then divide by nine to find the number of grams of total fat allowed. (You divide by nine because each gram of fat provides nine calories.) Multiply your total number of calories per day by .10 and divide by nine to find the number of grams of saturated fat allowed each day.

For example, if you're on a 2,000-calorie-per-day diet, 66.6 grams of fat and 22 grams of saturated fat should be your daily limit. On average, Americans will eat about twice that much.

How much food brings you 22 grams of fat? One serving of "Choice" beef contains from 12 to 15 grams of fat; a serving of "Select" contains four to ten. One tablespoon of butter is just under seven grams, while many brands of low-fat margarine contain only two grams per tablespoon. Whole milk has a whopping eight grams per cup; skim milk has none. You can add up the grams as the day goes along. If you choose low-fat options, maybe you'll have enough saturated fat calories left in your daily budget to indulge in some low-fat frozen yogurt, a cup of which may contain as little as two grams of saturated fat.

Get radical. Just because the American Heart Association says that no more than 30 percent of your daily calories should come from fat, doesn't mean that 30 percent should be your ultimate goal. Some heart specialists believe it's better to go even lower than that. (The average American derives about 37 to 40 percent of her calories from fat.) It is considered safe to go down to 20 grams of fat per day. This amount would be ten percent of a 2,000-calorie-per-day diet.

Go veggie-crazy. Animal products are the only source of dietary cholesterol. They also happen to be the foods that are higher in fat, especially saturated fat. Skim-milk products are exceptions to this. Plant products contain no cholesterol and are generally lower in fat than animal products. If they contain any fat at all, it is usually the polyunsaturated and monounsaturated kinds, which are healthier than the saturated kind. There are a few exceptions: Coconut oil, palm oil, palm kernel oil, and partially hydrogenated oils contain higher amounts of saturated fatty acids. Try to get your protein from vegetable sources, such as beans, whole grains, and tofu, and keep servings of high-fat animal products to a minimum. Your arteries will thank you for it.

Eat something fishy. In recent years, you may have heard news about fish oil reducing cholesterol. Fish oil does have high levels of omega-3 fatty acids, which have been associated with lower cholesterol levels. However, the people who received the greatest benefit from adding more fish to their diet frequently had the fish in their day-to-day routine instead of higher-fat meats. Also, fish oil itself tends to be high in fat, something you don't need much of. If you want to reap the benefits of fish oil in your diet, the best thing to do is add more servings of fish as substitutes for some of the meat dishes.

Try carbo loading. Try adding extra servings of complex carbohydrates to your diet. Complex carbohydrates, such as fruits, vegetables, pasta, whole-grain bread, rice, and other grains, will fill you up and make you feel more satisfied, reducing the desire for fatty meats and desserts.

Become a heart-healthy cook. Frying foods adds unnecessary fat. Try heart-smart ways to cook food, such as grilling, broiling, and steaming.

Take it off. If you're watching your fat intake, poultry skin, which contains high amounts of saturated fat, is out of the question.

Just say "no" to pastries. Those tempting pastries—Danish, pie crusts, eclairs, and so on—are a source of saturated fat. Pastry dough is usually made with shortening or butter—two significant sources of saturated fat. Snack on whole-grain breads and rolls, and read labels to be sure there's no saturated fat hiding in any packaged products.

Be discriminating about your eggs. You may think that eggs are loaded with fat and cholesterol; you are half right. Egg yolks are more than 50 percent fat and contain high amounts of cholesterol, but egg whites are fine. Be careful, though; egg yolks may also be hidden inside processed foods—read labels carefully. The American Heart Association suggests having no more than three yolks per week, including those found in processed foods or used in cooking.

Cut your serving size. You don't have to give up steaks altogether if you are trying to cut down on your saturated fat intake. Just go with smaller portions—about three ounces per serving (which is a piece about the size of a deck of cards). If you skip the meat at lunch and also avoid cheese and other high-fat dairy products, you can increase your portion to six ounces at dinnertime.

Leave the giblets. Organ meats, like egg yolks, are not part of a cholesterol-reducing diet. Even though they are rich in iron and protein, liver (including pâté), headcheese, and the rest are also very high in fat and cholesterol.

Add fiber to your diet. Soluble fiber, the kind of fiber found in fruits and brans, has been effective in lowering cholesterol levels. The problem is that it must be consumed in large amounts to have a cholesterol-lowering effect. It would take about a quarter-pound of oatmeal per day to get ten grams of soluble fiber, the amount that can lower cholesterol. A psyllium-husk powder, such as Metamucil, is a more effective provider of soluble fiber. A teaspoonful a day is sufficient. Psyllium may even help you cut the amount of LDL ("bad" cholesterol) in your blood by eight to ten percent. Fiber is not the ultimate answer, though, so don't overdo it. After you pass 10 grams per day, you receive diminishing returns; 20 grams per day won't double the decrease in your cholesterol level. And remember to introduce fiber into your diet gradually so as not to shock your system.

The following are foods that are high in soluble fiber. You should consider incorporating them into your day-to-day diet to help keep your cholesterol level down:
• Barley
• Dried beans and peas
• Fruits, especially apples, apricots, figs, mangos, oranges, peaches, plums, rhubarb, strawberries
• Lentils
• Oats/oatmeal
• Vegetables, especially broccoli, brussels sprouts, cabbage, carrots, okra, potatoes (white and sweet), turnips

Get moving. According to studies, a regular schedule of aerobic exercise can boost levels of HDL in the blood. Exercise can also be useful in reducing weight, which helps control cholesterol levels, as well. You should get 30 to 45 minutes of moderate exercise five days per week. Try walking or biking—any activity that accelerates your heart rate and keeps it up for at least 20 minutes. You can also add exercise into your daily routine by parking your car a quarter-mile away from work and walking the rest of the way, taking the stairs instead of the elevator, and so on. Check with your doctor before beginning any exercise program, especially if you have been sedentary.

Kick the cigarette habit. Of course, we all know that smoking can cause lung cancer and raise the risk of a heart attack. But did you realize that smoking can actually affect your cholesterol levels? When you stop smoking, your HDL ("good" cholesterol) levels rise significantly. When a two-pack-a-day smoker quits, she may experience an eight-point rise in HDL cholesterol.

Don't get discouraged. Don't give up, even if you've already had a heart attack or other evidence of heart disease. You can dramatically reduce your risk of a recurrence with some changes in lifestyle. At one time, heart specialists thought that once someone had heart disease, lifestyle changes wouldn't make much difference. They now believe that drastically lowering cholesterol—to as low as 160 or 170—may have a protective effect.

Follow the rules. The American Heart Association recommends certain dietary guidelines that are designed to prevent heart attacks, stroke, and other manifestations of cardiovascular disease from occurring in healthy adults. Here they are:

1) Your total fat intake should be less than 30 percent of daily calories.

2) Your saturated fat intake should be less than 10 percent of daily calories.

3) Your polyunsaturated fat intake should not exceed 10 percent of daily calories.

4) Your cholesterol intake should not exceed 300 milligrams per day.

5) Your carbohydrate intake should constitute 50 percent or more of daily calories, with an emphasis on complex carbohydrates.

6) Your protein intake should provide the remainder of the calories.

7) Your sodium intake should not exceed three grams (3,000 milligrams) per day.

8) Your alcohol consumption should not exceed one to two drinks per day. (One ounce of hard liquor, four ounces of wine, or 12 ounces of beer are each considered to be one drink.)

9) Total calories should be sufficient to maintain the individual's recommended body weight, as defined by the Metropolitan Tables of Height and Weight (Metropolitan Life Insurance Company, New York, 1983).

10) A wide variety of foods should be consumed.

AT THE DOCTOR'S

Since the condition is completely asymptomatic, the only way to know whether you have high cholesterol is to take a "fasting" blood test—a test conducted on a blood sample that is taken after you have not eaten or drunk anything for 12 to 16 hours.

If you are diagnosed as having borderline or high blood cholesterol, your physician will make a recommendation regarding your treatment. Most likely, the first step will be to make dietary and lifestyle changes, such as those described above. However, if your cholesterol level is very high, or if you have already unsuccessfully tried to lower it with lifestyle changes, your physician may prescribe a cholesterol-lowering medication, such as lovastatin or gemfibrozil.

If your cholesterol is on the high side, depending on your other risk factors for heart disease, your doctor may choose to refer you to a cardiologist, or heart specialist. The cardiologist may ask you to take an exercise-tolerance test, where you will exercise with an electrocardiograph attached to you. The electrocardiograph is a device that records the electrical impulses in the heart and can indicate whether areas of the heart are damaged or are receiving inadequate blood supply (due to a blocked artery, for example). If your doctor determines that you do have a blockage, you may be asked to submit to an angiogram, a test that will determine the location and severity of the blockage.

If drugs do not successfully lower your cholesterol and you are found to have heart disease that continues to progress despite treatment, your physician may recommend balloon angioplasty—a procedure where a tube with a balloon attached to it is inserted into the blocked heart artery. The balloon is then inflated, pressing the fatty deposits against the walls of the artery so that blood can flow more freely.

If the blockage is extremely severe or if it cannot be treated with balloon angioplasty, your cardiologist may recommend an arterial bypass operation. In this procedure, a section of a vein from the patient's leg or a section of artery from the chest is grafted onto the blocked artery (below the obstruction) and to the aorta (the main heart artery). In this way, blood flow is allowed to bypass the obstruction.

Sources: Henry Blackburn, M.D., Mayo Professor of Public Health and Professor of Medicine, University of Minnesota, Minneapolis, Minnesota. W. Virgil Brown, M.D., Past President, American Heart Association; Professor of Medicine, Director, Division of Arteriosclerosis and Lipid Metabolism, Emory University School of Medicine, Atlanta, Georgia. William P. Castelli, M.D., Director, Framingham Heart Study, Framingham, Massachusetts. Peter F. Cohn, M.D., Chief of Cardiology, State University of New York at Stony Brook Health Sciences Center, Stony Brook, New York. Basil M. Rifkind, M.D., F.R.C.P., Chief, Lipid Metabolism and Atherogenesis Branch, National Heart, Lung, and Blood Institute, National Institutes of Health, Bethesda, Maryland.

•HIGH BLOOD PRESSURE

How to Get It

Under Control

and Keep It

Under Control

IF YOU'VE BEEN DIAGNOSED WITH HIGH blood pressure, you're probably pretty nervous, maybe even a little scared. And with reason—high blood pressure is potentially a very dangerous condition. But, with your doctor's help, you can manage your blood pressure and have a long, active life.

The statistics are stark: At last count, 62,770,000 Americans—almost one-quarter of our country's population—had or were being treated for high blood pressure. Every year, 31,630 of these individuals die as a direct result of the condition. An additional 147,470 deaths every year occur from stroke (a blood clot that travels to the brain), making it the number-one fatality related to high blood pressure. Another 2,980,000 Americans have had a stroke and lived. Many of these people are now severely disabled and unable to care for themselves. In addition to strokes, high blood pressure can cause blindness, kidney failure, and a swelling of the heart that may lead to heart failure. That's why it's important to follow the treatment your doctor prescribes if you have high blood pressure.

High blood pressure during pregnancy causes special problems: First, the condition is extremely dangerous, posing a risk of stroke, preeclampsia (a condition that causes sudden weight gain, extreme water retention, blurred vision, and other symptoms), stillbirth, premature delivery, and low birth weight. Second, blood pressure may be difficult to control without medication, and many medications may pose a danger to the developing fetus.

High blood pressure, or hypertension, is defined as a persistently elevated pressure of the blood within the arteries that carry blood from the heart throughout the body. The exertion of excessive force upon the artery walls may cause damage to the arteries themselves and thereby to the heart, kidneys, and brain, leading to heart attack, kidney failure, or stroke.

So what exactly constitutes high blood pressure? A blood-pressure reading equal to or higher than 160 systolic (the top number) over 95 diastolic (the bottom number) is considered high. Between 140 and 159 systolic over 90 to 94 diastolic is considered "borderline" high. Blood pressure below these numbers is considered normal.

When no underlying cause of high blood pressure is present, the disease is called primary, or essential, hypertension. If another disease, such as kidney or heart disease, causes the elevated blood pressure, the condition is labeled secondary hypertension.

SYMPTOMS

The reason that high blood pressure has been dubbed "the silent killer" is that it very often has no symptoms. A person may suffer from the condition for years without feeling any different at all. However, high blood pressure may cause some nonspecific symptoms, such as headaches, fatigue, dizziness, flushing of the face, ringing in the ears, thumping in the chest, and frequent nosebleeds.

While high blood pressure itself has very few symptoms, a stroke can cause very severe ones. If you are experiencing any of the following stroke symptoms, call your doctor or an ambulance at once. Waiting too long or not recognizing the signs could mean the difference between life and death. If you experience any of these symptoms and then feel better within 24 hours, you may have had a transient ischemic attack, or TIA. A TIA is a warning sign that a full-blown stroke is on its way. Call your doctor at once.

- Sudden weakness or numbness of the face, arm, or leg on one side of the body.
- Sudden dimness or loss of vision, particularly in only one eye.
- Loss of speech, or trouble talking or understanding speech.
- Sudden, severe headaches with no apparent cause.
- Unexplained dizziness, unsteadiness, or sudden falls, especially accompanied by any of the previous symptoms.

CAUSES

There is no typical hypertensive person. Although many people believe that hypertension is caused by extreme activity or tension, this theory has not been proven. What scientists do know, however, is that some people are more susceptible to developing the condition than others. Heredity appears to play a role; persons whose parents are hypertensive are at greater risk of becoming hypertensive themselves. In the past, hypertension was attributed to aging, but current evidence indicates that age is not a primary factor. The incidence of hypertension in black persons—both children and adults—is about twice that of white persons (whether this is due to heredity, diet, lifestyle, or socioeconomic factors is unclear).

Overweight, prolonged stress, smoking, drinking, and excessive sodium in the diet (which causes fluid retention) may increase blood pressure, especially in persons prone to hypertension. There are also indications that the use of oral contraceptives may contribute to increased blood pressure. However, this is more likely to occur in women who are overweight, whose parents are hypertensive, or who have other hypertensive risk factors.

Lastly, pregnancy is associated with a higher risk of developing high blood pressure. During pregnancy, your blood volume triples, placing a great deal of additional strain upon the heart. Perhaps because of this increase in blood volume, many women who never had a problem with blood pressure become hypertensive, a condition called pregnancy-induced hypertension.

AT-HOME TREATMENT

You've heard the bad news. The good news is that, together with your doctor, you can control your condition. It won't be easy—you'll have to change the way you think and act. You may have to take medication for the rest of your life. You'll definitely have to cut out some bad habits and begin new, more healthful ones. However, your efforts are likely to pay off in a longer, healthier, happier life. Here's where to start:

Accept it. Doctors say that many people who are diagnosed with hypertension just refuse to believe it (and refuse to make the changes that will help them control their condition). Realizing that you actually have a blood pressure problem is harder than it sounds, especially when you feel perfectly fine. Do yourself a favor: Choose life over denial. Follow your doctor's instructions carefully.

You also have to take your medicine faithfully. If you stop taking your blood pressure medication, you'll probably feel fine, but the disease will continue to progress unchecked. Your kidneys, your heart, the arteries in your eyes, and many other vital organs may be damaged. In addition, discontinuing your medication can actually raise your blood pressure to levels higher than they were before you started taking the drug—a rebound phenomenon.

Take home readings. Your doctor may prescribe a home blood-pressure monitor for you if you have been diagnosed as being hypertensive, or if he or she wants more blood-pressure readings before making a definitive diagnosis. There are a number of advantages to monitoring your blood pressure at home. For example, you will have early warning if your pressure becomes dangerously high, so you can get medical attention. A monitor can also save you money by saving you trips to the doctor, and if your doctor has prescribed at-home monitoring, chances are your insurance company will pay for the device. Make sure the equipment is calibrated and

you know how to use it. Talk to your doctor if you're not sure.

Shed excess pounds. Overweight is directly linked to increased blood pressure. In most people, weight loss can help reverse the trend—by about two blood-pressure points for each pound lost. If you are severely hypertensive, weight loss is a necessity. If you are only slightly hypertensive, losing some weight may enable you to stay off of medication. Even some weight loss is better than none. A loss of only 10 pounds may completely cure most people who suffer from borderline hypertension—140 to 159 systolic and 90 to 94 diastolic—a level of blood pressure that increases the risk of stroke by three times.

Get moving. Exercise has various benefits for those with high blood pressure, not the least of which is helping with weight loss. People with severe hypertension shouldn't exercise until their blood pressure is controlled; however, for those with only mild hypertension, aerobic exercise (20 to 30 minutes per day, three times per week) may result in a blood-pressure reduction of about eight points that will last at least half a day.

Not all exercises are beneficial for all people. In fact, anaerobic exercise, such as weight lifting, push-ups, and chin-ups, may actually be dangerous for people with high blood pressure. These types of exercise should not be done without the explicit consent of your doctor. Aerobic exercise is the kind most likely to help lower blood pressure. Aerobic exercises are those that raise your pulse rate and sustain that rate for at least 20 minutes. These include walking, jogging, stair-climbing, aerobic dance, swimming, bicycling, tennis, skating, and cross-country skiing. Of course, it is always best to get your doctor's OK before beginning any exercise program, especially if you have been inactive for a while.

Cut down on salt. Americans are accustomed to foods that are far too salty to be healthy. On average, we consume eight to ten grams of salt a day. And excess salt intake has been linked with high blood pressure.

Recent research indicates that blood pressure can be significantly reduced by simply eating a third less salt. Ideally, your short-term goal should be to cut your intake down to six grams per day; your long-term goal should be about four-and-a-half grams per day. Tastes are adaptable. After awhile on a low-salt diet, you will become much more sensitive to the taste of salt and need less to make something taste salty.

So how do you know how much salt you're eating? One teaspoon of table salt contains over two grams—almost half the recommended daily amount. The average American adult unknowingly takes in somewhere between one-and-a-half to two extra teaspoons of salt a day from sources like

> ## 10 STEPS TO LOWER BLOOD PRESSURE
>
> - Accept your condition.
> - Try to lose any excess weight.
> - Monitor your blood pressure at home.
> - Start a program of aerobic exercise, with your doctor's permission.
> - Eliminate excess salt from your diet.
> - Drink no more than one alcoholic drink per day.
> - Increase your intake of dietary potassium and calcium, with your doctor's permission.
> - Substitute polyunsaturated fats for saturated ones in cooking.
> - Quit smoking.
> - Learn to relax.

frozen entrees, canned vegetables, and even antacid medications. To avoid this extra salt, read labels before you buy. Many labels express the amount of sodium in milligrams (1,000 milligrams equals 1 gram). To calculate the amount of sodium chloride, or salt, multiply the amount of sodium by two-and-a-half.

Stick to one drink a day. While one alcoholic drink a day is not harmful and may even lower blood pressure, more than one may cause a rise in blood pressure. What constitutes a drink? A 1.5-ounce shot of hard liquor, a 4-ounce glass of wine, or a 12-ounce beer, all of which contain about 1 fluid ounce of alcohol.

Eat a handful of raisins. There are some things you can take that do not require a prescription: raisins, bananas, currants, milk, yogurt, and orange juice. All

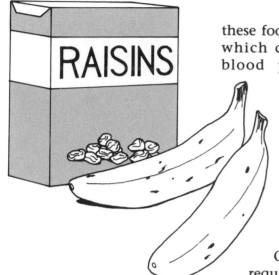

these foods contain potassium, which can help lower your blood pressure. Although potassium supplements might help, you shouldn't take them without the permission of a doctor, because they may be hazardous to individuals with certain medical conditions.

On average, a person requires three or four servings of potassium-rich fruits and vegetables per day. Doubling that amount may benefit your blood pressure, some experts believe.

Have some milk, especially during pregnancy. Although not shown to have any significant effect on blood pressure, extra dietary calcium may have some other benefits for the hypertensive. In any case, though, some extra skim milk, low-fat yogurt, or leafy green vegetables in your daily diet certainly won't hurt you.

There is more evidence that calcium can significantly reduce high blood pressure in pregnant women. Some researchers suggest that pregnant women should almost double the recommended daily allowance of calcium to maintain safe blood pressure levels. Of course, pregnant women should always consult with their doctors before taking any supplements or exceeding the recommended amount of any

nutrient. The recommended daily allowance for calcium during pregnancy is about the amount contained in eight servings of low-fat milk, yogurt, or broccoli (1,200 milligrams).

Switch to canola oil. It's pretty common knowledge that substituting polyunsaturated oils for saturated fats in your diet can help you reduce your level of blood cholesterol. But did you know that polyunsaturated oils can also help reduce blood pressure? Some physicians believe that substituting canola and safflower oils for saturated fats in cooking may cut your blood pressure by about ten points.

Kick the nicotine habit. Cigarette smoking is not at all acceptable for people with high blood pressure. Nicotine raises your blood pressure and greatly increases your risk of having a stroke. The American Heart Association says that cigarette smoking thickens the blood, facilitating the formation of clots. In the arteries leading to the heart, blood clots can cause a heart attack. In the arteries leading to the brain, blood clots can cause a stroke.

The good news is that you can improve your health almost immediately by kicking the habit right now. Two years after you quit smoking, your risk of developing coronary artery disease will be the same as if you had never smoked. The same cannot be said for a person's risk of other smoking-related diseases, such as lung cancer.

Besides nagging, your doctor can do other things to help you quit smoking. Nicotine gum and nicotine skin patches, prescribed by your doctor, can reduce the discomfort of withdrawal. Your local Heart Association can provide you with more information on quitting.

Lighten up. Many people with high blood pressure have the classic "Type A" personality—aggressive, hostile, frustrated, or angry. Relaxation is one of the prescribed treatments for these workaholic go-getters. Relaxation can take the form of prayer, yoga, biofeedback, or just resting, among other things (you may need to experiment a bit before you discover what works best for you). If you're chronically stressed-out, you may release a lot of adrenaline into your system. When the adrenaline rush hits, arterioles (tiny blood vessels) constrict and go into spasm. The heart must work harder to push blood through the narrowed arterioles, and the effect is higher blood pressure.

AT THE DOCTOR'S

High blood pressure must be diagnosed by a physician (it is recommended that everyone have their blood pressure checked at least once a year). One high reading alone is not enough to make the diagnosis; the doctor will usually take several readings, on both arms, during your visit.

The reading is taken with a stethoscope and a sphygmomanometer, or blood-pressure meter. The blood pressure is measured in a main artery of the arm by shutting off and then releasing the flow of blood in the artery with the inflatable cuff of the sphygmomanometer while listening to the arterial pulse with the stethoscope.

If you are diagnosed with high blood pressure, your physician may want you to make certain lifestyle changes (many of which are outlined above). He or she may also prescribe medications, depending on the severity of your hypertension, your age, and whether you have other illnesses. Commonly prescribed high-blood-pressure drugs include diuretics, which eliminate excess fluid from the body, and beta-blockers, which reduce the force with which the heart pumps blood throughout the body.

If you have been diagnosed as having high blood pressure and you become pregnant, you should see your doctor as soon as possible to discuss ways to control your condition during pregnancy.

Sources: David B. Carmichael, M.D., Medical Director, Cardiovascular Institute, Scripps Memorial Hospital, La Jolla, California. **William P. Castelli, M.D.,** Director, Framingham Heart Study, Framingham, Massachusetts. **Jeffrey A. Cutler, M.D.,** Hypertension Specialist and Chief, Prevention and Demonstration Research Branch, National Heart, Lung, and Blood Institute, National Institutes of Health, Bethesda, Maryland. **James A. Hearn, M.D.,** Assistant Professor of Medicine, University of Alabama at Birmingham, Birmingham, Alabama. **Robert A. Phillips, M.D., Ph.D.,** Director, Hypertension Section, Associate Director, Cardiovascular Training Program, Division of Cardiology, Mount Sinai Medical Center, New York, New York. **John T. Repke, Ph.D.,** Associate Professor of Obstetrics and Gynecology, Johns Hopkins University, Baltimore, Maryland.

•HIVES

Get Rid of

the Itch

YOU'VE JUST ENJOYED ONE OF SUM-mer's gifts—soft, sweet cakes heaped with luscious, fresh strawberries and topped with mounds of whipped cream. Then it happens. Your skin begins to tingle. Tiny bumps appear that quickly form raised red areas. You begin to itch like mad. You've got hives.

Almost anything can give you hives—skin eruptions and intense itching doctors call "urticaria." Foods like peanuts, eggs, nuts, beans, chocolate, strawberries, tomatoes, citrus fruits, fish, and pork are common culprits. But hives can also be caused by nonfood factors, such as drugs like penicillin or aspirin, heat, cold, sunlight, exercise, fever, stress, or even scratching or rubbing the skin. In very sensitive people, dust, molds, animal dander, and even some plants can raise the welts.

CAUSES

Hives are most often a sign of an allergic reaction in which something causes the body to release histamine, which, in turn, causes the skin to leak plasma. The plasma causes the skin to erupt with raised, smooth patches or welts known as "wheals." These skin eruptions vary in size and can appear in just a few areas or all over the body.

In sensitive people, it doesn't take much of the offending substance to cause a reaction. For example, if you're allergic to a particular fish and you order a different food that was cooked in the pan used previously to cook the fish, you could break out in hives.

Fortunately, hive outbreaks generally don't stick around. In some people, the welts last no more than a few minutes; in others, a few days. In rare cases, people have been known to suffer chronic, recurrent outbreaks or have hives that persist for years. In addition to itching and welts, some people also experience fatigue, fever, nausea, and difficulty breathing if the allergic reaction causes swelling in the mucous membrane lining the respiratory tract. If you have any of these symptoms, get medical help immediately.

AT-HOME TREATMENT

It's not always possible to identify what's causing your hives, especially if they're chronic. In 70 to 80 percent of cases, you just have to live with an unknown cause and treat the symptoms.

Kill the itch with antihistamines. Over-the-counter antihistamines such as Benadryl are effective in treating the intense itching and swelling of hives. They can prevent the released histamine from triggering more hives. Be aware, however, that they also cause drowsiness and dry mouth. Never drive an automobile or operate heavy equipment or power tools after taking antihistamines. You may find they are most effective at night when the itching is more annoying. (If you have glaucoma, enlarged prostate, or heart disease, talk with your doctor before taking antihistamines.) Prescription antihistamines often cause less drowsiness. They cost more, but are worth it if you have to drive while taking the medication.

Nix the scratch. Scratching makes hives itch more and can make you susceptible to secondary infection. Resist the urge!

Try P.M. gloves. Many people scratch their hives while they sleep, increasing inflammation and causing even more hives. If you're bothered by nocturnal scratching, try wearing soft cotton gloves to bed.

Wrap up. Another way around nighttime scratching is to wrap hives in an elastic bandage (not too tight) or cover them with clothing.

Milk it. Cool inflamed tissues with cold milk compresses. The milk soothes angry tissues and eases itching. Wet a cloth in cold milk and place it on your skin for 10 to 15 minutes at a time.

Go for the cold. Ice packs or ice cubes can temporarily stop the itching and reduce the swelling. Place the ice in a towel (not directly on the skin) for five minutes at a time, three or four times a day.

Soothe it in a bath. Soak in a soothing anti-itch bath. Add one to two cups of Aveeno powder (available over the counter in pharmacies), one-half to one cup of baking soda, or one to two cups of finely ground oatmeal (you can buy "colloidal oatmeal" at your pharmacy or grind your own in a coffee grinder) to your bath. Be sure to keep the water cool or warm (not hot, which stimulates the release of more histamines).

Cortisone it. Some people get itch relief using one-percent corti-sone preparations, available over the counter.

Be careful with the anti-itch "-caine" type products such as benzocaine and topical Bena-dryl. Some people experience allergic reactions to them. If your hives appear to get worse after using these products, discontinue their use immediately.

Loosen up. Hives often appear in places where clothing constricts—bra straps, waistbands, etc. Relieve the pressure by wearing looser garments.

Keep it moist. Sometimes dry skin contributes to the itchiness of hives. If your skin is dry, avoid long baths and moisturize your skin several times a day.

Uncover the infection. Sometimes hives aren't an allergic reaction at all, but a symptom of a chronic infection such as a tooth infection, yeast infection, or intestinal parasite infection. Consider these possibilities if your hives don't clear up or if they've become recurrent, and check with your doctor.

Call the doctor. Most hive episodes are just temporary inconveniences that don't last more than a day or two. However, in addition to infection, chronic or recurrent hives may indicate a more serious health problem

11 TIPS TO TREAT YOUR HIVES

- Take an over-the-counter antihistamine.
- Don't scratch.
- Wear soft gloves at night.
- Cover the hives with bandages or clothing.
- Use cool milk compresses.
- Place ice on the hives.
- Soak in a cool or warm Aveeno, oatmeal, or baking-soda bath.
- Try topical cortisone.
- Loosen up your constricting clothing.
- Treat underlying infections.
- Call the doctor if you have warning symptoms or the hives persist.

such as lupus, hepatitis, tuberculosis, thyroid disorders, a sexually transmitted disease, or even some forms of cancer. See your physician or visit an emergency room if, in addition to hives:

- You have facial or throat swelling.
- You have difficulty breathing.
- You have a fever.
- You're losing weight or suffering from malaise (a general feeling of not being well).
- Your hives persist for four to six weeks.

PREVENTION

The real key to fighting hives is prevention. Since the problem is an offending source, the solution is avoiding that source.

Keep a diary. It's important to identify the cause of your allergic reaction whenever possible. Keep a diary of the foods you eat, the medications you take, your activities, etc., and your hive outbreaks. Include vitamins and herbs, over-the-counter drugs, and wine (even aspirin can be a cause of hives).

Try an elimination diet. If you suspect your allergen is a food but haven't been able to identify it with your food diary, try an elimination diet. Start eliminating the foods you think may be causing your symptoms. Then eat one of the foods. If you have no reaction, add another and another until you have a reaction.

Steer clear of the trigger. Once you've identified your allergy trigger, avoid it. If it's an ingredient like monosodium glutamate or mustard, get into the habit of asking about ingredients and additives and how foods are cooked in restaurants. At the grocery store, read labels carefully. With drug sensitivities, inform your physician and pharmacist and consider wearing a "Medic-Alert" bracelet to let others know of your allergy in an emergency.

Manage your stress. Many people find they experience hives under stress. Manage your stress with meditation, biofeedback, progressive relaxation, or some other stress management technique.

Sources: Philip C. Anderson, M.D., Chairman of Dermatology, University of Missouri-Columbia School of Medicine, Columbia, Missouri. Larry Borish, M.D., Staff Physician, National Jewish Center for Immunology and Respiratory Medicine, Denver, Colorado. Judy Jordan, M.D., Spokesperson, American Academy of Dermatology; Dermatologist, San Antonio, Texas. Anne Simons, M.D., Coauthor, *Before You Call the Doctor*; Family Practitioner, San Francisco Department of Public Health; Family Practitioner and Assistant Clinical Professor, Family and Community Medicine, University of California San Francisco Medical Center, San Francisco, California.

●INCONTINENCE

How to

Relieve an

Embarrassing

Problem

INCONTINENCE: IT'S A PROBLEM THAT can be difficult to discuss. But, rest assured—you're far from being the only one who has troubles with bladder control. At least 12 million, and perhaps as many as 20 million, people in the United States and Canada are suffering right along with you—oftentimes in silence. Incontinence is a problem that has only been recognized relatively recently in America as a treatable condition and not merely as an unavoidable symptom of aging. Other cultures in times past seem to have been much more aware of the problem and open to creative solutions. The ancient Egyptians developed products for incontinence, and in Great Britain around the turn of the century, it was perfectly acceptable for a woman to hold what was called a "slipper" under her dress to relieve herself during a long church service.

SYMPTOMS

There are different types and degrees of urinary incontinence. You may leak urine when exercising, lifting heavy objects, laughing, coughing, or sneezing. You may leak urine when your bladder is too full. You may find yourself rushing to the bathroom, only to make it too late. You may not even be aware that you have to go when, suddenly, you are wet.

CAUSES

The loss of bladder control is not a disease but a symptom, with a plethora of possible causes. It can affect anyone at any age—from children to the elderly, both women and men. Women, however, are three times more likely than men to be incontinent.

The cause of incontinence may be as minor as an infection triggered by a cold, bladder irritation, or the use of certain prescription or over-the-counter medications. In women, incontinence is often the result of sagging pelvic-floor muscles. This set of muscles at the bottom of the pelvis supports the lower internal organs and helps them maintain their shape and proper function. Childbirth and certain types of surgery, such as a hysterectomy (removal of the uterus), can cause these muscles to become deficient, allowing urine to leak out when you laugh, sneeze, exercise, or when your bladder is overly full.

Incontinence can manifest in a number of ways, and one person can suffer from more than one form of it. Stress incontinence occurs from rigorous or spontaneous activity, like jumping, running, coughing, laughing, or sneezing. Urge incontinence is marked by a need to go so suddenly that you may not be able to make it to the bathroom in time. Overflow incontinence is a full bladder that begins to dribble. And reflex incontinence is marked by an unawareness of the need to urinate, resulting in leakage.

AT-HOME TREATMENT

You will probably want to talk to your doctor about your incontinence problem. Meanwhile, and along with any treatment the doctor prescribes, try the strategies below. They should help you feel drier and more secure.

Strengthen your pelvic floor. The muscles that make up the pelvic floor support the lower internal organs, such as the bladder and the uterus, and control the sphincter muscles that, in turn, regulate the urethra and rectum. You use these muscles to stop and start your urine stream. Incontinence can occur when the pelvic-floor muscles become weak, but since you can control these muscles voluntarily, you can do exercises to help strengthen

---

16 WAYS TO STAY DRY AND CONFIDENT

- Do exercises to strengthen the pelvic-floor muscles.
- Ask your doctor about resistive exercise.
- Contract your pelvic-floor muscles when coughing or sneezing and when carrying or lifting something.
- Be wary of exercise gimmicks.
- Avoid foods and beverages that may irritate your bladder.
- Try juices that control the odor of your urine.
- Keep up your fluid intake.
- Shed any excess pounds.
- Quit smoking.
- Buy pads, briefs, liners, or inserts to absorb leakage.
- Invest in an external collecting device for traveling.
- Always empty your bladder before going on a trip of an hour or more.
- To empty the bladder completely, urinate, then stand up, sit down again, and lean forward.
- Don't wear clothing that takes a long time to take off.
- Bring a change of clothing with you when you go out.
- Call 1-800-BLADDER for information.

---

them. This, in turn, can help control leakage, especially in the case of stress incontinence. You must do the exercises correctly for them to have the proper effect, however.

Help for Incontinent People (HIP), a not-for-profit organization in Union, South Carolina, recommends a few simple exer-

cises. For best results, do them on a daily basis. If you need further instruction, HIP has manuals and tapes, and your doctor is always a good resource. Your doctor may, in fact, suggest that your exercise regimen be a little more difficult, depending on your specific case.

1) Lie on your back with your knees bent and feet slightly apart. Contract all the openings in the pelvic floor—the rectum, the urethra, and the vagina. To help you isolate the muscles, first squeeze as if trying to keep from passing gas. Next, contract the vagina as if trying not to lose a tampon. Then, proceed forward as if trying to stop urinating. Hold the tension while slowly counting to three. Then slowly release the tension. Repeat five to ten times. You should feel a "lift" inside you. Be sure to breathe smoothly and comfortably and do not tense your stomach, thigh, or buttock muscles; otherwise, you may be exercising the wrong muscles. Check your abdomen with your hand to make sure the stomach area is relaxed.

2) Repeat the first exercise while using a low stool to support the lower part of your legs. Raising your legs will help further relax the pelvic floor muscles for the exercise.

3) Repeat the first exercise while kneeling on the floor with your elbows resting on a cushion. In this position, the stomach muscles are completely relaxed. If you are unable to

kneel, roll up a blanket and place it under your groin while you lie on your stomach.

Another exercise is to lie on the floor on your back and lift one leg at a time. Over time, this tightens the pelvic floor muscles.

Aside from the exercises outlined above, resistive exercise can be applied to the sphincter muscles of the urethra and rectum to help restore continence. The term resistive exercise describes force exerted against a weight. In this case, the exercise is done with cones that are about the size of a tampon and that come in varying weights for use inside the vagina. When a cone is inserted, the sphincter muscles must contract in order to hold the weight and not let it drop. Over a few months, with the use of progressively heavier weights, the pelvic-floor muscles gradually get stronger. These weight sets are available from physicians, who can guide your use of the cones, or from medical supply stores. Be sure to carefully read and follow the accompanying instructions on proper use for best results. Start by holding in the lightest weight for 15 minutes, two times a day. Once successful at that weight, try the next heaviest weight for the same amount of time. Some versions of these cones come with an electronic biofeedback system, called a perineometer, which tells you the amount of pressure you're applying.

You can also try contracting the pelvic-floor muscles to pre-vent leakage when coughing or sneezing or when carrying or lifting something. To do this when lifting, stand close to the object to be lifted with your feet slightly apart, one foot just in front of the other. Then, bend your knees but keep your back straight. Lean forward slightly as you contract, or tighten, your pelvic muscles. Then lift the object.

Avoid bladder irritants. Experts are not entirely sure why some foods and beverages seem to irritate the bladder lining and, as a result, cause bladder leakage. Try eliminating the following substances from your diet, or at least decrease your intake of them to see if your urine control improves.
• Hot spices and the foods they are used in
• Tomato-based foods
• Sugars
• Chocolate
• Coffee
• Tea
• Acidic fruits and acidic fruit juices, such as grapefruit and tomato. (Surprisingly, orange juice is not an irritant, because it is metabolized by the body into a more alkaline, or less acidic, fluid before it reaches the bladder. Grape juice, cranberry juice, cherry juice, and apple juice do not irritate the bladder either and may, in

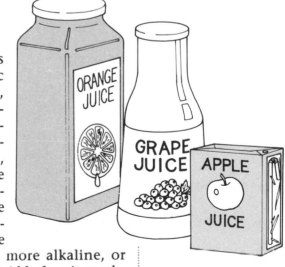

fact, control urine odor. Also, a few drops of lemon or lime juice added to a glass of water probably will not be enough to irritate the bladder.)
• Carbonated sodas—except seltzer, which is not highly carbonated
• Alcoholic beverages

Take precautions. Before going on a trip that will last more than an hour, empty your bladder completely whether you have the urge or not. After voiding, stand up and sit down again, and then lean forward to squeeze the abdomen and bladder to help make sure you have voided completely.

Plan an escape route. Some women's clothing—especially jumpsuits and bodysuits—can often be difficult to take off in a hurry. Don't wear bodysuits, or look for ones with a snapped opening at the crotch for quick-and-easy removal. Always bring a change of clothing with you just in case, and if an accident does stain your clothes, a three-hour soak in a mixture of one gallon of water and one cup of dishwashing detergent should remove any urine stains.

Don't be taken in by gimmicks. Be suspicious of exercise contraptions claiming to help decrease incontinence. A gadget that is advertised to tone the pelvic-floor muscles may actually exercise an unrelated muscle group, if it does anything at all. For example, the muscles of the pelvic floor will probably not benefit from an exerciser for use between the thighs. Don't waste your time and money if you're not sure whether a certain exerciser will help you with your incontinence problem.

Don't restrict your fluid intake. People who suffer from incontinence often limit their fluid intake. But cutting back on liquids may have the opposite effect to what's intended, since becoming dehydrated can lead to constipation, which in turn can irritate nearby nerves that will trigger the bladder to void.

Instead of cutting down the quantity of fluids you drink, schedule the times that you drink. You can regulate the fullness of your bladder by drinking liquids at set intervals, allowing you to better predict when you'll have to urinate.

A normal bladder holds about two cups of fluid; problem bladders may hold as little as a half-cup or as much as a quart and a half. If you can't sleep through the night because you have to go to the bathroom, try tapering off your fluid intake between dinner and bedtime, but try to get the recommended total fluid intake of six to ten eight-ounce cups a day before that.

Lose the spare tire. Obesity can interfere with bladder control, because the excess weight makes the muscles of the pelvic floor sag.

Say goodbye to cigarettes. Smoking has two adverse effects on bladder control: Nicotine irritates the bladder, and a smoker's cough can only cause problems for the person with stress incontinence.

Check your pharmacy. Many products are available at your drugstore to contain any accidents, whether urine or a bowel movement.

You can also buy external collecting devices for traveling or bedside use. They can make a long car trip more comfortable. Look for these devices at medical-supply stores and pharmacies or through medical-specialty mail order catalogs.

More good news: A urethral plug that can be inserted directly into the urethral opening should be available within the next year or two. This new product, already in use in Europe, will block the flow of urine during everyday activities.

Get some support. A free information packet to guide you to products and services for incontinent people is available by calling 1-800-BLADDER. This toll-free number is sponsored by Help for Incontinent People.

At the Doctor's

Since incontinence is often caused by an underlying medical condition, it's probably a good idea to talk to your doctor about any problems you have with bladder control. There are many medical treatments available, depending on the type and severity of incontinence you suffer from.

Most treatment regimens for women involve strengthening the muscles of the pelvic floor. While these muscles may be strengthened by exercise (see above), other methods, such as electrical pelvic-floor stimulation, may be more effective in severe cases. Sometimes, surgery is necessary to correct incontinence. There are also drugs used to treat certain types of medical conditions that cause incontinence.

When you do see the doctor, take along a list of any prescription or over-the-counter medicines you have been taking, because some medications can cause incontinence. You can also aid your physician's diagnosis by bringing along a diary of your urinary and leakage patterns. The diary should include the time of day of urination or leakage; the type and amount of fluid intake that preceded it; the amount voided in ounces (pharmacies carry measuring devices that fit right inside the toilet bowl); the amount of leakage (small, medium, or large); the activity engaged in when leakage occurred; and whether or not an urge to urinate was present. Keep such a diary for at least four days before you see your doctor.

Sources: **Katherine F. Jeter, Ed.D., E.T.,** Executive Director, Help for Incontinent People, Union, South Carolina. **Peter K. Sand, M.D.,** Associate Professor of Obstetrics and Gynecology, Northwestern University School of Medicine; Director, Evanston Continence Center, Evanston Hospital, Evanston, Illinois. **Thelma Wells, Ph.D., R.N., F.A.A.N., F.R.C.N.,** Professor of Nursing, University of Rochester School of Nursing, Rochester, New York.

○INFERTILITY

How to Improve Your Chances of Becoming Pregnant

THEY SAY THERE'S A BABY BOOM GOING on. And, since you've turned to this page, chances are you plan on joining the crowd of proud, diaper-changing, sleep-deprived new parents. The statistics stack up in your favor: About 85 percent of all couples who try to conceive will succeed within one year. More than one-fifth of the women will get pregnant within the first month of trying.

However, the plan of action is not always foolproof. Things can go wrong along the way, interfering with the process of conception, where the sperm unites with the egg and forms the embryo.

The definition of infertility is a couple who, with proper frequency of adequate sexual intercourse, does not conceive after one year of trying. The problems can range from a man having defective sperm or a low sperm count to a woman who doesn't produce eggs, has a deformed uterus, or whose fallopian tubes are blocked, preventing the egg's passage into the uterus.

This chapter does not attempt to address or remedy the various reasons for infertility. No at-home treatment can compete with the tremendous advances of medicine in this area. In general, the experts interviewed for this chapter recommended that couples try the steps outlined below for one year to maximize their chances of conception. After that time, they recommend seeking medical help.

There are some women who should see a physician before the one-year mark, however. This includes those who are over 40; these women should probably get a doctor's advice before trying to con-ceive in the first place. Women over 35 should see a physician if they haven't conceived after six months of trying. You should also see a doctor before the year is up if you have reason to believe that you may have had some damage to your reproductive tract as a result of an infection, if you have irregular periods or no periods at all, if you notice milk coming from your breasts but are not nursing a child, or if you have had an operation on your reproductive tract (the latter goes for your partner, too).

Keep in mind that your chances of conceiving are extremely high. Most of all, do not become discouraged. Hundreds of thousands of couples who thought they could not conceive are now parents. With any luck, you will be, too.

AT-HOME TREATMENT

The following tips will help increase your chances of getting pregnant. Good luck!

Get a clean bill of health. If you've decided you want to get pregnant, your first step should be a thorough physical examination. Your doctor will need to check for any physical problems, such as masses or cysts in the pelvic area. You should also make sure that you don't have any sexually transmitted diseases or low-grade vaginal infections. Ovarian cysts, fibroids, and endometriosis, an inflammation of the lining of the uterus, can all interfere with pregnancy.

Calculate the date of ovulation. The woman's egg must be fertilized within 24 hours after its release from the ovary. The man's sperm can survive in the woman's reproductive tract for 48 to 72 hours. To ensure that the egg and sperm will have a chance of coming together to create an embryo, a couple must try to have sex at least every 72 hours around the time of ovulation. Every 48 hours is even better. However, the man's sperm count may drop too low if he ejaculates more than once every 48 hours.

You maximize your chances of getting pregnant by calculating your approximate date of ovulation and concentrating your attempts at getting pregnant around that date. There are four methods of estimating the ovulation date.

The first technique is dubbed the calendar method. It involves figuring out the length of your menstrual cycle and making an educated guess about the approximate date of ovulation. The average woman ovulates 14 days before the onset of her next menstrual period, making the time fairly simple to calculate. In a 28-day cycle, for example, ovulation would occur on day 14 (the cycle starts with day one, the first day of menstrual flow). In a 35-day cycle, ovulation would occur on day 21. In a 21-day cycle, ovulation would occur on day 7, and so on.

Start by charting your period for three months. Add five days before and three days after the approximate date of ovulation in your longest cycle. If you have sex every 48 hours within this period, you'll probably be on target. Of course, this method may not be helpful if your periods are irregular.

The second method of ovulation prediction is called the basal body-temperature method. This requires a little more work on your part than the calendar method. You keep track of your basal body temperature every day for a few months (basal body temperature is your body temperature before you get out of bed in the morning). This method is based on the fact that your body temperature will rise slightly around the time of ovulation. After a few months of keeping track of your basal body temperature, you will soon be able to predict which days of your cycle you will be most fertile. A rise of one degree Fahrenheit means that ovulation is near. Your best bet for conceiving is to have intercourse every 48 hours for a few days on either side of the expected date of ovulation. Basal body thermometers, which have more markings and are easier to read than standard thermometers, are available at most pharmacies.

The third method is the mucus method of ovulation prediction. This requires you to study your vaginal secretions throughout the month (some women may feel a little squeamish about this). Right before ovulation occurs, the vaginal mucus becomes more slippery, profuse, and stretchy, telling you that it's time to begin having intercourse every 48 hours. Continue until about three days after the slippery-mucus phase has ended.

Finally, you can buy an ovulation-prediction test kit at your local pharmacy or drugstore. These are relatively effective, but they are also expensive (some run as high as $25 per kit, and you may need more than one kit per cycle).

Keep up the supply. While men should have sex no more often than once every 48 hours to keep up their sperm count,

they should also try to ejaculate at least once every two to three days throughout the month. Less frequent ejaculation may also cause the sperm count to drop.

Try clean living. A generally healthy lifestyle is perhaps the best way to enhance your chances of getting pregnant. This is also the best thing for the health of your baby.

Relax. Severe stress can interfere with reproductive function. When you're under too much stress, your sex drive suffers. In an extreme case, you may stop menstruating. Try exercise, meditation, yoga, or anything that helps you ease stress.

Tell your partner to chill out. Extreme heat is sperm's enemy. Heat kills sperm. (That's one of the reasons the testicles are outside of the body—to keep them cool.) Your partner may want to switch to boxer shorts, if he finds them comfortable. He should also avoid hot tubs and whirlpools. Beaded seat covers may benefit taxicab and truck drivers because they allow air to circulate. Testicular varicose veins can also increase temperature; your partner should check with a urologist if he suspects this problem.

Savor the afterglow. You might try to relax and linger in bed for half an hour after sex. Staying horizontal will minimize any leakage of sperm from the vagina. This tip may not really make much of a difference, but it certainly can't hurt

13 STEPS TO MOTHERHOOD

- Get a thorough physical examination before trying to conceive.
- Have sex at least every 72 hours for five days before and three days after your estimated ovulation date.
- Have sex at least once every two to three days throughout the month, but not more often than once every 48 hours.
- Maintain a healthy lifestyle.
- Eliminate excess stress from your life.
- Give your partner advice about keeping his testicles cool.
- Remain lying down for a half-hour after sex.
- Place a pillow underneath your hips after intercourse.
- Don't smoke cigarettes.
- Eliminate as many medications as you can.
- Avoid the use of vaginal lubricants if possible.
- Have sex in the "missionary" position.
- Try not to become overly obsessed with your efforts.

your chances of getting pregnant or your relationship with your partner—if he stays there with you.

Defy gravity's pull. Placing a pillow under your hips after intercourse may also prevent sperm leakage. Like lying down for a half-hour, this has not been proven to be effective—but it can't hurt.

Quit smoking. Cigarette smoking can lower a man's sperm count and interfere with a woman's fertility. Also, if you do become pregnant, a developing embryo may be harmed by your smoking—even in the first few days after conception. So, the sooner the two of you quit, the better.

Check your medications. Many medications can impair fertility. This includes some common over-the-counter analgesics. Eliminate those that you can and check with your doctor about any prescription drugs that you are taking.

Don't lubricate. Some products designed to lubricate the vagina may be impeding your efforts to get pregnant. Certain gels, liquids, and suppositories can impair the sperm's ability to move through the woman's reproductive tract and fertilize the egg. If you really need a lubricant, your physician can tell you which products are not detrimental.

Be conventional. The "missionary" position, with the man on top, minimizes sperm leakage from the vagina. It may not provide a tremendous fertility boost, but it certainly won't do any damage.

Keep it light. Of course, you are trying to conceive, but don't try too hard. Worrying and fretting about it can take over your lives, ruin your lovemaking, and add stress to your relationship—all of which can be counterproductive to your efforts.

Sources: William C. Andrews, M.D., Executive Director, American Fertility Society; Professor of Obstetrics and Gynecology, Eastern Virginia Medical School, Norfolk, Virginia. **Paul A. Bergh, M.D.,** Assistant Professor of Obstetrics and Gynecology, Division of Reproductive Endocrinology, Mount Sinai Medical Center, New York, New York. **Edmond Confino, M.D.,** Associate Professor, Director of Gynecology, Department of Obstetrics and Gynecology, Mount Sinai Hospital Medical Center, Chicago, Illinois. **Sanford M. Markham, M.D.,** Assistant Professor of Obstetrics and Gynecology, Georgetown University Medical Center, Washington, D.C.. **Richard J. Paulson, M.D.,** Associate Professor of Obstetrics and Gynecology, Director, In Vitro Fertilization Program, University of Southern California School of Medicine, Los Angeles, California.

•INGROWN TOENAILS

Easing the

Pain

YOU BOUGHT A NEW PAIR OF HIKING boots for a trip with some friends. As you walk along, your new boots feel tighter and tighter as your feet swell. Your big toe begins to hurt. At the five-mile point, you're limping, and you stop to check your feet. The nail of your big toe has pressed into the inner soft tissue on either side of the toenail bed, which is now reddish-blue. The toe is swollen and there's pus coming from the side of your toenail.

Better call off your hike. You've got an ingrown toenail, a common infection of the tissue surrounding the toenail. The good news is that most ingrown toenails can be relieved with a minimum of pain and discomfort. The bad news is that if you don't treat your nail infection properly, it can lead to more serious complications.

CAUSES

Ingrown toenails occur when the sharp edge of a toenail cuts into the skin walls surrounding it. They're usually caused by cutting the nail too short on the sides. Ingrown toenails can also be caused by an injury to the toenail, improperly fitting shoes, or an inherited nail deformity.

Real problems can develop when bacteria enter the toe wound and an infection develops. This can cause pain, swelling, inflammation, and sometimes an abscess.

AT-HOME TREATMENT

Once you've developed an ingrown toenail, you need to treat it promptly to prevent an infection. If you are diabetic or have vascular disease or some other condition that affects circulation, don't try to self-treat your ingrown toenail; see your doctor.

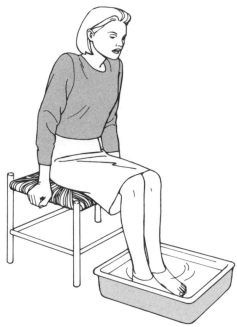

Go for the soak. You can relieve soreness by soaking your foot in warm (not hot) water with Epsom salts (one to two teaspoonfuls of Epsom salts to one quart of water). Soak your feet for five to ten minutes, once or twice a day.

Another excellent foot soak that works against bacteria and inflammation is Domeboro. It's available over the counter in pharmacies. Soaking in this solution for 20 to 30 minutes each night can help bring down inflammation enough so that the nail can grow out naturally.

Try topical. Antibiotic topical ointments like Neosporin applied to the wound can help, too.

Take off your surgical hat. You're not a foot surgeon, so forget bathroom toe surgery. The instruments you would use are probably contaminated with bacteria, so you run the risk of introducing more bacteria into your wound or otherwise complicating the situation.

Forget "V" surgery. An old home remedy suggests cutting a "V" at the top center of the nail. It's supposed to relieve the pressure. Forget it. Nails grow from the bottom, not the top. You'll just end up with a silly-looking nail that's ingrown and maybe a worse infection.

Change your shoes. If you've developed an ingrown toenail, you're going to want shoes that give your toes plenty of room and don't put pressure on your injury. One option is open-toed shoes or sandals. Airy footwear allows your ailing toe to breathe, which will help your infection heal.

PREVENTION

You can prevent ingrown toenails and avoid the hassles they cause. Try these tips:

Cut straight. People who cut their toenails in a rounded or angled fashion are asking for ingrown toenails. Cut your toenails straight across. If needed, use a file to soften sharp corners.

Watch out for short cuts. Another mistake is cutting nails too short. Skin can get pushed up in front of the toenail when you stand, so the nail can imbed itself into the skin when it grows out. Get in the habit of cutting the nail longer, at least to the end of the skin, not below the end of the toe.

Grab your toe guards. Some ingrown toenails result from injuries to the toenails. If you lose your nail as a result of an injury, the nail may grow inward when it comes back. Wear shoes to protect your feet.

---

6 TIPS FOR PROTECTING YOUR TOES

- Cut your nails straight across.
- Don't cut your nails too short.
- Protect your feet with proper shoes.
- Be careful not to stub your toes.
- Be careful with pedicures.
- Wear shoes that fit.

If you're working in dangerous conditions, wear steel-toed boots to keep your tootsies safe.

Watch where you're going. Everybody has "stubbed" a toe before. It hurts like the devil and can make the nail grow in thicker, causing an ingrown condition.

Say "no" to some pedicures. A pedicure can be luxurious, but be sure your technician is trained and uses proper instruments. Don't let him or her use metallic instruments to remove skin from your toes. Pumice stones are safe.

Wear shoes that fit. Women often suffer from ingrown toenails because they wear tight-fitting shoes that pinch the toes or heels that push the toes into pointed toe boxes. Buy shoes that are long enough and have plenty of room in the toe area. Try not to wear heels higher than an inch.

Sources: **Raymond Merkin, D.P.M.,** Podiatrist, Rockville, Maryland. **Rock G. Positano, D.P.M., M.Sc., N.P.H., F.A.C.P.R.,** Codirector, Foot and Ankle Orthopedic Institute, Hospital for Special Surgery, New York, New York. **Donald Skwor, D.P.M.,** Past President, American Podiatric Medical Association; Podiatrist, Memphis, Tennessee.

●INSOMNIA

How to Get a

Better Night's

Sleep

YOU'VE COUNTED SHEEP, PORSCHES, and ceiling tiles. You've counted backward from 1,000 and made it all the way to zero. You've gone over tomorrow's business presentation in your mind five times. You've even tried to psych yourself out by telling yourself: "I don't need sleep. I can function perfectly well without it." It didn't work. Nothing worked. You're still awake—and the sun is beginning to peek over the horizon.

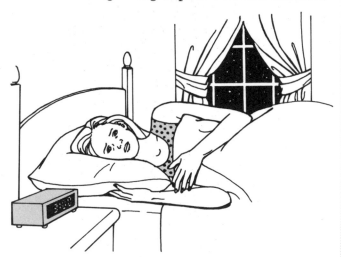

Insomnia is the most common sleep disorder in North America and in Europe. One-third of the people in the United States are not getting enough sleep at night to function well the next day. Half of those people only have one or two bad nights a week. The other half lie awake staring at the ceiling night after night, and spend their days yawning and tired.

CAUSES

Insomnia is one of the least understood sleep disorders. Sleep experts often speak of the frustration they experience at not being able to help many of the patients who come to them, desperate for a little shut-eye.

Almost anything can cause insomnia. Some of the more common culprits are poor sleep habits, too much caffeine, depression, anxiety, certain medications, restless leg syndrome (chronic leg twitches), alcohol, and drugs.

AT-HOME TREATMENT

After nights of not sleeping, many insomniacs get into bed with a sense of dread. They have developed a fear of not being able to sleep. This can set up a catch-22 situation, where the fear of not sleeping actually begins to keep you awake. This type of insomnia can escalate into a nightly problem that may last weeks, months, or years. The tips that follow were designed to break you out of this cycle, or to put a stop to your insomnia before it gets underway. These suggestions should put you on the road to better sleep—starting tonight.

Don't torture yourself. Tossing and turning and allowing your frustration to build is the worst thing to do. If you can't sleep, read in bed, watch television, just do something restful. Even without falling asleep, lying comfortably in bed all night allows your body to recover as much as if you had slept. Your brain won't get its needed rest, but if your body is recovered, you're still better off than if you spend the night staring at the clock and agonizing. You might even consider putting the clock out of view.

Get good and sleepy. One cardinal rule for insomniacs: Don't nap. If you do, you'll have more trouble sleeping the next night, continuing the cycle of insomnia. For the same reason, you shouldn't stay in bed late the morning after you had trouble sleeping. Even if you drag a bit during the day, it's better to let yourself get good and sleepy.

Try not to worry about it. You may have some misconceptions about sleep that make you fret about your insomnia, making it harder for you to sleep. For example, often when you wake up out of what seems like a deep sleep, you feel wide awake. Because you feel so wide awake, you think you're through sleeping for the night. This is usually not the case. You feel so alert because your insomnia has woken you from your REM stage (REM stands for Rapid Eye Movement, the stage of sleep in which you dream). At this point in your sleep cycle, your brain is very active. Just relax and give it about 30 minutes; you will probably fall back to sleep quite easily. Oftentimes when you wake up, you feel as though you never slept at all. Actually, most people sleep longer than they think. So you may be better rested than you realize.

Block out the noise. It's possible that you are being repeatedly awakened by loud noises. In many cases, you're not aware of what woke you up—you just know that you're awake again. If you live near an airport or a busy freeway, this could be your problem. Cut down ambient noise as much as you can.

Failing that, invest in a good pair of earplugs.

Try a sleeping pill. Don't be ashamed to ask your doctor for a prescription sleeping pill, or check your pharmacy for an over-the-counter remedy. Do not, however, use prescription pills for more than a month at a time. Also, avoid them if you are at high altitudes, because your insomnia may be a sign that you are having trouble breathing and need more oxygen. Sleeping pills, which slow your breathing rate even further, can increase your oxygen debt and may be dangerous. (If you often suffer insomnia at high altitudes, your doctor can prescribe a medication called Diamox.)

Your doctor may not be in favor of over-the-counter sleeping pills. They can have side effects. Some sleep aids contain antihistamines that dry out your mucous membranes and make you drowsy the next day. Pregnant or nursing women and women with a serious medical problem should consult their doctor before taking any drugs. You should also know that if you snore, sleep medications may make it worse. Also if you suffer from sleep apnea, or labored breathing during sleep, sleeping pills can be dangerous.

Finally, only take sleeping pills before you go to bed. Don't pop one when you wake in the middle of the night, because the effect will last well into the next day.

Check your comfort level. An uncomfortable bed may keep waking you and you probably don't realize it. Soft beds are more forgiving and usually better for sleeping than firm ones.

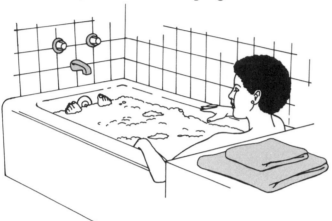

Soak yourself to sleep. Try taking a 20-minute hot bath two hours before bedtime to relax your body and make it ready for sleep. Don't wait until right before bedtime, because a bath can actually be temporarily stimulating and delay sleep. Make this soaking bath really hot, like a hot tub, but remember, do not bathe in very hot water if you are pregnant or have any significant health problems.

Teetotal it at bedtime. A drink may seem like a good idea just before bed, since alcohol can make you feel drowsy and may actually put you to sleep. Unfortunately, you'll probably pay for it later when you wake up in the night with a headache, a full bladder, or an upset stomach. Even worse, alcohol's sedative effect only lasts a short time, and then there is a rebound effect that actually makes you more likely to have trouble going back to sleep.

No caffeine after the sun's over the yardarm. Of course you know that too much coffee, tea, or soda with caffeine can keep you up at night. Limit your caffeine intake to two cups of coffee or other caffeine-containing beverage in the morning and don't have any after noon.

Let your bed do its job. Regularity is important to help you get to sleep. That is why you should associate your bed—and only your bed—with sleep. So don't move to the couch or to the guest-room bed to try to get to sleep. Even animals seem to choose the same location for sleeping every night.

Same time to bed, same time to rise. Sleep specialists agree that sticking to a specific sleep schedule, even on weekends, may be the crucial rule for insomniacs. It's best to try to get your body onto a schedule, so that it will expect sleep at the same time every day. Get up at your usual time each day and resist the temptation to nap, even if you didn't get a wink of sleep the night before. The next night you'll be ready for a good night's sleep.

Leave your work at the bedroom door. If you bring work to bed, you're in danger of forming unpleasant, anxiety-provoking associations with your bed. It's important to have positive, restful associations with your bed. Reading a book and watching television are good, relaxing bedtime activities. (Of course, sex is also an acceptable activity for bedtime, and it may even help you get to sleep afterward.)

Make bedtime a ritual. For children, bedtime stories or bedtime baths are the signal that it is now time for sleep. Parents reinforce this behavior by ritualizing the bedtime process and sticking to it. Ritual may also be helpful for adults—especially for insomniacs, who tend to have problems relaxing prior to bedtime, since they are worried about not sleeping. You can try meditation, relaxation exercises (such as tensing, then relaxing, each muscle in sequence), or listening to relaxing music. Repeat your ritual every night before you retire.

Try an old favorite. Drinking warm milk or a malted-milk drink before bed won't necessarily make you drowsy, but it can be comforting and help you get into the mood for sleep. Unless you are allergic to milk or are lactose intolerant, give it a try; it can't hurt.

Get out of bed. One piece of advice that sleep experts give their patients is to cut the amount of time they spend in bed. About 90 percent of people spend too much time in bed, they say. As you lengthen the time you spend in bed, your sleep is spread thinner and becomes less efficient. If you only need seven hours of sleep, but you sleep for ten hours, you'll be more tired than if you had slept for only seven hours, because your sleep will not have been high quality. For one week, try staying in bed for two hours less than you do now; this may improve the restorative power of your sleep, making you feel more rested in less time.

Check your medications. Some prescription medications may keep you awake at night. Drugs prescribed for asthma, thyroid problems, and other conditions may be responsible for your sleep problem. Ask your doctor about any medications that you are taking.

Try everything. Not everyone has the same way of falling asleep; there is no right or wrong method. The key is not to give up too soon. You should stick with any technique you try for at least a week or two, not just one night. Be your own sleep scientist, and see what works for you. Think back to before you had a problem with insomnia; try to remember how much you used to sleep and what helped you get to sleep. You can also try keeping a sleep log to help you keep track of what you've tried and what works.

Don't try to sleep. Falling asleep is something that requires the opposite of effort. Effort is work, and work keeps you awake. The harder you try, the harder it will be. Don't struggle to get to sleep; simply lie still, relax, and let sleep come.

Cool down. High-quality sleep requires a lower body temperature than waking hours. A lack of proper body-temperature regulation may be the cause of insomnia in many people. Try lowering your body temperature artificially. You might want to try keeping the bedroom a little cooler than the rest of the house. A hot bath taken about two hours before bedtime can do the trick because after your body's temperature has been raised, it drops back down within a couple of hours. Exercising at least six hours before bedtime will also lower your body temperature just in time for sleep.

Have a midnight snack. Maybe your mother told you that eating before you go to bed will give you nightmares, but mom's not always right. In fact, going to bed on a full stomach may actually help you sleep. This could help explain the powerful urge to nod off after a big holiday dinner.

Rethink how much sleep you need. It is thought that on average, adults need eight hours of sleep per night. However, sleep researchers agree that this is not the case for everyone; different individuals have very different sleep needs. Interestingly, the amount each person needs remains amazingly constant. One expert tells the story of a 70-year-old nurse who slept only one hour each night, took no naps during the day, and said that she never felt tired. In fact, she said she didn't understand why other people wasted so much time in bed. She had averaged the same amount of sleep each night since she was a child. Other people may need 9, 10, or even 11 hours of sleep per night. There is no "norm."

Studies demonstrate that people can think just as well if they have slept well or if they have been sleep deprived. The problems come when people are worried about how little they sleep. If you sleep for 90 minutes and when you wake up you are told that you have

---

22 TIPS TO HELP YOU GET YOUR "ZZZZZS"

- Pass sleepless hours reading in bed, watching television, or relaxing.
- Don't take naps.
- Keep your mind off the problem as much as possible.
- Cut down ambient noise or use earplugs.
- Take a prescription or over-the-counter sleeping pill.
- Invest in a comfortable bed.
- Don't drink alcohol before bed.
- Have no more than two cups of caffeine-containing beverages per day, and drink them before noon.
- Sleep only in your bed.
- Try to go to sleep and get up at the same time every day.
- Never work in bed.
- Take a hot bath two hours before bedtime.
- Develop a nightly relaxation ritual.
- Drink a cup of warm milk before bed.
- Stay in bed for fewer hours every night.
- Find out whether your medication could be causing the problem.
- Use trial and error to find out what works for you.
- Don't try to go to sleep, just let it come.
- Lower the temperature in your bedroom.
- Exercise six hours before bedtime.
- Eat something before you go to bed.
- Change your perception of how much sleep you really need.

slept for eight hours, you will feel great. But if you sleep for eight hours and are told that you have only slept for 45 minutes, you'll feel exhausted.

The point is: You may not need as much sleep as you think you do. Let your body, not your perception, be your guide.

AT THE DOCTOR'S

Most garden-variety cases of insomnia can be greatly helped with the tips in this chapter. Try them out, and see what works for you. If nothing has helped after six months, consult your doctor for a recommendation for a sleep clinic near you, or call the National Sleep Foundation at 213-288-0466 for a referral to a sleep specialist.

A sleep specialist will ask you questions about your lifestyle and sleeping habits. She may ask you to stay overnight in a sleep laboratory, where she can observe you and, possibly, monitor your brain waves as you slumber (or toss and turn, as the case may be). She will probably ask you to make certain changes in your lifestyle. If you need them, she may prescribe sleeping pills for use on a short-term basis.

Sources: **Karl Doghramji, M.D.**, Director, Sleep Disorders Center, Jefferson Medical College, Thomas Jefferson University, Philadelphia, Pennsylvania. **J. Christian Gillin, M.D.**, Professor of Psychiatry, Director, Mental Health Clinical Research Center, University of California at San Diego; Staff Psychiatrist, Veterans Administration Medical Center; Adjunct Professor in the Department of Psychology, San Diego State University, San Diego, California. **Peter Hauri, Ph.D.**, Author, *No More Sleepless Nights*; Professor of Psychology, Director, Mayo Clinic Insomnia Program, Rochester, Minnesota. **German Nino-Murcia, M.D.**, Founder and Medical Director, Sleep Medicine and Neuroscience Institute, Palo Alto, California.

⊙Irritable Bowel Syndrome

Fend Off the

Abominable

Abdominal

You never know when it's going to hit—just when you're sitting down to a meal with friends, right before a big presentation to your board of directors, as you meet someone special for that first date. The unpleasant constipation, diarrhea, bloating, and cramping of irritable bowel syndrome often comes without warning and seemingly at the worst times.

Irritable bowel syndrome, also known as IBS, is one of those personal health problems most of us have difficulty talking about with anyone, even our doctor. You may find some comfort in the fact that an estimated 40 million people suffer from it. In fact, the National Institutes of Health in Bethesda, Maryland, say that as many as half the people who complain of a digestive disorder probably have irritable bowel syndrome. For unknown reasons, women tend to experience IBS more often than men do and often suffer more symptoms around their menstrual periods.

Symptoms

IBS, which is also often called "spastic colon," "mucous colitis," and "functional bowel disorder," isn't a disease, but a collection of symptoms that includes both constipation and diarrhea, often alternating. Other symptoms may include gas, bloating, nausea, headache, and fatigue.

Doctors classify IBS into two types. The first, spastic colon, is characterized by cramps, or a dull aching in the lower abdomen that often begins before a meal and disappears after a bowel movement. The second type features diarrhea and an urgent need to defecate, particularly after a meal or on awakening at night.

Causes

Doctors aren't sure what causes or what cures irritable bowel syndrome. Normally, after you eat and your food has been digested, the remains pass in liquid form into the large intestine (also known as the colon or bowel). It's here that most of the water is removed. Then the semi-solid waste products move via a wavelike action called "peristalsis" into the rectum and out the anus. In IBS, peristalsis does not function properly. In a normal colon, the wavelike action is gentle, rarely noticeable. However, with IBS, the contractions become uncoordinated—sometimes forceful, other times weak. The result is pain, cramping, diarrhea, constipation, and other symptoms.

IBS can be particularly frustrating because people who have it often go through extensive—and expensive—tests, X rays, and invasive exams only to be told, "We don't know what's causing the problem." Their colons usually look normal, without ulcers, polyps, tumors, or other structural problems.

Doctors believe irritable bowel syndrome does have an emotional component. Feelings of nervousness, anxiety, guilt, depression, or anger may bring on or aggravate IBS symptoms. Other possible causes include foods such as coffee and raw fruits and vegetables, drugs such as hormones, overuse of laxatives, and intolerance of milk sugar (lactose intolerance).

At-Home Treatment

Since doctors often can't help with IBS, it's up to you to treat your symptoms with home remedies. Once you've had your symptoms diagnosed by a physician, these remedies can help you:

Keep track. Play detective in order to discover what's causing your IBS symptoms. For about two weeks, keep a diary: your moods, foods you eat, stress you may be under, and digestive distress. Be sure to include notes about where you are in your menstrual cycle. After a couple of weeks, review your diary and see if you detect any patterns. Do your symptoms come on after you eat certain foods? Do you notice an increase in symptoms when you're under certain stresses? What seems to make symptoms better or worse?

Foods that are common problems for IBS sufferers include: milk (for those with lactose intolerance), gas-producing foods such as cole vegetables, spicy foods, wheat products, citrus fruits, sugar, chocolate, and foods artificially sweetened with sorbitol.

Take a break. Stress is part of life and a certain amount of it is productive and healthy. However, if stress is exacerbating your IBS symptoms—and more than one in three IBS sufferers say it does—consider it a clue that you're not managing your stress as well as you could.

Often people aren't even aware that they're feeling stressed. When you're stressed, your muscles tense. Improve your awareness and learn to relax your muscles using pro-gressive relaxation: Sit in a quiet place where you won't be disturbed. Close your eyes and, beginning with your face, tense and relax each muscle group in your body. Try practicing progressive relaxation for ten or 15 minutes, twice a day, or whenever you feel tense.

Progressive relaxation is just one of many stress management techniques. You might also try meditation, yoga, biofeedback, visualization, relaxation tapes, deep "belly" breathing, or other techniques. Try several and see what works best for you.

Exercise regularly. When you're afraid to get too far from a bathroom, exercise is probably the last thing on your mind. But a regular program of moderate exercise can help the digestive system work more efficiently by increasing peristalsis motility. It can also help you manage stress and give you a more positive outlook.

Loosen up. Negative attitudes can have disastrous results on the digestive system. Examine your own attitudes. Do you see the world in absolutes? Do you demand perfection from yourself and others? Are you hostile or critical? What fears and concerns are keeping you stuck in negative attitudes? You may want to seek help from a pro-

19 Tips for Keeping IBS at Bay

- Keep an IBS diary.
- Manage your stress.
- Eliminate negative attitudes.
- Exercise regularly.
- Chew your food thoroughly and eat more slowly.
- Eat small meals more frequently.
- Increase your dietary fiber.
- Cut out caffeine.
- Decrease the fat in your diet.
- Don't eat gas-producing foods.
- Be careful with spicy foods.
- Quit smoking.
- Try hot baths or heating pads to relieve abdominal pain.
- Don't delay going to the bathroom.
- Find out whether you are lactose intolerant.
- Cut out sorbitol.
- Limit your alcohol intake.
- Don't reach for laxatives.
- Get support.

fessional counselor to help you make some positive changes in your mental outlook.

Don't gobble your food. Eat slowly and chew your food thoroughly. Gobbling food can make you swallow air, which can cause gas. Chewing gum can have the same effect.

Eat less, more often. Smaller, more frequent meals are easier on the digestive system.

Load up on the fiber. Fiber can help normalize bowel movements by increasing the bulk and softening hard stools and by absorbing excess water in loose stools. Cereals and breads made from whole grains and fresh fruits and vegetables are excellent sources of fiber. However, increase your fiber intake slowly. Increasing fiber too quickly can cause gas, cramping, and bloating. Additional gas that you may experience when you up your fiber intake should go away within two to four weeks. Be sure to drink plenty of water to keep the fiber moving efficiently through your digestive tract.

Nix the caffeine. When you've got IBS, you don't need to stimulate your digestive tract, which is what caffeinated coffee does. It can also cause heartburn and abdominal cramping. Caffeine is found in coffee, black tea, chocolate, some sodas, and some herbal teas like mate and guarana.

Cut the fat. Dietary fat is difficult for the body to digest. Steer clear of high-fat foods like butter, heavy cream, hot dogs, sausage and other fatty meats, pizza, and fast foods. Eat a low-fat, high-fiber diet.

Turn off the gas. For some IBS sufferers, gas and bloating is a problem. If you're bothered by flatulence, you don't need to compound your problem by eating gas-producing foods. Stay away from onions, broccoli, brussels sprouts, cabbage, red and green peppers, and carbonated beverages, along with any other offending foods you've identified in your food diary.

Watch the spice. You may find that a plate of spicy Mexican or Asian food is just what your digestive tract doesn't need. Some spices can aggravate the digestive tract and stomach lining. Pay attention to which spices worsen your symptoms and eliminate them from your diet.

Heat it up. If you have abdominal cramping, try taking a hot bath or applying a heating pad to the lower abdomen to relieve the pain.

Go when the urge strikes. Don't wait if you feel the urge to go to the bathroom. Delaying may cause constipation.

Lay off dairy. As nursing babies, our bodies produce an enzyme called lactase that enables us to digest our mother's milk. After we are weaned, unlike many other mammals, we continue to drink milk and consume dairy products. The problem is that some of us are no longer able to digest milk sugar (lactose). If you suspect that you are one of those people, read the chapter on lactose intolerance and talk to your doctor. Until you are certain, consider laying off dairy products for a while, since they cause symptoms similar to IBS in lactose-intolerant people.

Nix the sorbitol. Your irritable bowel symptoms may be due to an intolerance to the artificial sweetener sorbitol. Eliminate sorbitol from your diet (read labels carefully) and see if it helps.

Go easy on the booze. Alcohol in any quantity isn't good for any-one, but it can be a diarrhea disaster for someone with IBS. If you do drink, limit your alcohol consumption.

Quit smoking. Cigarette smoking irritates the digestive system and affects your normal digestive movement. Having IBS is another good reason to quit.

Forget the laxatives. Some people reach for laxatives to relieve the constipation of IBS. Don't do it! Laxatives, especially when overused, can make your IBS symptoms worse. If you abuse laxatives due to an eating disorder, get professional help.

Get support. Suffering from IBS can make you feel frustrated and alone. You're not alone! There are plenty of others who feel exactly as you do, and it helps to have their support. Call hospitals in your area to find a local IBS support group or write to the Intestinal Disease Foundation, Inc., Attn: HR, 1323 Forbes Ave., Suite 200, Pittsburgh, PA 15219, to find out how to start one.

Sources: **Barbara Greene**, Clinical Psychology Doctoral Candidate, State University of New York, Albany, New York. **Douglas A. Grossman**, **M.D.**, Professor of Medicine and Psychiatry, Division of Digestive Diseases, University of North Carolina, Chapel Hill, North Carolina. **Gary R. Lichtenstein, M.D.**, Assistant Professor of Medicine, University of Pennsylvania School of Medicine, Philadelphia, Pennsylvania. **Suzanne Rose, M.D.**, Assistant Professor of Medicine, University of Pittsburgh Medical Center, Pittsburgh, Pennsylvania. **William Whitehead, Ph.D.**, Professor of Medical Psychology, Johns Hopkins University School of Medicine, Baltimore, Maryland.

•Knee Pain

How to Get

Rid of It—for

Good

Knees are one of those things we often take for granted. And it's not as though we don't use them; we do—constantly. In fact, we tend to give these joints quite a beating, especially if we walk, run, ski, or use a stair climber for exercise. But it's not until they start grinding, clicking, or aching that we remember that they're there. Even then, sometimes we try to ignore the pain until it grows so intense that we just can't ignore it anymore.

Causes

Because of their complex design, the knees are one of the most injury-prone joints in the body. Unlike the more stable hip joint, which is a ball in a deeply cushioned socket, the knee joint is more exposed—and more vulnerable.

The knee joint consists essentially of two bones, one rounded and the other relatively flat. The thighbone (femur) ends in two rounded knobs (condyles), which sit on the relatively flat shinbone (tibia). The knee's other component is the kneecap, a small, rounded bone sitting in a groove between the thighbone and the knobby ends. The kneecap gives strength to the joint. As the knee bends and straightens, the kneecap slides up and down in the groove. A tendon attaches the kneecap to the thigh muscles above, and a ligament connects it to the shinbone below.

The kneecap acts like a pulley, increasing the power of the muscles attached to it. The upper and lower leg bones act like long levers on the joint, increasing power and force. A small change in the levers is magnified many times over in the knee. This intricate design can cause problems, especially for the kneecap, which accounts for about 20 percent of all knee pain, say knee experts.

It's not the alignment of the bones in the knee, but rather the alignment of the surrounding structures that keeps this complex joint functioning properly. The kneecap is pulled in different directions by the muscles, tendons, and ligaments around it. As long as all of these pull in just the right way, the kneecap moves back and forth smoothly in its track. If any one muscle, tendon, or ligament pulls too strongly or not hard enough, the kneecap is pulled out of its track and can no longer glide easily against the thighbone. This can cause pain and may even damage the kneecap.

Because women have wider hips than men, the upper-leg bone of a woman enters the knee at a greater angle, which twists the knee. This makes women more vulnerable to certain types of kneecap injuries, such as chondromalacia patella, in which the smooth layer of cartilage that undercoats the kneecap becomes roughened or cracked, resulting in chronic pain.

Other problems arise when the large muscles in the thigh (quadriceps) are inflexible due to disuse or lack of stretching before exercise or if these muscles are overused. In this case, inflammation of the knee tendons (patellar tendinitis), sometimes called "jumper's knee," can result. Difficulties can also come about when one group of muscles is stronger than another and pulls harder.

There are many other potential causes of knee problems, including injuries like falls, automobile accidents, and athletic injuries, or diseases like arthritis. But by far the majority of knee problems are caused by overstressing the joint. This may come in the form of increasing a certain type of exercise too quickly, or by putting the wrong type of force on the knee. Overuse injuries of the knee are also common. These generally come about when you do one type of exercise, such as high-impact aerobics, running, or climbing. Constant kneeling can cause the same problem.

AT-HOME TREATMENT

The following tips may help ease your pain and prevent it from returning:

Maintain a normal weight. Extra pounds put stress on all the body's joints, particularly the knees. With every step you take, you put one-and-a-half times your body weight on your knee. Running increases that to five times your body weight.

If you're twenty, thirty, forty, or more pounds overweight you might be adding a great deal to the stress on your knees. If you jog, for every 20 pounds that you are overweight, you're putting 100 pounds of extra force on each knee with each step. The additional force can increase the likelihood that knee pain will develop. If you are overweight, you will need extra muscle strength to prevent injuries.

Get some support from your feet. When your feet are not supporting you properly, it can cause problems all over your body, including your knees. One common cause of knee problems is overpronation, or excessive rolling inward of the foot. This rolling also rotates the lower leg and can throw your knee out of alignment. When the knee is misaligned, the kneecap tracks wrong and can grind, causing pain.

If overpronation is your problem, you can try supportive shoes designed to prevent pronation, or orthotics, which are special shoe inserts. Over-the-counter, preformed orthotics are available, or a podiatrist, orthopedist, chiropractor, or sports-medicine specialist can make one specifically for you.

Over-the-counter athletic insoles can also help to soften the blow of your foot's landing on hard ground. You can purchase them at an athletic-shoe store, sports-supply store, or even in some grocery stores.

Get your feet some support, too. Wearing the right shoe can help prevent many kinds of knee problems. You should wear the lowest heel possible—under one inch, if possible. Higher heels, which tend to throw the body forward, can cause your knee extra stress.

If you tend to overpronate, try to buy shoes that tout anti-pronation properties. Some athletic shoes have higher density materials on the inside edge of the sole, but softer, cushioning material on the outside edge. Because the inside edge will not "give," the shoe inhibits pronation.

A stiff heel counter, the part of the shoe that cups the heel, can also stabilize the heel and help prevent overpronation. And of course, you should look for a good fit (with at least a thumb's-width of room at the toe and the heel held firmly) and good cushioning (especially in the forefoot, for an aerobics shoe).

Don't get too worn out. That old running shoe may look fine, but the supportive structure inside may be worn out, leaving your foot—and by association, your knee—unsupported. After 400 to 600 miles, it's time to get new running shoes; walking shoes last a little longer—600 miles or more.

Keep yourself in line. Being bowlegged or knock-kneed could put you at greater risk for knee problems. You can check your alignment by standing with your ankles touching. Your ankle bones and your knees should touch. If your knees touch, but your ankles don't, you're knock-kneed. If your ankles touch, but your knees don't, you're bowlegged. If you are very far out of alignment, you may be better off avoiding certain activities that stress the knees. Instead of running, try swimming or working out on a cross-country ski machine for your exercise routine.

Be cautious about drugstore products. The only thing an over-the-counter knee brace does is remind you that your knee is injured and that you should avoid overtraining. It does not really correct or prevent problems. If you do use a knee brace, however, use the one-piece neoprene or elastic braces. The elastic wraps don't apply pressure to the knee evenly. Also, be careful that you don't become dependent on a knee brace. Besides, if you're in enough pain to go out and purchase a knee brace, you really should see a doctor about your problem.

---

18 WAYS TO LEAVE KNEE PAIN IN YOUR PAST

- **Shed excess body weight.**
- **Buy the right kind of shoes for your feet and for your activity.**
- **Try orthotics or athletic insoles.**
- **Replace running and walking shoes at appropriate intervals.**
- **Check your body's alignment.**
- **Avoid over-the-counter knee braces.**
- **Avoid deep knee bends, squats, and kneeling.**
- **Don't try to "run through" knee pain.**
- **Vary your running route, changing sides of the street frequently.**
- **Don't run on hard surfaces.**
- **Don't run downhill.**
- **Vary your physical activities.**
- **Use rest, ice, compression, and elevation.**
- **Take an over-the-counter analgesic or anti-inflammatory.**
- **Avoid heat during the first 48 to 72 hours following a knee injury.**
- **Get a professional massage.**
- **Do gentle exercises for muscles around the knees.**
- **Listen to your body's signals.**

Avoid the culprits. If you've got knee pain, you'd do well to avoid activities that stress the knee joints. Deep knee bends, pliés, and squats—especially with weights—are three of the worst. Kneeling on hard surfaces is another "no-no."

If you lift weights, try not to fully flex your knee, and keep the amount of weight you ask your knees to lift to a minimum. When you kneel (to do gardening, for example), use foam kneeling pads and take frequent breaks to rest your knees.

Don't be a stoic. Some people, especially athletes, believe that if you "run through" knee pain, it will work itself out. They are probably doing themselves more harm than good. When you feel pain, your body is trying to tell you something—listen to it. Don't continue to stress the part of your body that is in pain. Rest is how the body heals itself, not adding extra workload.

Change your running path. If you run the same route every day, you may be setting yourself up for knee problems. Roads are "canted," or slanted from the center. Running on the same side of the road can overstress the knees. Try running or walking on the flattest part of the road and switch sides frequently, if you can.

Soft-step it. Roads and sidewalks may be the most convenient surfaces on which to walk or jog, but concrete and asphalt can be too hard, increasing the

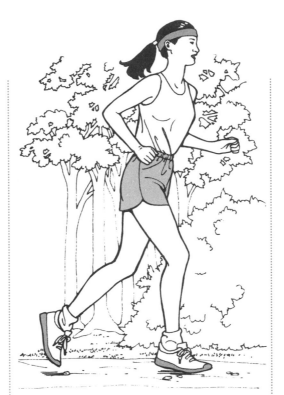

beating your knees take. The best surfaces are soft tracks and forest pathways. Avoid sand, however; it's too soft and can stress the knees.

Take an uphill route. Running or walking downhill is very hard on the knees, as well. Your knees tend to brake your momentum as you go downhill, a function that can overstress them. If you must go downhill, try to traverse down, but it's best to avoid downhill training altogether.

Cross-train. Too much repetitive action is a prime cause of knee problems. You strengthen one set of muscles, but not the counterbalancing muscles. Try to vary your exercise routine with numerous types of physical activities, rather than just one or two. Instead of just walking all the time, try biking, swimming, dancing, aerobics, weight training, or any other activity you might enjoy. If you choose biking as a regular exercise activity, raise the seat up so that your leg is almost fully extended on the downward stroke.

Try some advanced therapy. Let's say that you've gone ahead and overworked your knee, and now it hurts. Give it R.I.C.E.—rest, ice, compression, and elevation. First, take the weight off your knees. For the first 24 to 48 hours, use an ice pack (20 minutes on, 20 minutes off) to limit the swelling. Then, wrap your knee (not too tightly) in an elastic bandage and prop up that leg.

As far as icing goes, there are several options: You can freeze water in a paper cup and massage the area with it for the 20 minutes. You can also try icing the area with a bag of frozen vegetables, such as peas or corn kernels.

Get some OTC help. Over-the-counter analgesics, such as aspirin and ibuprofen (the ingredient found in Advil and Motrin-IB), are very effective in relieving knee pain. The reason is that these medications serve as anti-inflammatories, bringing down the swelling and inflammation that may come with knee injuries.

Acetaminophen, the ingredient found in Tylenol and Anacin-3, may ease the pain but probably won't do much for inflammation. However, you should stick to this drug if you have an ulcer, a bleeding condition, or a sensitive stomach, since anti-inflammatories can aggravate these conditions. Of course, if you are pregnant, nursing a baby, or have any special medical conditions, you should consult your doctor before taking any drugs, nonprescription or otherwise.

Stay cool. Cold prevents fluid buildup and swelling, but heat can promote it. Stick with cold treatments for the first 48 to 72 hours after a knee injury. Stay away from hot tubs and hot packs during this initial phase.

Get a rubdown. Even though a massage does not affect the bony structures of your knee, a rubdown can improve your circulation and loosen any tight muscles that surround the knee. If your knee is already in pain, you should only submit to a professional massage; don't just ask a friend to oblige.

Exercise your knees. Rest is the prescription for an injured knee. However, when the muscles around the knee become weak from disuse, the whole structure can become unstable and susceptible to future problems. Gentle exercises can break this cycle.

Exercises can also correct imbalances and increase flexibility. However, not just any exercise will do. Some exercises can be damaging to your knees. For example, avoid loading the knee with weight when it's in a fully flexed, 90-degree position, especially if you have kneecap pain. In fact, the only time your knee should be bearing any weight in a 90-degree, flexed position is when you're getting up from a chair.

Try performing these exercises regularly to improve the strength and flexibility of your knees:

1) Hamstring stretch. Lie on your back, raise your right leg, and hold the thigh up with your hands. Gently and slowly straighten the knee until you feel a stretch in the back of the thigh. Don't bounce. Hold the stretch for 10 to 20 seconds. Repeat three to five times on each leg.

You can also perform this hamstring stretch in a standing position with your leg on a chair. Slowly lean forward, reaching down the shin until you feel a stretch in the back of the thigh. Hold for 10 to 20 seconds.

2) Quadriceps stretch. Stand with your right hand on the back of a chair. With your left hand, pull your left heel toward your left buttock and point your left knee to the floor until you feel a stretch in the front of the thigh. Hold for 10 to 20 seconds. Repeat the stretch, using the right hand and right leg.

If you can't reach your ankle, loop a towel around your foot to pull back the leg, or do the stretch lying on your stomach on a bed or the floor.

3) Calf stretch. Stand two to three feet from a wall and lunge your right foot forward. Keep your left leg straight, with your heel on the floor and your toes pointed forward; keep your right leg slightly bent. Lean into the wall with both hands on the wall supporting you until you feel a stretch in the left calf. Hold for 10 to 20 seconds. Repeat, with your left leg bent and your right leg straight.

4) Hip-extensor strengthener. This exercise strengthens the muscles in the back of the hip. Lie on your stomach, tighten the muscle at the front of your right thigh, then lift your right leg eight to ten inches from the floor, keeping the knee locked. Hold for five to ten seconds. Do ten repetitions. Repeat with the left leg.

5) Hip-abductor strengthener. This exercise strengthens the muscles at the outside of the thigh. Lie on your left side, tighten the muscle at the front of your right thigh, then lift your right leg eight to ten inches from the floor. Hold for five to ten seconds. Do ten repetitions. Repeat on opposite side.

6) Hip-adductor strengthener. This exercise strengthens the muscles at the inside of the thigh. Lie on your left side, with your head supported by your left hand and your right leg crossed over in front of your left leg. Tighten the muscle at the front of the left thigh, then lift the left leg eight to ten

245

inches from the floor. Hold for five to ten seconds. Repeat ten times. Switch legs, and repeat ten times.

7) Quadriceps strengthener. Lie on your back with your right leg straight and your left leg bent at the knee to keep your back straight. Tighten the muscle at the front of your right thigh, and lift your right leg five to ten inches from the floor, keeping the knee locked. Hold for ten to twenty seconds. Repeat ten times. Switch legs, and repeat ten times.

Tune in to your body. The biggest reason people get overuse injuries is that they don't pay attention to the signals their bodies give them. If you're running and you start to feel pain, your body is giving you the signal to back off a bit on the pace or the distance.

At the Doctor's

If your knees are overstressed by too much exercise, or if they hurt because you've just started a new exercise program and you're moving ahead too quickly, you can follow the home-care suggestions outlined in this chapter. However, if you have a serious knee injury or if your pain persists, you should see a physician who can evaluate your condition and recommend appropriate medical treatment. Remember: You depend on those joints, and they require proper care to function well. Don't wait until you've severely damaged your knees before you seek help.

Sources: **Michael Baskin, M.D.**, Assistant Clinical Professor, Department of Orthopedics, Oregon Health Sciences University, Portland, Oregon. **Kathleen Galligan, D.C.**, Chiropractor, Lake Oswego, Oregon. **Ellen Nona Hoyven, P.T.**, Owner and Director, Ortho Sport Physical Therapy P.C., Clackamas, Oregon. **Chrissy Kane, L.P.T.**, Physical Therapist, Outpatient Physical Therapy Department, Providence Medical Center, Portland, Oregon. **Michael Martindale, L.P.T.**, Physical Therapist, Sports Medicine Center, Portland Adventist Medical Center, Portland, Oregon. **Elliot Michael, D.P.M.**, Director, Residency Program for Podiatric Medicine, Holladay Park Hospital, Portland, Oregon. **Louisa Silva, M.D.**, General Practitioner, Osteopath, Acupuncturist, Salem, Oregon.

•Lactose Intolerance

How to Avoid

Unpleasant

Symptoms

YOU MAY BE SOMEONE WHO LOVES dairy products. But your body could have some decidedly different ideas about foods such as pizza, ice cream, and milk. These foods taste great going down, but may leave you with indigestion, bloating, diarrhea, or gas. Such symptoms may be signs of lactose intolerance—an inability to digest the milk sugar lactose.

About 50 million Americans suffer from this condition. It does not affect them all to the same degree, however. Some people may be bothered only by large amounts of milk products; for others, it only takes a little lactose.

Lactose intolerance is not an equal-opportunity problem. It affects some ethnic groups much more than others. About 75 percent of African-American, Jewish, Native American, and Mexican-American adults and 90 percent of Asian-American adults have this condition. Only about 10 to 15 percent of non-Jewish white adults are lactose intolerant. These figures concern only adults because the inability to tolerate lactose affects adults more than children. The reason is that we all lose some of our ability to digest milk sugar as we grow older.

Some people discover their lactose intolerance themselves; others find out from a doctor. People who belong to the ethnic groups that are most likely to suffer from lactose intolerance may have a greater awareness of the problem, since it may be common in their families.

If you suspect that you are lactose intolerant but you are not sure, your physician may be able to help you rule out other problems. You can also try this simple test: Lay off all milk products for a few weeks and see if you feel any better. This is not a definitive test; if your symptoms don't improve, you may still be lactose intolerant and reacting to the lactose in nondairy products you consume. However, if your symptoms do lessen, you may be lactose intolerant and might benefit from cutting down on milk products in your diet. Always keep in mind, however, that if you plan to reduce the dairy in your diet, you should make certain you are getting sufficient calcium and vitamin D from other food sources. Talk to your doctor if you're not sure you're getting enough of these important nutritional elements.

If things don't improve, you may be suffering from another digestive disorder, such as irritable bowel syndrome or caffeine intolerance, both of which cause similar symptoms. It's always a good idea to play it safe and get a physician's opinion, especially if you notice a major change in your bowel patterns.

CAUSES

Lactose intolerance is usually caused by a shortage of the enzyme lactase, which normally breaks down milk sugar in the intestine into simple parts that can be absorbed into the blood stream. Without lactase, lactose is not properly digested, resulting in the unpleasant symptoms of lactose intolerance.

AT-HOME TREATMENT

Lactose intolerance cannot be cured, but its symptoms can be easily managed at home. Once you know for sure that you are lactose intolerant, you can try the following tips:

Gauge the severity of your problem. The first thing you need to know in order to manage lactose intolerance is how much lactose your body can tolerate; this will vary from individual to individual. Cut all dairy food and lactose from your diet for about three to four weeks so that your system is free from lactose. Then start to add small amounts of milk and cheese to your diet. Gradually increase your intake and carefully monitor your symptoms. Knowing what your body can and can't handle will keep you from overloading the system.

Break up your consumption. Drinking eight ounces of milk in one sitting might be too much for you. But you might be able to have a half cup of milk with your cereal in the morning and another half cup with your dessert after dinner. Sticking with small serving sizes may keep your symptoms to a minimum. Trial and error will tell you just how small those servings should be.

Don't let dairy go solo. If you do consume small amounts of dairy products, make them part of a snack or meal with other foods. Having more food in your stomach slows down the digestive process and may help prevent lactose intolerance symptoms.

Drink chocolate milk. One study has shown that adding cocoa and sugar to milk can help the body to digest more lactose and can reduce bloating and cramps in lactose-intolerant people. Some experts believe that chocolate may slow the rate at which the stomach empties. A slower emptying rate may mean that less lactose enters your system at once; hence, fewer symptoms.

Put back what nature left out. You can buy lactase-enzyme supplements in tablet or liquid form without a prescription. These can supply your body with the lactase you need to digest dairy food properly. Chew the tablets with or right after consuming a dairy product; you add the drops directly to a carton of milk. You can also buy lactose-reduced and lactose-free milk. Two common brands are Lactaid and Dairy Ease.

Eat some live food. Yogurt that contains active cultures is usually well tolerated by lactose-intolerant people. Read the container to find out whether the product you are buying contains active cultures (you may have to go to a health-food store to find a yogurt with active cultures). Yogurt is an excellent source of calcium, which you're probably lacking if your dairy intake is limited.

Then, try some old cheese. If you're a cheese lover, stick to aged, hard cheeses such as Swiss, cheddar, or Colby, because they have lower amounts of lactose than soft cheeses.

Be a lactose detective. Many prepared and processed foods contain lactose as an ingredient. And looking for the word "lactose" on the label won't always help, since it is often listed as whey, curds, milk by-products, dry milk solids, nonfat dry milk power, casein, galactose, skim milk powder, milk sugar, or whey protein concentrate. Some examples of hidden sources of lactose are bread, cereals, pancakes, chocolate, soups, puddings, salad dressings, sherbet, instant cocoa mix, candies, frozen dinners, cookie mixes, and hot dogs. While the amounts of lactose in these foods may be small, people who are very sensitive may experience symptoms.

Check your medications. Drug manufacturers include lactose as a filler in about 20 percent of prescription medications and in about 6 percent of over-the-counter drugs, and sometimes it is not listed as an ingredient on the label. If you only take medication occasionally, you may not be troubled, but if you take a lactose-containing medication on a regular basis, it could cause problems. Ask your doctor or pharmacist for information on any drug's ingredients. If they can't help, write directly to the drug manufacturer.

Don't forget about calcium. If you are lactose intolerant, it is easy to avoid most dairy prod-

10 WAYS TO MANAGE SYMPTOMS OF LACTOSE INTOLERANCE

- Figure out how much dairy food you can comfortably handle.
- Eat small servings of dairy products at a time.
- Eat dairy products with other foods.
- Try drinking chocolate milk.
- Take lactase-enzyme supplements.
- Eat yogurt that contains active cultures.
- Eat only hard, aged cheeses.
- Check for lactose in processed foods.
- Find out if your medication contains lactose as a filler.
- Make sure you get enough calcium from other sources.

ucts. Allowing your calcium intake to drop, however, is a mistake. Calcium is a vitally important nutrient for women, especially during pregnancy, while nursing a baby, and after menopause. Green, leafy vegetables, such as collard greens, kale, turnip greens, and Chinese cabbage (bok choy), as well as oysters, sardines, canned salmon with the bones, and tofu, are all good sources of calcium. You can also talk to your doctor about taking a calcium supplement. See the chapter on osteoporosis for more information on adding calcium to your diet.

Sources: **David Alpers, M.D.,** Professor of Medicine and Chief of the Gastroenterology Division, Washington University School of Medicine, St. Louis, Missouri. **Elyse Sosin, R.D.,** Supervisor of Clinical Nutrition, Mount Sinai Medical Center, New York, New York. **Jane Zukin,** Author, *The Dairy-Free Cookbook,* and Editor, *The Newsletter for People with Lactose Intolerance and Milk Allergies.*

●Lupus

Strategies for

Coping

A DIAGNOSIS OF LUPUS ERYTHEMATOSUS often strikes terror in the heart of the sufferer. Lupus is a chronic inflammatory disease that can affect the skin, joints, blood, kidneys, and other parts of the body. In its mildest state, it causes a red skin rash. In its most severe, it can cause death. However, for most people, lupus is a mild disease. With the lifestyle strategies presented here, as well as regular medical care, most people with lupus can live long and active lives. The key is to be well informed about the disease and not be panicked by the diagnosis.

Lupus is an immune system disorder. Normally the body makes antibodies that protect against invaders like bacteria and viruses. When you have lupus, something has gone wrong with the body's natural immunity and it becomes unable to distinguish between foreign invaders and its own cells and tissues. The immune system begins manufacturing antibodies (called "auto-antibodies") that are directed against the body. Inflammation, pain, and injury to the tissues result from this malfunction.

If you've been diagnosed with lupus, you're not alone. The Lupus Foundation of America estimates that 500,000 Americans have the disease and 16,000 new cases are diagnosed every year. It's often called a "women's disease" because it occurs 10 to 15 times more often in women than in men. About ten percent of lupus sufferers have close family members who have the disease and children have about a five-percent risk of inheriting the disease from lupus-affected parents.

Lupus is divided into two types: discoid—the milder type—and sys-temic. Discoid lupus is a chronic disease of the skin that is characterized by a red rash on the cheeks and nose and other parts of the body. It often appears for the first time after exposure to the sun. This form of the disease is limited to the skin; it usually doesn't involve other organs. In one in ten people with discoid lupus, the disease evolves into systemic lupus. Unfortunately, there's no way to know whether or not discoid lupus will become systemic lupus and there is no known treatment to stop the disease's progression.

Systemic lupus is more serious. It can affect any organ or bodily system. It commonly attacks the blood vessels, connective tissues, joints, and skin and can involve the heart, lungs, liver, intestines, and kidneys. A red "butterfly" patch may appear on the cheeks and nose.

No two cases of systemic lupus are the same. In one individual, it may affect only the skin and joints; in another, it may be the kidneys, lungs, or joints. The disease may come and go without warning.

At one time, doctors insisted that women with lupus shouldn't become pregnant and bear children. Now, however, they know that 50 percent of lupus pregnancies are completely normal and 25 percent of women with lupus deliver normal babies prematurely. In the remaining 25 percent of the pregnancies, there is miscarriage or death of the fetus. Any woman who has lupus and becomes pregnant is considered "high risk," which means that problems may occur and must be anticipated. If you have lupus and are pregnant, be sure to get early and regular prenatal care.

Symptoms

Because many of the lupus symptoms mimic other health problems, diagnosis can be difficult. Unfortunately, there isn't a single test or cell culture that will definitively identify lupus. The American Rheumatism Association has issued a list of 11 signs and symptoms that help distinguish lupus from other diseases. If you answer "yes" to four or more of these symptoms, suspect lupus (the symptoms don't have to occur all at the same time).

- Do you have a red rash over your cheeks?
- Do you have red raised patches on your skin?
- Does your skin react to sunlight with a skin rash?
- Do you have painless sores (ulcers) in your nose and/or mouth?
- Do your joints feel achy and swollen?
- Has your doctor told you that you have inflammation of the lining of the lungs (pleuritis) or that you have inflammation of the heart sac (pericarditis)?
- Have your urine tests shown elevated protein levels and/or "cellular casts" (abnormal elements in the urine from red and/or white blood cells and/or kidney tubule cells)?
- Have you experienced seizures?
- Are you anemic?
- Has your doctor informed you that your immunologic tests are positive?
- Are your tests for antinuclear antibodies (ANA) positive?

Causes

No one really knows what causes the immune system to go awry and develop lupus. Researchers point to a genetic predisposition to the disease and to certain environmental "triggers" such as infections, antibiotics (especially sulfa drugs and penicillin-type drugs), exposure to ultraviolet light, extreme stress, and certain medications.

Doctors also suspect some type of hormonal involvement, probably estrogen, which would account for the large number of women who have lupus. Women often say they have an increase in symptoms before their menstrual periods and/or during pregnancy. However, medical experts still don't know exactly how hormones are involved.

At-Home Treatment

Since there really isn't an effective treatment for lupus, this section should perhaps be called "Coping." There are plenty of strategies that can help you cope with and minimize your symptoms.

---

7 Strategies for Coping with Lupus

- Maintain a positive attitude.
- Manage your energy carefully.
- Learn about lupus.
- Take nonsteroidal anti-inflammatories.
- Try acetaminophen if you can't take aspirin.
- Develop good communication with your doctor.
- Join a support group.

Adopt a positive "wellness" attitude. Living well with any chronic disease, including lupus, can be difficult, but it's possible and worth the effort. One of the first steps is to decide you're going to be the best you can be and then take responsibility for doing what helps or hinders your life. Focus on your abilities rather than your disabilities. It's up to you whether you choose to see yourself as a victim of a chronic disease or as someone who is active and responsible for her life.

Conserve your energy. When you've only got a limited amount of energy, you don't want to waste it. Begin by planning your days. Prioritize what's important and what you can let go of. What can you simplify or eliminate? Spread out activities. Plan activities that take the most energy during times when you're feeling the best and most energized. You don't have to do everything today or even tomorrow. When you can, delegate tasks.

Think about your daily and weekly commitments and determine where you can insert energy-saving shortcuts. Perhaps you can use some devices like book holders or convenience foods to conserve valuable energy.

Develop good doctor/patient communication. To enhance your communication with your health team:

- Take lists of questions you would like answered when you go for an appointment.
- Keep a medical diary.
- Ask your doctor about medications and dosages.
- Tell your doctor immediately whenever you have an adverse drug reaction.

Learn about your disease. Understanding what lupus is and what you can expect can help diminish your fears about it. It can also help you learn to recognize early symptoms of disease activity and get help when you need it.

Take NSAIDs. Nonsteroidal anti-inflammatories like aspirin and ibuprofen can help reduce inflammation and ease pain. If aspirin upsets your stomach, ask your pharmacist for enteric-coated brands or take it with meals.

Try acetaminophen. If you can't take aspirin, acetaminophen is an effective over-the-counter pain reliever. (It's not as effective in reducing inflammation, however.)

Get support. Living with a chronic disease like lupus can bring up a wide range of feelings. It's helpful to talk with others who share your problem. Ask your doctor or hospital about chronic-illness or lupus support groups in your area or contact the Lupus Foundation of America, Inc. (1-800-558-0121).

PREVENTING FLARE-UPS

Lupus symptoms can come and go seemingly at random. You can help prevent flare-ups and minimize symptoms by using these strategies:

Get immunized to protect against specific infections. Often, infections precipitate outbreaks of lupus. Talk with your physician and make sure your immunizations are up-to-date.

Avoid sun exposure. Protect your skin from exposure to ultraviolet light by wearing protective clothing like hats and long sleeves and by wearing sunblock.

Exercise. Regular exercise can help prevent muscle weakness and fatigue, one of the most common effects of the disease. If you have joint pain or other symptoms that make exercising difficult, ask your doctor to provide specific exercises for your condition.

Manage your stress. First outbreaks and successive flare-ups of lupus often occur during times of stress. Excessive stress depresses the immune system. Manage your stress with a regular stress reduction program.

Avoid cigarette smoking. Studies have demonstrated that cigarette smoking depresses the immune system. If you smoke, stop.

Limit alcohol. Excessive alcohol consumption isn't healthy. Limit yourself to no more than one or two ounces per day.

Eat a well-balanced diet. Give your body the best possible opportunity to stay healthy. While there are plenty of so-called lupus diets, none have been shown to be effective against the disease. Stay away from fad diets that advocate eating or avoiding particular foods or taking excessive amounts of vitamins or minerals. Your immune system's cells can be adversely affected by nutritional imbalances or deficiencies. Choose a balanced diet with a wide variety of foods from all food groups and that are low in fat and high in fiber.

Some of the drugs commonly used to treat lupus may stimulate appetite and, if you're not careful, you could end up gaining unwanted weight. Eating a diet that is rich in low-fat, high-fiber foods and exercising regularly should help you keep your weight within a desirable range.

Get plenty of rest. Fatigue is one of the biggest problems lupus sufferers face. Adequate rest can go a long way toward fighting fatigue. In addition to getting enough sleep at night, try to schedule mini-rest periods throughout the day.

---

7 TIPS FOR PREVENTING FLARE-UPS

- Avoid exposure to the sun.
- Get regular exercise.
- Protect yourself against infections.
- Learn to manage your stress.
- Don't smoke cigarettes.
- Limit your alcohol intake.
- Eat a well-balanced diet.

Source:
Lupus Foundation of America, Inc.
4 Research Place, Suite 180
Rockville, MD 20850
301-670-9292

•MENOPAUSE DISCOMFORTS

Easing the

Transition

FIRST, YOU NOTICE SOME CHANGES IN your menstrual cycle. You're bleeding less and your period is a day or two shorter than normal. Then you begin to experience moments of intense heat and sweating that come and go quickly and unexpectedly. You're on the threshold of a new phase in your life. You're beginning menopause, the cessation of the menstrual cycle.

Every woman has heard menopausal horror stories—everything from weight gain and loss of sex drive to thinning hair. Relax. Most of what you've heard simply isn't true. Many women confuse natural aging changes with menopausal symptoms. Menopause is a natural transition period in your life that's exciting and challenging and actually has few symptoms associated with it.

Menopause, also called "the climacteric," or the "change of life," is a period of four to five years, usually two years before the last menstrual period and two to three years after. For most women, menopause occurs between ages 45 and 55. However, some women experience it earlier; some, years later. You'll probably experience menopause at about the same age that your mother did.

CAUSES

Women's health experts aren't really sure what triggers menopausal changes. During a woman's fertile years, her ovaries produce hormones and an egg each month at ovulation. As menopause approaches, egg production and menstrual periods become less regular until they stop altogether. These changes start when the ovaries stop responding to sex hormones secreted by the pituitary gland. The resulting decline in the ovaries' production of the female hormone estrogen causes the symptoms we associate with menopause.

Although the drop in estrogen usually begins in a woman's late 30s, she usually doesn't notice symptoms until she experiences changes in her menstrual cycle, most often around age 45. The menstrual cycle will become longer or shorter, and the bleeding might be heavier or lighter than normal. Eventually, the periods cease altogether. It's important that women keep track of the changes in menstrual bleeding so that the doctor can determine if, in fact, these changes are normal menopausal changes or if they might be caused by a health problem. It's also important for women to note that although ovulation becomes sporadic during menopause, it still may occur and contraception is still necessary. In fact, even after menstrual bleeding ceases, most doctors recommend women continue using birth control for another year.

"Hot flashes," periods of intense heat and flushing over the face, neck, and chest are a common complaint of women going through menopause. It is one of the few menopausal "symptoms" that can actually be traced to the hormonal changes of menopause. For one in four menopausal women, the bone thinning of osteoporosis is a problem. The female hormone estrogen plays a large role in keeping a woman's bones strong and healthy. As estrogen production declines with menopause, women begin to increasingly lose calcium from their bones. Osteoporosis can cause compressed vertebrae, which can lead to back pain, a humpbacked look ("dowager's hump"), loss of height, vertebral fractures, and increased risk of bone fractures, particularly in the wrists and hips. Both men and women experience increased bone loss with age, but osteoporosis is more common among women. You are at greater risk for osteoporosis if:

- You're Caucasian or Asian.
- You're thin-framed.
- You smoke cigarettes.
- You don't exercise regularly.
- You have a family history of osteoporosis.
- You drink excessive amounts of alcohol.
- You take steroids.

Another symptom often associated with menopausal hormone shifts is vaginal dryness. As estrogen production decreases, the walls of the vagina become thinner and drier, which can make intercourse uncomfortable. It can also lead to a vaginal inflammation called "atrophic vaginitis" that causes abnormal discharge, burning, and itching, as well as vaginal pain or soreness during intercourse.

Some women say they experience pounding heartbeat, joint pains, headaches, itching skin, increased facial hair, and decreased armpit and pubic hair with menopause, but researchers haven't been able to demonstrate that these changes are due to the hormonal fluctuations of menopause. Mood swings and depression during this time are also often blamed on hormonal changes. However, experts say these psychological changes aren't related to menopausal hormone fluctuations. They may, in fact, have more to do with fatigue caused by sleep disturbances due to hot flashes or with anxiety a woman may have about her changing role in life. You may or may not notice any or all of these menopausal symptoms as you move through this important life transition. One in four women experiences no symptoms; one in four experiences very uncomfortable symptoms. The rest experience some mild physical or emotional symptoms.

Women who have their uterus removed in a hysterectomy, but retain one or both ovaries, stop menstruating after the surgery. However, they continue to go though the hormonal changes of menstruation. Women who have had their ovaries and uterus removed during hysterectomy experience "surgical menopause," which tends to have more severe symptoms than normal menopause. These women often require hormone therapy to lessen symptoms and lessen the health risks of too little estrogen.

AT-HOME TREATMENT

It's important to keep in mind that menopause is a natural transition, not an illness. Postmenopause is a time of freedom— from the discomfort and hassles of menstruation, from contraception, and in many cases, from child-rearing responsibilities. It's a time when you can concentrate on your own agenda and on what you want to do with your life.

Home remedies can help you manage some of the uncomfortable symptoms you may experience during menopause. It's important that you not confuse natural aging changes with menopausal symptoms. Menopause is a good time to have a complete physical examination and to discuss your body's changes with your doctor. Ask your doctor to give you a blood test to ensure you're not becoming anemic (this test should be repeated several times throughout your menopausal cycle). Talk with your doctor about osteoporosis, and if you have any of the risk factors, request a bone density study. Also, discuss the pros and cons of hormone replacement therapy (HRT), also known as estrogen replacement therapy (ERT). If you start to bleed between your menstrual periods, bleed excessively, or begin periods six months or more after period cessation, see your doctor immediately.

Dress the part. Eighty percent of menopausal women experience the intense heat, flushing, and sweating of hot flashes. Since these episodes come without warning, the best advice is to dress for them. Wear loose clothing that can easily be removed, such as cardigan sweaters. Keep a spray bottle filled with cool water and "spritz" your face when hot flashes hit. Or blot your face with a cool washcloth for instant heat relief.

Fan it. Carry a small wood-and-paper fan or one of the battery-powered types that's small enough to fit in your purse. When the heat hits, reach for your fan.

Nix the caffeine and alcohol. Many women find that alcoholic or caffeinated beverages trigger hot flashes. If you find that's your situation, avoid them completely. Substitute herbal teas or decaf coffee. (Be ready for a couple of days of headache and fatigue from caffeine withdrawal.)

Caffeinated beverages also cause the kidneys to excrete more calcium, a factor in the bone thinning of osteoporosis. So even if your hot flashes aren't triggered by caffeine, it's a good idea to cut your consumption.

Turn down the thermostat. Keeping your home and office temperature at 68 degrees Fahrenheit or less will make you more comfortable. If you're bothered by nighttime hot flashes, consider turning down the heat even further and keeping a window open.

Use your mind. When you feel a hot flash coming on, cool it by using your mind's eye. Visualize a cooling wave of air or water enveloping you, washing away the heat.

Be a creative lover. Many women experience vaginal dryness during menopause. That's because lower levels of estrogen cause the mucous membranes of the vagina to thin and secrete less moisture. The result can be painful or difficult intercourse. Some of this dryness can be overcome by taking more time with foreplay during lovemaking or exploring other ways of giving one another pleasure.

Bring on the lubricant. Another way to combat vaginal dryness is with vaginal lubricants. Inexpensive, effective options include plain vegetable oil, unscented cold cream, or water-based lubricants like K-Y Jelly (available over the counter in pharmacies). Many gynecologists recommend a product called Astroglide, a long-lasting, water-based lubricant, because it's most like a woman's natural secretions. Do not use Vaseline or other petroleum-based products.

Get out and move. Mood swings and depression haven't been linked to the hormonal changes of menopause. The emotional roller coaster some women find themselves on at this time may have more to do with a negative view of aging. After all, menopause is a milestone, a harbinger of change, and some women see menopause as an ending rather than the exciting beginning it can be. One way to combat these negative emotions is with exercise. Regular aerobic exercise lifts spirits because it releases endorphins, the body's own "feel good" chemicals. It also makes you feel healthier and more in control and gives you more energy.

In addition, any "weight-bearing" exercise like walking, running, aerobic dancing, or weight lifting can help combat the bone thinning of osteoporosis, a problem for many menopausal women. With regular exercise, bones become

---

15 Ways to Treat Your Menopausal Symptoms

- Wear loose, easily removed clothing.
- Carry a personal fan.
- Avoid caffeine and alcohol.
- Keep the thermostat below 68 degrees Fahrenheit.
- Use visualization to cool hot flashes.
- Take more time and be creative in lovemaking.
- Use a vaginal lubricant.
- Exercise regularly.
- Eat enough calcium.
- Eat a low-fat diet rich in complex carbohydrates and low in animal protein.
- Get support.
- Don't be too thin.
- Stop smoking.
- Live a healthful premenopausal lifestyle.
- Consider hormone therapy carefully.

---

stronger and more dense and have less risk of fracturing. (Nonweight-bearing exercise like swimming doesn't increase bone density.)

Go for the calcium. With aging, everyone loses calcium, one of the major components of bones. As estrogen levels drop in menopausal women, calcium loss speeds up. Nutritionists say that menopausal women need more calcium. Postmenopausal women who are undergoing hormone replacement therapy need 1,000 mg of elemental calcium per day; women who are not receiving hormone therapy need 1,500 mg per day. The quantity of elemental calcium is not the same as the milligrams of calcium listed on calcium supplements. For example, it takes

1,200 mg of calcium carbonate to get 500 mg of elemental calcium.

Women often mistakenly believe that if they eat a lot of dairy products, they'll get enough calcium. But diets high in animal protein cause the body to excrete even more calcium. A better alternative is to eat a diet rich in vegetables, fruits, and complex carbohydrates. When you do eat dairy products, opt for nonfat or low-fat varieties like skim milk, nonfat yogurt, and low-fat cheeses. Be sure to include plenty of these calcium-rich foods in your diet: almonds, brewer's yeast, broccoli, cheese (low-fat varieties), collard greens, dandelion greens, ice milk, kelp, mackerel (canned), milk (skim or low-fat), mustard greens, oysters, salmon (canned with bones), sardines (canned with bones), spinach, tofu, and yogurt (nonfat or low-fat varieties). To ensure that they get enough of this important mineral, many health experts recommend women begin taking calcium supplements at age 35.

Talk about it. Experts call menopause the "climacteric," because it's a big life change. It's a signal that one phase of your life is over and another is beginning. Often, it's a time when we begin to notice changes in our bodies—new wrinkles, aches, and pains. As your roles in life change at this time, it can bring up questions, concerns, and insecurities about how you see yourself. It's helpful to talk with other women who are going through the same thing. One great way to get support is through a menopause support group. Often local hospitals, community colleges, or professional groups sponsor such groups. Or you can start your own with friends who are experiencing menopause.

Watch your diet. Heart disease is the number one killer of women over the age of 55. At menopause, a woman's risk for coronary heart disease increases. Estrogen has a protective effect on the heart. As estrogen levels drop, that protection disappears and the risk for heart disease escalates. At menopause, a woman's levels of LDL (so-called "bad" cholesterol) begin to rise. Within ten years, she has the same risk of heart disease as a man.

Diet has the potential to affect significantly your risk of serious health problems like heart disease, osteoporosis, and even cancer. An ideal diet for menopausal women is one that is low in fat (high-fat diets have been associated with heart disease and some cancers) and lower in animal protein (too much animal protein causes excretion of calcium). Plant foods, especially complex carbohydrates, are low in fat and provide calcium and many anticancer elements like beta carotene.

Don't get too thin. There's an old saying, "A woman can never be too rich or too thin." When it comes to osteoporosis, you can be too thin. You may have dieted all your life to stay thin, but your slim figure may contribute to osteoporosis. A moderate amount of body fat actually helps to fight osteoporosis. "Pleasingly plump" (not obese) is the healthiest postmenopausal figure for a woman.

Get rid of the cigarettes. Women who smoke cigarettes are more likely to develop osteoporosis (and lung cancer, among other health problems).

Plan ahead. Unfortunately, most of us eat the typical American diet—40 percent of our calories come from fat, 20 percent from sugar, and 5 percent from alcohol. On top of that, many of us don't exercise. When menopause comes, we find we have to go to the doctor for medical intervention in the form of hormones just to help undo what we've been doing to our bodies for years.

Many health authorities believe that if women prepare for menopause by exercising and eating right for the 20 years before it starts, only a small percentage of menopausal women would need to take hormone therapy.

Consider hormone therapy carefully. One of the biggest decisions facing menopausal women is whether or not to take hormone replacement therapy (HRT), also called estrogen replacement therapy (ERT).

HRT can reduce or eliminate hot flashes and vaginal dryness and soreness and, in some women, decrease the risk of osteoporosis. Some women who take HRT also report less fatigue and depression.

However, HRT may increase the risk of breast cancer and gallbladder disease. Some experts believe that hormone therapy promotes the growth of tumors that may already be present. Others believe that hormone therapy has no effect on the large percentage of women who are not "hormone sensitive." If you have any of the following, you should not take estrogen: history of breast, ovarian, or uterine cancer; history of blood clots; high blood pressure; gallstones or gallbladder disease; or large uterine fibroids. Talk with your physician about the pros and cons.

Sources: **Amanda Clark, M.D.**, Assistant Professor of Obstetrics and Gynecology, Oregon Health Sciences University, Portland, Oregon. **Sonja Connor, M.S., R.D.**, Coauthor, *The New American Diet;* Research Associate Professor, School of Medicine, Oregon Health Sciences University, Portland, Oregon. **Sadja Greenwood, M.D., M.P.H.**, Author, *Menopause Naturally;* Assistant Clinical Professor, Department of Obstetrics, Gynecology, and Reproductive Services, University of California, at San Francisco, San Francisco, California. **Anne Simons, M.D.**, Coauthor, *Before You Call the Doctor;* Family Practitioner, San Francisco Department of Public Health; Family Practitioner and Assistant Clinical Professor, Family and Community Medicine, University of California San Francisco Medical Center, San Francisco, California. **Susan Woodruff, B.S.N.**, Childbirth and Parenting Education Coordinator, Tuality Community Hospital, Hillsboro, Oregon.

●Menstrual Cramps

Yᴏᴜ ᴡᴀᴋᴇ ᴜᴘ ꜰᴇᴇʟɪɴɢ ᴛᴡɪɴɢᴇꜱ ɪɴ your lower abdomen and your back feels stiff and achy. As the morning wears on, your abdominal pain and discomfort get worse. It's that time of the month again, and you've got menstrual cramps.

During the reproductive years, most women experience some discomfort around their menstrual periods. It's not a serious condition, but, as any woman who has experienced cramps knows, it's uncomfortable and annoying. For some women who have severe menstrual cramping, it can even be incapacitating.

CAUSES

Menstrual cramping (also called "dysmenorrhea") that occurs for one to two days, often accompanied by congestive, bloating-type symptoms, is called primary menstrual cramps. It's hereditary and usually begins with the onset of menstruation in adolescence. Sometimes primary cramps lessen after pregnancy, perhaps due to the stretching of the cervix. Some women find their menstrual cramps are worse before age 30 and then become progressively less severe. Other women find no age-related changes.

For years, women have been told by the medical community that their menstrual cramps were "all in their heads." Women were treated as if they exaggerated their pain and discomfort and were often given strong tranquilizers or analgesics. Finally, medical science has confirmed what women have known for centuries—menstrual cramps do have a physiologic basis. They are caused by the release of a large amount of the hormone prosta-

glandin just before the onset of menstruation. This hormone, which is produced in various parts of the body, including the uterine lining after ovulation, causes the uterus to contract. Like any muscle, when the uterus contracts, its blood supply is temporarily cut off and pain results. Prostaglandin production is also responsible for the nausea, vomiting, hot and cold sensations, headaches, diarrhea, backaches, dizziness, and even fainting that some women experience around their menstrual period.

Secondary menstrual cramps begin later in life, after a woman has been menstruating for several years. They can be caused by an underlying condition such as fibroid tumors, pelvic infection, pelvic lesions, endometriosis, pelvic congestion, or pelvic varicose veins. Pain from secondary cramps is usually more severe than the pain from primary cramps and can be accompanied by nausea, vomiting, and diarrhea. Secondary cramping also tends to last longer and occur at different times than primary cramps. The following are some of the more common underlying causes of secondary dysmenorrhea:

Endometriosis. This is a condition in which pieces of the uterine lining (endometrial tissue) grow outside the uterus and cause adhesions and bleeding in the pelvic cavity and bowel area. When cramping is caused by endometriosis, pain may be severe and may even occur throughout the month.

Fibroids. These are noncancerous growths in the uterine wall. They usually cause no problem until they become too large or interfere with the uterine function. They can cause menstrual cramps when they've outgrown their blood supply and degenerate. The cramps caused by fibroids tend to occur during ovulation. If you have fibroids and are experiencing discomfort, see your doctor.

Cervical stenosis. "Stenosis" means narrowing. Cervical stenosis causes menstrual cramping because the cervical opening isn't large enough to allow menstrual blood to pass through. It is sometimes caused by an abortion or other surgical procedure.

Pelvic inflammatory disease (PID). This is a serious infection of a woman's uterus, fallopian tubes, or ovaries that can cause scarring of the fallopian tubes and infertility. In addition to cramping, PID symptoms include fever, chills, back pain, spotting, pain during or after intercourse, and puslike vaginal discharge. PID symptoms often come on suddenly. If you suspect you have PID, contact your physician immediately.

AT-HOME TREATMENT

Home remedies are often effective for primary cramps. They can relieve some of the symptoms of secondary cramps, too, but the underlying condition that causes them must be treated by a physician for ongoing relief. If self-care doesn't provide sufficient relief, or if your cramping occurs at times other than before or at the onset of menstrual bleeding, consult your doctor for proper diagnosis and treatment.

Try antiprostaglandins. Since prostaglandins cause cramps and other menstrual-related

---

10 TIPS FOR BEATING THE CRAMPS

- Take aspirin or ibuprofen.
- Try a heating pad or hot water bottle.
- Stay warm.
- Exercise regularly.
- Switch to menstrual pads.
- Soak in a hot bath.
- Drink plenty of water.
- Do pelvic tilt exercises.
- Lie on your back with your knees bent.
- Reconsider your birth control.

---

symptoms, it makes sense to take a prostaglandin inhibitor like aspirin or ibuprofen. However, women with a history of ulcers should not take aspirin or ibuprofen.

Heat it up. When cramps strike, lie down and place a heating pad or hot water bottle on your lower abdomen. The heat increases blood flow to the area and helps relax cramped muscles.

Stay warm. Women who stay warm during their menstrual cycle suffer less severe cramping than those who work in cold environments.

Exercise regularly. When you're feeling crampy and bloated, the last thing you want to do is exercise, but a regular program of exercise during the rest of the month can help lessen cramping during the menstrual period. Regular exercise increases circulation in the pelvic region and helps clear out excess prostaglandins.

Try menstrual pads. For some women, tampons contribute to menstrual cramping. Consider using pads instead.

Soak in a hot bath. A hot bath relaxes muscles and promotes circulation to the pelvic area. It can also help relieve lower back pain.

Drink plenty of water. When the body becomes dehydrated, it produces a hormone, vaso-pressin, that contributes to uterine contractions.

Tilt your pelvis. So-called "pelvic tilt" exercises provide relief for some women. Get on all fours with your elbows on the ground. Now rock back and forth. This exercise is especially helpful for women who have a "retroverted" uterus, one that is swollen and puts pressure on the back.

Lie on your back with your knees bent. Some women find this position eases their cramps and backache.

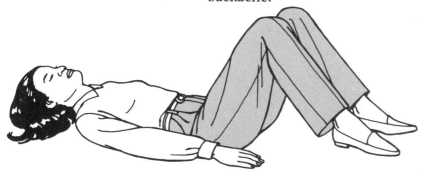

Reconsider your birth control. If you're using an intrauterine device (IUD), it could be contributing to your menstrual cramping. Consider an alternative form of birth control like a diaphragm, condoms, or the Pill.

Birth-control pills help many women who suffer from menstrual cramps because they suppress ovulation, decreasing the production of prostaglandins. The Pill also tends to shorten the length and decrease the flow of menstrual blood, which may also decrease cramping. Some health conditions make birth-control pills a poor contraceptive choice. Don't take birth-control pills if you have liver disease (hepatitis, cirrhosis, or benign liver tumors), have a history of heart disease or angina, have ever had a stroke, have a history of breast cancer, or if you smoke.

Other conditions such as diabetes, high blood pressure, gallbladder disease, varicose veins, and uterine fibroids make birth-control pills a questionable choice. Be sure that your physician has a thorough health history from you and discuss with him or her the pros and cons of birth-control pills before taking them.

Sources: Phyllis Frey, A.R.N.P., Nurse Practitioner, Bellevue, Washington. Sadja Greenwood, M.D., Assistant Clinical Professor, Department of Obstetrics, Gynecology, and Reproductive Services, University of California at San Francisco, San Francisco, California. Anne Simons, M.D., Coauthor, *Before You Call the Doctor*; Family Practitioner, San Francisco Department of Public Health; Family Practitioner and Assistant Clinical Professor, Family and Community Medicine, University of California San Francisco Medical Center, San Francisco, California. Harold Zimmer, M.D., Obstetrician and Gynecologist, Bellevue, Washington.

Strategies to

Ease the Hurt

IT'S THE FIRST SKI OF THE SEASON. THE snow is beautiful, the air is crisp, and you feel terrific. You're Wonder Woman! You effortlessly slice down the mountain again and again.

That was yesterday. Today, you can barely move. Every muscle in your body is screaming in pain. What happened?

You overdid it. Too much, too soon. Now your muscles are letting you know and you're paying the price with muscle pain.

Muscle pain from overuse is an all-too-common problem, especially at the beginning of a season of activities like gardening or sports or when we suddenly decide to "get into shape."

CAUSES

When you overuse your muscles, you actually break down muscle fibers, causing tiny tears. The torn fibers swell slightly and an accumulation of muscle-breakdown products, like enzymes, makes you feel stiff and sore.

Another common source of muscle pain is cramping. You're jogging or doing aerobic dance when suddenly your calf (or foot or thigh) is gripped with an incredible, incapacitating spasm that sends you writhing to the ground howling in pain. When a muscle cramps, it suddenly—and painfully—shortens and knots up. Muscle cramps can be caused by anything that interferes with the mechanisms that cause muscles to contract and relax—drugs, vigorous exercise in hot weather, even electrolyte (sodium/potassium) imbalance.

For a muscle to contract and relax properly, it needs adequate supplies of oxygen, fat, and sugar and the right concentrations of minerals like potassium, sodium, and calcium. When the brain wants a muscle to contract, it sends an electric "contract" signal down the nerves to the muscle. When the electric impulse reaches the muscle, the minerals calcium and sodium inside the muscle and potassium outside the muscle move, causing the brain's signal to flow along the muscle, causing it to contract.

A variety of factors can interfere with this complicated electrical message system. A muscle may spasm if you've worked it for too long and depleted its glycogen, its energy supply. Or there may be too many waste products in the muscle.

A muscle cramp is a clear signal from your body: "Stop. You've traumatized me." Any time you have a muscle cramp, your muscle isn't getting enough blood (and oxygen and fuel). To let you know it has a problem, the muscle spasms. The spasm, in turn, dramatically decreases the blood flow to the muscle, which causes pain.

Some women (and men) suffer painful nighttime leg cramping, especially in the calf. In fact, leg cramps at night are the most common form of muscle cramps. They are usually caused by a pinched nerve or an exaggeration of the normal muscle-tendon reflex. When you turn over in your sleep, nerves can become pinched and cause muscles to cramp. Or sometimes when you turn over, you contract the muscles, and the tendons attached to the muscles stretch. The stretched tendon sends a message to the spinal cord, which, in turn, sends a message to the muscle, causing it to contract painfully.

Muscle pain can also be caused by more serious injuries to the muscles like a strain or a tear. A muscle strain or "pulled muscle" occurs when you've stretched the muscle beyond its normal limit. A strain injures the muscle fibers, causing them to contract, bleed, and swell. Usually you'll feel a sharp stabbing pain when you try to move the muscle. Or, sometimes, the pain will be dull and throbbing.

A muscle tear occurs when the muscle has been so hyperextended that all of its fibers rupture and actually tear. A torn muscle is a serious injury that needs professional care.

AT-HOME TREATMENT

You can't always prevent muscle soreness, stiffness, or cramping. But when they do hit, you can use these home remedies to help ease your suffering.

Halt! Pain is your body talking to you. Listen! If you develop muscle cramps while exercising, stop immediately. Don't try to "exercise through it." If you do, you could end up with a muscle strain or tear.

Give it the old one-two. When a cramp strikes, take these two steps: 1) Stretch the cramped muscle with one hand; 2) At the same time, using your other hand, gently knead and squeeze the center of the muscle where you can feel the knot. Be sure to stretch the cramped muscle in the direction opposite from the way it's contracted. For example, if the cramp occurs in your calf muscle, stand on the leg and lean forward with your foot flat on the ground. If you can't stand on your leg, sit on the ground and pull your toes up toward your knee.

Take a walk. Once the muscle cramp has eased somewhat, take a few moments to walk around and get the blood flowing back into the muscle.

Cool it. OK, you know you've overdone it with activity. Now what? A cold shower or a cold bath right away can reduce trauma to your muscles and prevent muscle soreness and stiffness. Many world-class runners have their legs hosed off with cold water after a grueling workout.

You can also use ice packs to reduce the inflammation and soreness. Apply cold packs for 20 to 30 minutes at a time every hour. The cold shunts blood away from injured muscles and numbs the area, which reduces pain. It also brings about a "reflex inhibition" of the muscles, which causes them to relax.

Say no to heat. You're stiff and sore and a hot tub sounds great, right? Wrong! Heat can make muscle soreness and stiffness worse, especially within the first 24 hours after the injury. Hot tubs, showers, or heating pads increase blood circulation to the area, which causes the blood vessels to dilate, fluid to accumulate, and tissues to swell. When heat is used for too long, it causes the area to become congested and makes you feel even more sore and stiff.

If you can't say no to heat, don't overdo it. Never use heat on sore muscles for more than 20 minutes at a time. A better option is "contrast therapy," in which you alternate a hot pad for four minutes with an ice pack for one minute.

Reduce the pain. Some of the best anti-inflammatory drugs ever invented—aspirin and ibuprofen—are available over the counter. Follow the directions on the label. Over-the-counter aspirin creams also work well for reducing pain and inflammation.

Go for the stretch. You're so sore you can barely move, but moving is exactly what you should do. Light exercise, especially gentle stretches, the day after overexercising can really help. Try 20 minutes or so of stretching or easy walking.

Get into the swim of it. Another way to ease those sore muscles is to take a leisurely swim. The cool water will reduce muscle inflammation and the stretching will ease the stiffness.

Try massage. When you're sore and stiff, it's not the time to try deep tissue massage, but a gentle stroking will bring circulation to the area and feel terrific.

Nix "hot" and "cold" creams. You've heard the ads for them,

---

11 TIPS FOR TREATING MUSCLE PAIN

- If your muscle cramps, stop.
- Stretch and squeeze cramped muscles.
- After a cramp starts to loosen up, take a walk.
- Use cold on sore muscles.
- Don't use heat.
- Take anti-inflammatories.
- Stretch gently.
- Take a swim.
- Get a gentle massage.
- Don't use topical sports creams.
- Use R.I.C.E.

"They relieve sore, aching muscles instantly." Don't believe it. Those topical creams create a chemical reaction on the skin, but they don't actually heat or cool the tissues.

If you do use one of these products, test it first on a small area to make sure you're not allergic. Also, never use such a cream with a heating pad or hot water bottle because it can cause serious burns.

R.I.C.E. it. If you've pulled a muscle, try R.I.C.E.—rest, ice, compression, and elevation. Stay off the injury. Put a bag of ice cubes on it (20 minutes on; ten minutes off). Wrap it in an elastic bandage to reduce swelling. Keep the injured area elevated above your heart.

PREVENTION

Muscle pain usually isn't serious, but it can be bothersome and quite uncomfortable. Often, you can prevent muscle cramps before they strike. Try these tips to head off painful muscle cramps:

Start slowly, gently. You don't have to "go for the burn" to get into shape. In fact, if you have muscle soreness or stiffness a day or two after a workout, you've done too much. It's better to start slowly and build up your endurance over time; this is especially true if you've been inactive for a while. If you're pregnant or if you haven't been exercising and you're over 40, talk with your doctor before beginning an exercise program.

Check out your calcium/magnesium. Some health authorities believe that if you get muscle cramps often, you may not have enough calcium and magnesium in your muscles. Women, in particular, can become calcium deficient, especially as they get older and calcium loss increases. To stay healthy, most women need about 1,500 mg of calcium every day. Most women consume about half that amount in their daily diet. Consider taking calcium supplements. You can also increase your dietary calcium by eating calcium-rich foods such as almonds, brewer's yeast, broccoli, nonfat or low-fat dairy products, canned salmon, and dark, leafy vegetables like mustard and collard greens.

Yes, we have no bananas. If you're prone to muscle cramps, you may have a potassium deficiency. Try eating more foods that are rich in potassium like bananas, potatoes, oranges, and tomatoes. You probably don't need to take a potassium supplement unless you're also taking diuretics or "water pills" for water retention problems. If you're on such medication, talk with your doctor about the amount of potassium supplementation you need.

Get the muscles ready. One of the most effective ways to prevent muscle pain, cramping, and injuries like strains and tears is to warm up the muscles before exercising. Many people stretch first, then warm up. But exercise experts say it's better to warm up first, then stretch before exercising. Take five or ten minutes to walk or gently pedal your bike to "pre-warm" the muscles.

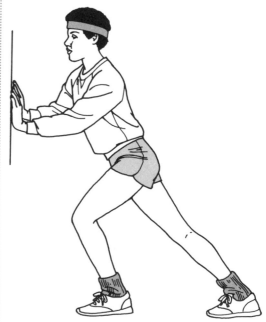

Stretch it out. Stretching after your pre-warm-up and before exercising increases muscle, tendon, and ligament flexibility. Do a series of stretches appropriate for your activity. Stretch gently. If any stretch hurts, stop immediately; you're stretching too far. Hold each stretch for at least 30 seconds and breathe deeply while holding. Never do "bouncing" exercises, which can actually cause muscles to contract rather than stretch.

Stay warm. You may notice you have more cramping on chilly days. Wrap up with layered clothing and keep those muscles warm to help prevent muscle cramps.

Drink, drink, drink. It's not uncommon to see runners or bicyclists on warm days suddenly seize up in pain from muscle cramps. The problem? Dehydration. One of the most common causes of muscle cramping, especially when it is hot out, is not drinking enough fluids. Drink before, during, and after exercising. Try to drink at least four ounces of water for every half mile in distance you cover.

Bouillon, please. If you're going to be exercising for more than an hour in hot weather, your body will lose not only water, but also valuable sodium. Some sports enthusiasts opt for expensive sports drinks, so-called electrolyte replacement fluids. But our experts recommend drinking a cup of beef or chicken bouillon before exercising as an effective and inexpensive way to replace lost sodium.

Try nighttime stretches. If the P.M. cramps are your problem, try stretching a few minutes before you go to bed. Pay particular attention to stretching out the

---

10 STRATEGIES TO PREVENT MUSCLE PAIN

- Start slowly and build endurance.
- Increase your calcium intake.
- Eat potassium-rich foods.
- Do "pre-stretch" warm-ups.
- Stretch before exercising.
- Stay warm.
- Drink plenty of fluids.
- Try drinking some bouillon before exercising.
- Stretch before you go to bed.
- Don't use heavy bed covers.

---

calf muscles. Try this "runner's stretch": Stand two to three feet from the wall and lean your chest against it, keeping your heels touching the floor. Can you feel the stretch in your calves?

Kick off those covers. The culprit in cramping of the feet and legs at night may be as close as your covers. Replace heavy blankets and quilts with an electric blanket set on low to keep your muscles warm and take some of the weight off.

Sources: **Ellen Nona Hoyven, P.T.**, Owner and Director, Ortho Sport Physical Therapy P.C., Clackamas, Oregon. **Chrissy Kane, L.P.T.**, Physical Therapist, Outpatient Physical Therapy Department, Providence Medical Center, Portland, Oregon. **Michael Martindale, L.P.T.**, Physical Therapist, Sports Medicine Center, Portland Adventist Medical Center, Portland, Oregon.

●NAUSEA AND VOMITING

How to Calm a

Queasy

Stomach

NAUSEA AND VOMITING ARE TWO symptoms that require very little introduction. Unfortunately, almost everyone has experienced them at one time or another. Although these symptoms can make you feel absolutely awful, they are usually not a sign of serious illness and almost always disappear within a day or so.

CAUSES

A variety of illnesses and ailments can cause nausea and vomiting. Some of the most common causes are food poisoning, bacterial or viral infections, allergic reactions to certain foods or drinks, overconsumption of alcohol, pregnancy, motion sickness, migraine headaches, ulcers, and the consumption of certain drugs.

AT-HOME TREATMENT

If you suspect that your queasiness is due to an ulcer, a headache, or morning sickness, see the corresponding sections in this book. Otherwise, try the suggestions that follow. They are designed to reduce your discomfort and to help your symptoms go away as quickly as possible.

Try a liquid diet. If your stomach is upset, it probably doesn't need the additional burden of digesting food. It's best to stick with fluids until you feel a little better. However, don't start replenishing fluids until you have stopped vomiting. Because cold liquids can irritate the stomach, make the first drink a warm one. A fluid containing sugar is most easily absorbed by the body.

Liquids are also necessary to prevent the dehydration that may occur as a result of vomiting or diarrhea. A good choice is a diluted, noncitrus fruit juice, such as apple juice, which may be drunk warm or cold.

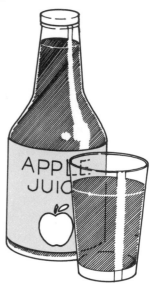

Go with the flow. Doctors agree that the best idea for ridding yourself of a 24-hour stomach bug is bed rest. You may feel miserable, but there is no choice except to let the illness run its course. The more rest you get, the more energy your body will have to devote to fighting the bug.

Avoid stomach irritants. As anyone who has suffered from a hangover knows, alcohol can be very irritating to the stomach. Fatty or highly seasoned foods, caffeine, and cigarettes are all hard on the stomach. These substances are best left for when you are feeling better.

Stick with the bland and the mushy. When you are ready to move from fluids to more solid food, start with soft foods, such as bread, unbuttered toast, steamed fish, or bananas. You should stay away from fats and stick to a low-fiber diet.

Add foods back gradually. When you do start eating again, begin with very small amounts of food. Gradually build up to larger meals.

Don't fight it. When you feel the urge to vomit, don't resist it. Trying to hold it back can damage your esophagus. Remember, vomiting is your body's way of trying to get rid of infection. For your own good, just go along with it.

Coat your stomach. Some over-the-counter stomach medications that contain bismuth, such as Pepto-Bismol, can coat the stomach and provide some relief. However, avoid Alka-Seltzer, because the aspirin in it can irritate the stomach.

Use a soothing compress. When vomiting, put a cold compress on your head. It won't stop your vomiting, but it may help you feel a little better.

Replace what you lose. Not only do you need to replace fluids you have lost through vomiting, but you must keep the proper balance of electrolytes (sodium and potassium) in your system. You can do this by taking a sports drink, such as Gatorade, that contains the electrolytes you need and is gentle on the stomach.

AT THE DOCTOR'S

If your vomiting is violent or persists for more than 24 hours or if the vomit contains blood, you should

9 STEPS TO A CALMER STOMACH
• Stick with clear liquids.
• Rest in bed until you recover.
• Avoid stomach irritants.
• When you start to eat again, begin with bland, soft foods.
• Start with small amounts of food and build up to larger meals.
• Never fight the urge to vomit.
• Take an over-the-counter medication containing bismuth.
• Place a cold compress on your forehead.
• Try a sports drink to replace electrolytes.

probably see a doctor, since you may be suffering from a potentially serious illness. The physician will ask you questions about the circumstances preceding your symptoms in an attempt to ferret out the cause of your discomfort. She may also conduct blood tests and cultures for viruses or bacteria. If she determines that your stomach upset is caused by a bacterial infection, the doctor may choose to prescribe antibiotics. She may prescribe other types of medication for nausea and vomiting that are caused by infectious diseases, food poisoning, or parasites.

Sources: **Cornelius P. Dooley, M.D.**, Gastroenterologist, Santa Fe, New Mexico. **Steven C. Fiske, M.D.**, Past President, New Jersey Gastroenterological Society; Associate Professor of Medicine/ Gastroenterology, Seton Hall University School of Postgraduate Medicine; Assistant Clinical Professor of Medicine and Gastroenterology, University of Medicine and Dentistry of New Jersey, Newark, New Jersey. **Albert B. Knapp, M.D., F.A.C.P.**, Adjunct Assistant Attending Physician, Lenox Hill Hospital, New York, New York; Instructor in Medicine, New York Medical College, Valhalla, New York. **Neville R. Pimstone, M.D.**, Chief of Hepatology, Division of Gastroenterology, University of California Davis, Davis, California.

•NECK PAIN

ANY NUMBER OF THINGS CAN BRING ON that persistent pain. A long, hard day at the office, a frustrating argument with one of your kids, or a night's sleep in an awkward position can leave you with a stiff, sore neck. At work or at home, any area of your life that causes you stress can become a literal "pain in the neck."

CAUSES

Plenty of things can contribute to neck pain, including emotional tension. Worrying about your job, your relationship or family, or holding back feelings of anger, sadness, and fear can cause you to tense the muscles in your neck, resulting in pain and stiffness.

Poor posture can cause neck pain, too. To function properly—and painlessly—the head and spine must balance in a straight line against the pull of gravity. Poor posture, obesity, weak stomach muscles, or too much sitting can all pull the curve of the lower back forward. To compensate, the upper back curves further backward and the neck is forced painfully forward. People with jobs that require them to lean forward often develop a pain in the neck commonly known as "desk neck." Even sleeping on a too-soft mattress or in a neck-straining position such as facedown or on a pillow that's too high, can leave your neck with "kinks."

Of course, injuries like those common in sports, neck sprains ("whiplash") caused by auto accidents, or anything that causes the neck to be snapped backward (hyperextended), can bring on neck pain and stiffness, too. So can diseases and "wear and tear" problems like arthritis. But by far the most common cause of neck pain is simple muscular tension.

It's no wonder neck pain is common. Just look at the neck's construction. The neck is a slender stack of seven small bones called the vertebrae, which are held in place by 32 complex muscles. Eight nerves carry movement and sensation (including pain) messages and four major arteries and veins transport blood between the head and heart. To make this engineering nightmare even more complex, the neck is more mobile than any other part of the body and holds up a 20-pound head.

When muscles become tense due to physical or emotional stresses, the blood supply to the muscles shuts down. The neck muscles object by sending pain messages via the nerves. The pain, in turn, causes even more tension, less blood flow, and more pain. To relieve this tension-pain-tension cycle, you have to eliminate what's causing the muscle tension and then relieve the muscle spasms.

AT-HOME TREATMENT

Try these strategies to break the tension-pain-tension cycle:

Take the weight off. Lying down is one of the simplest and most effective ways to relieve the neck of its heavy burden and give it a chance to recover. Be sure the pillow you're using lets your head lie flat, in line with the rest of your spine.

Cool it. Ice decreases inflammation and soothes painful nerves. You can use an ice substitute or fill a plastic bag with ice, cover it with a pillowcase, and apply it to your neck for 15 minutes at a time.

Go for heat. Once the ice has brought down the inflammation and calmed irritated nerve endings, heat can ease stiff muscles. Heat increases circulation to the area and feels great. Apply a warm towel or hot-water bottle, or stand in a hot shower and let the water hit your neck. Be careful not to overdo it, though. Too much heat can inflame your symptoms and worsen the pain.

Massage it out. Massage is great for easing tense muscles and can provide temporary relief from muscle-tension pain. Take a hot bath or shower first to relax your muscles. Then have someone use oil or lotion and gently rub your neck and shoulders using small, circular motions. Next, have them use a firmer pressure and rub your neck and shoulders with long, downward strokes. Or, you can give yourself a neck massage for 10 or 15 minutes. If you have your massage just before retiring, it'll help you sleep.

Try anti-inflammatories. Aspirin, ibuprofen, and acetaminophen are effective over-the-counter anti-inflammatories that can help ease your neck pain. If your stomach is bothered by aspirin, ask your pharmacist for enteric-coated brands.

---

6 WAYS TO RELIEVE A PAIN IN THE NECK

- Lie down.
- Use ice.
- After icing, try some heat.
- Use massage to relax your muscles.
- Take over-the-counter pain relievers.
- Call the doctor.

Call your doctor. Usually minor neck pain and stiffness can be effectively handled at home with the remedies listed here. In most cases, the pain disappears within a day or two. However, some types of neck pain require professional help. See your doctor if:
- your pain is caused by an injury.
- your neck pain is accompanied by fever, headache, or muscle aches.
- you have tingling or numbness in your arms or hands.
- you have vision problems.
- the pain increases or persists for several days despite home remedies.

PREVENTION

It's best to prevent the tension-pain-tension cycle before it starts. Try these strategies for protecting your precious neck.

Schedule neck breaks. At work or play, try not to stay in any one position for too long, especially if you're in a neck-straining position. Set a timer to remind yourself to take a break once or twice every hour. Stretch and walk around for a few minutes before returning to your activity.

Make your work "on the level." Do you find yourself rubbing a sore neck by late afternoon? Chances are your work area is contributing to your neck problems. When you lean over, look down, or reach up for long periods of time, you strain your neck and shoulder muscles. Keep you work at eye level. Change the height of your chair, computer screen, or desk. Use stands to hold up reading material. Don't reach up, use a stepladder.

8 TIPS FOR PREVENTING NECK PAIN

- Take frequent breaks.
- Work at eye level.
- Stay fit.
- Do neck exercises.
- Strengthen your stomach muscles.
- Improve your posture.
- Sleep on a firm mattress.
- Learn to relax.

Keep in shape. A strong, flexible neck can withstand a great deal of strain without pain or injury. Keep your neck strong with the neck exercises listed in this chapter. You can also strengthen your neck and back by swimming.

Exercise that neck. There are two types of neck exercises that are terrific for increasing neck flexibility and strength: range-of-motion exercises and isometric exercises. Range-of-motion exercises stretch stiff neck muscles. If your neck feels sore or stiff, apply moist heat before doing the exercises. Perform them slowly, breathing out as you stretch, and repeat them three times per day, five times each session.

1) *Head to shoulder.* Sit up straight, but relaxed. Slowly turn your head to the right as far as you can, hold, then return it to center. Repeat in the opposite direction.

2) *Head to chin.* Drop your chin slowly onto your chest, hold, relax.

3) *Ear to shoulder.* Tilt your head toward your left ear, hold, and return to center. Repeat on the opposite side.

4) *Head back.* Tilt your head backward so that you're looking at the ceiling. Hold, then bring it back down.

Isometric exercises are performed against resistance. The key is not to move your head during resistance.

1) *Palm/Forehead press.* Sit up and relax, press your forehead into your palm, resisting the motion.

2) *Side head press.* Sit erect and relaxed, press your hand against the right side of your head, trying to bring your ear to your shoulder. Resist the motion. Repeat on the opposite side.

3) *Back of neck press.* Tilt your head forward. Press both hands against the back of your head. Try to pull your head up, but resist the motion.

4) *Temple press.* As you press your hand against your temple, try to turn your chin to your shoulder. Resist the motion.

Break your bad habits. Most of us have developed pain-in-the-neck habits such as talking with the phone "crimped" between our neck and shoulder, shampooing hair in the sink, or sleeping with a fat pillow. Be aware of the activities that cause your neck strain and avoid them or replace them with neck-healthy ones.

Look to your stomach. If you have poor muscle tone in your abdominal muscles, it forces the upper-back curve backward and the neck painfully forward. Strengthen stomach muscles with exercises like bent-knee situps.

Check your posture. Poor posture can pull the curve of the lower back forward, which, in turn, causes the upper back to curve farther backward and the neck to curve forward to compensate.

Check your posture with the "wall test." Stand with your back to a wall, heels several inches from the wall. Your buttocks and shoulders should touch the wall and the back of your head should be close to the wall. Keep your chin level. Now step away from the wall. Step back and check your posture again. This "wall posture" is the one you should maintain throughout the day.

Buy a new mattress. Do you wake up every morning feeling stiff and sore in your neck or back? Blame your too-soft mattress, pillows that are too high, or poor sleeping habits. Sleep on a firm mattress and use a pillow that keeps your head level. Don't sleep on your stomach; it forces your head up.

Learn to relax. Some people walk around with shoulders hunched, neck tense. It's a habit. They aren't even aware they're holding their body tensely. Become aware of your muscle tension with progressive relaxation. Sit in a quiet place. Starting with your head, alternately tense, then fully relax all the muscle groups in your body. By the time you've reached your feet, you should be feeling relaxed.

Pay attention to your muscle tension. What makes you tense up? When you're in a stressful situation, practice consciously relaxing tense muscles. Or whenever you feel your muscles tensing up, breathe deeply into your abdomen, pushing out your belly, and then let it all out completely.

Sources: **Robert Berselli, M.D.,** Orthopedic Surgeon, Portland, Oregon. **Kathleen Galligan, D.C.,** Chiropractor, Lake Oswego, Oregon. **Michael Martindale, L.P.T.,** Physical Therapist, Sports Medicine Center, Portland Adventist Medical Center, Portland, Oregon.

●OILY HAIR

Get Rid of the

Grease

NOTHING CAN RUIN A BEAUTIFUL HAIR-style faster than oily hair. Excess oil makes hair look stringy, dirty, and limp. With greasy hair, it's almost impossible to hold a styling shape. Oily tresses are a common problem that bedevils millions—men and women alike.

Oil—in moderation—is a natural and healthy part of hair. Everyone's scalp has oil (sebaceous) glands that secrete sebum, or oil, onto the hair shafts. Oil is what helps keep the hair moist and prevents it from becoming too brittle and breaking. Oil is also what gives hair its luster and shine. People with oily hair simply have too much of a good thing.

CAUSES

If you have oily hair, chances are you have oily skin, too. The oil is just appearing on a different part of the skin—the scalp. The same factors that bring about oily skin produce oily hair. One of these factors is genetics. If members of your family have oily hair (or oily skin), you probably will, too.

The texture of your hair can also determine how oily your hair is. Fine hair tends to be oilier than coarser hair. Because fine hairs are smaller in circumference and the hairs take up less room on the scalp, people with fine hair usually have more hair. The more hair follicles, the more oil glands (two or three per hair follicle) pumping sebum onto the hair. In fact, a person with fine hair may have as many as 140,000 oil glands. Since fine hair is more fragile, the additional oil helps protect it from breakage.

You've probably noticed that your hair feels oilier at certain times in your menstrual cycle. That's because hormones called androgens affect oil production. Most women say their hair is oiliest near the beginning and end of the menstrual period, and less oily during the middle of the period. Because of these hormones, young women in their teens and early 20s often complain of oily hair.

AT-HOME TREATMENT

You can't change your genes or your sex hormones, but there are some things you can do to combat greasy hair.

Bring on the shampoo. If you've got oily hair, go ahead and shampoo every day. Some women find that, at certain times of the month, they have to shampoo twice a day to control the oilies.

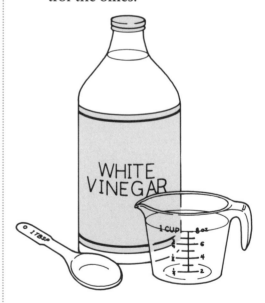

Try an acidic rinse. One way to make sure you've really rinsed the soap and excess oil from your hair is to use an acidic rinse after shampooing. Use two tablespoons of white vinegar to one cup of water, or use the juice of one lemon (strained) to one cup of water. Rinse through hair, then rinse with warm water.

Lather up. Your shampoo can remove only so much oil at one time, so don't be stingy with the shampoo.

One more time. Shampoo and rinse thoroughly once. Then repeat the process to make sure you get rid of the oil. If your hair is really oily, try leaving the shampoo on for five minutes or so before rinsing.

Go for a "solvent" shampoo. You can spend all kinds of money on shampoos with fragrances, conditioners, and additives, but they won't cut the grease. You need a "solvent" type shampoo that will wash out the excess oil. Some experts recommend adding a couple of drops of Ivory Liquid to your regular shampoo. Or you can use commercial solvent-type shampoos without additives, like Prell or Suave. Normal hair needs shampoos with a pH between 4.5 and 6.7. Oily hair needs more alkaline products—shampoos with a pH higher than 6.7.

Rinse, rinse, rinse. Regardless of the shampoo you use, rinse thoroughly. Soap residue collects dirt and oil quickly.

Nix conditioners. Dry hair needs conditioning, oily hair doesn't. Conditioners coat the hair shafts, something oily hair doesn't need. If you find your ends have become dried out, just apply a small amount of

9 WAYS TO BEAT THE "GREASIES"

- Shampoo daily.
- Use plenty of shampoo.
- Shampoo twice.
- Use "solvent" shampoos.
- Rinse your hair thoroughly after shampooing.
- Don't use conditioners.
- Try an acidic rinse.
- Don't overdo the brushing.
- Reconsider your birth control.

conditioner to the dry ends, not your whole head.

Forego the 100 brush strokes. "Brush your hair 100 times at night." That's the old advice for beautiful hair. Forget it if you've got oily hair. Too much brushing simply distributes oil from your scalp down the hair follicles.

Reconsider your birth control. Since sex hormones affect the scalp's oil production, you may find that birth control pills increase your hair's oiliness. If oiliness is a problem, talk with your doctor about it when choosing contraception. You may wish to use a barrier method such as a diaphragm.

Sources: **Paul Contorer, M.D.**, Chief of Dermatology, Kaiser Permanente; Clinical Professor of Dermatology, Oregon Health Sciences University, Portland, Oregon. **Rose Dygart**, Cosmetologist; Barber; Hair-Care Instructor; Manicurist; Owner, Le Rose Salon of Beauty, Lake Oswego, Oregon. **Nelson Lee Novick, M.D.**, Author, *Super Skin: A Leading Dermatologist's Guide to the Latest Breakthroughs and Treatments in Skin Care*; Associate Clinical Professor of Dermatology, Mt. Sinai School of Medicine, New York, New York.

●OILY SKIN

Tips for Grease

Relief

CREAMY MOISTURIZERS HAVE NEVER been your best friend. You put on your makeup at 8:00 A.M., but by 10:00 A.M., your forehead, nose, and cheeks are shining with an oily residue. You've got oily skin. Your only consolation is that years from now your skin will probably look better, and younger, than that of your drier-skinned friends because you'll wrinkle less.

If you have oily skin, it probably isn't the only oil-related problem you're dealing with. People with oily skin not only suffer from skin that has an oily appearance and feel (often less than an hour after washing), but they often also have more blackheads, whiteheads, and acne breakouts. Oily-skinned individuals also tend to have larger pores, which indicate large oil glands. These same people usually have oily hair and many have problem dandruff. That's because the same factors that cause oily skin cause oily hair.

CAUSES

If you trace your skin's genealogy, you'll probably find that others in your family—your mother, grandmother, father, perhaps an aunt—had oily skin too. It's a genetically inherited trait. Some people inherit so-called normal skin, while others inherit dry or oily skin.

Your hormones also play a big part in the oiliness of your skin. When you were a child, your facial oil glands (sebaceous glands) were very small and didn't produce much oil. When you hit puberty and the hormones started flowing, your oil glands grew larger and began secreting more oil. That's why so many teenagers and young women (and men) in their 20s have problems with oily skin. The amount of oil your sebaceous glands secrete depends on your inherited tendency toward oily skin and the amount and kind of hormones your body produces.

It's the male hormones (androgens) that control oil production in the skin. For women, this may sound contradictory, but a woman's body produces both male and female hormones. In women, these hormones are produced by the ovaries and the adrenal glands. Many women notice that their skin looks and feels more oily at certain times around their menstrual cycle and during menopause. This is due to the fluctuating levels of androgens.

Most women who have oily skin have a normal hormonal balance. A few, however, have too much oil because the ovaries or adrenal glands are producing too much hormone. If you have excessively oily skin, you may want to talk with your doctor and see if you need a blood test to determine if you need hormone-balancing therapy.

One of the myths about oily skin is that it causes acne. Acne is caused when oil becomes trapped below the skin's pores and becomes contaminated with bacteria. People with oily skin don't have blocked oil problems. The oil readily comes to the skin's surface. Acne problems can appear when excess oil isn't removed and it clogs the pores.

AT-HOME TREATMENT

You can't change your family genetics or your normal hormone output, but you can do plenty to get grease relief. These tips can help you with your oily skin:

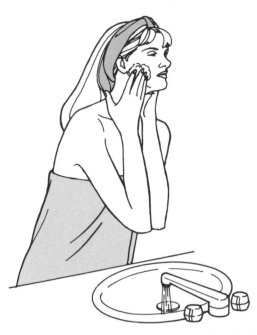

Cleanse, cleanse, cleanse. It's vital to keep oily skin squeaky clean. When your skin looks oily, it also looks and feels dirty. Cleansing removes excess oil and dead skin cells. Wash your skin at least twice a day—more if necessary.

Choose your soap carefully. Dry skin needs moisturizing-type soaps. Oily skin needs a detergent-type soap. Inexpensive bath soaps like Ivory work well to cut the grease. Some dermatologists recommend adding a couple of drops of Ivory Liquid dishwashing detergent to your regular cleansing soap to act as a solvent and clean the grease. Other skin-care experts believe that dishwashing liquid is too harsh—even for oily skin. A milder grease-cutting alternative is a glycerine soap.

Try wipes. Rubbing alcohol is a terrific degreaser. Astringent wipes that contain alcohol or a combination of acetone (Sebinil) and alcohol help remove oil and dead skin cells and make pores appear smaller. Use astringents every couple of hours between face washings. You can buy individual, pre-packaged alcohol towelettes, which are easy to carry with you, or you can simply blot your face with rubbing alcohol.

Pull out the facial tissues. If you don't have an alcohol wipe available, simply wipe off the excess oil with a paper facial tissue. Cosmetic companies like Estee Lauder also offer special oil-absorbing tissues that are very effective in removing oil between cleansings.

Cool it. Cold water is an excellent way to get rid of excess oil. Try splashing your face with cool water a couple of times a day.

Forget moisturizers. Save your money. You don't need moisturizers. Never go to bed with creams on your skin or you'll wake with an oily mess in the morning. Forgo oils, too. Don't use mineral oil or petroleum oil on your oily skin. Applying external oil to your skin can clog your pores and cause acne.

Try mist. People with oily skin often have to cleanse their faces several times a day. But all that soap, water, and drying can rob moisture from the skin. Since applying moisturizers isn't the answer, what can you do about dried-out oily skin? Try facial mists (available in health-food stores) that provide moisturizer without adding oil or chemicals. These usually contain mineral water, herbs, and sometimes vitamins.

Scrub-a-dub. Gentle facial scrubs are great for removing oils and dead skin cells from oily skin. You can make your own by mixing a small amount of finely ground almonds (almond meal) with honey. Then gently massage the almond-honey paste into your skin with a hot washcloth. Rinse thoroughly. You can also make a scrub from oatmeal and aloe vera gel. Rub gently onto the skin, leave on for 15 minutes, then rinse thoroughly.

---

11 TIPS FOR TREATING YOUR OILY SKIN

- Keep your skin clean.
- Use a grease-cutting soap.
- Wipe with astringents.
- Blot oil with facial tissues.
- Splash your skin with cold water.
- Don't use moisturizers.
- Mist your skin with facial sprays.
- Use facial scrubs.
- Try masques.
- Use no makeup or water-based makeup only.
- Call the doctor.

Put on a masque. Skin-care experts often use clay masques to remove excess oil. You can buy clay masques over the counter or make your own by mixing a little Fuller's Earth (available at pharmacies) and water to make a paste. Apply to your face and leave on for 20 minutes. Rinse thoroughly.

Go for water-based. If you have oily skin, you really shouldn't use makeup. Try to go without it as often as possible. If you do use makeup, use water-based rather than oil-based types. Look for "matte"-type makeup. Also, blot excess oil with powder or gel blushers.

Hello, doctor? Usually, you can effectively cope with oily skin using home remedies, but sometimes you need professional help. See your dermatologist if you get acne or if you notice any sudden change in your skin (e.g., from dry to oily).

Sources: **Vera Brown,** Skin-Care Expert; Author, *Vera Brown's Natural Beauty Book.* **Paul Contorer, M.D.,** Chief of Dermatology, Kaiser Permanente; Clinical Professor of Dermatology, Oregon Health Sciences University, Portland, Oregon. **Nelson Lee Novick, M.D.,** Author, *Super Skin: A Leading Dermatologist's Guide to the Latest Breakthroughs and Treatments in Skin Care;* Associate Clinical Professor of Dermatology, Mt. Sinai School of Medicine, New York, New York. **Frank Parker, M.D.,** Professor and Chairman, Department of Dermatology, Oregon Health Sciences University, Portland, Oregon. **Margaret Robertson, M.D.,** Staff Physician, St. Vincent Hospital and Medical Center, Portland, Oregon.

How to Keep

Your Bones

Healthy and

Strong

Perhaps your grandmother suffered from the problem: She walked with hunched shoulders and seemed to grow a little shorter every year. Now, maybe, your mother is starting to develop the same stoop. You're worried that you could be next.

Osteoporosis, or porous bones, plagues almost one-third of all women over 60 years of age. It is characterized chiefly by a decrease in the calcium content of the bones, which leaves them thin and brittle. Although its origins are largely unknown, osteoporosis is one of the most common disorders affecting women. The disease is not life-threatening, but may lead to bone fractures, which can result in serious complications.

As the disease progresses, the spinal column may decrease in length, causing a height loss of as much as several inches. It may also become curved, producing the characteristic "dowager's hump." These changes result from fractures caused by the pressure of body weight on the deteriorating vertebrae.

SYMPTOMS

Depending on the strength of the bones, osteoporosis may initially cause either no symptoms or extreme pain. If there is pain, it is most commonly in the lower back. Initially, sudden back pain may follow fractures of the vertebrae (the bones of the spine). Pain from the fracture itself may subside, but discomfort from osteoporosis may continue. The pain could lead to further inactivity, which in turn weakens additional vertebrae.

CAUSES

The chances of acquiring osteoporosis seem to increase dramatically with age. One prevailing theory maintains that the disease results from a loss of the female hormone, estrogen, which affects the calcium content of the bones. Menopause (cessation of menstruation) and hysterectomy (which induces menopause) may lead to osteoporosis, because the body's production of estrogen is linked to menstruation.

A diet deficient in nutrients, especially calcium, may also contribute to osteoporosis. So can being sedentary.

For reasons that are not entirely known, osteoporosis is more likely to affect white and Asian women than black women. In addition, slender women, especially those who have fair skin, run a higher risk of having the disorder than do stouter, darker-skinned women.

Osteoporosis is almost exclusively a women's disease. There are a number of reasons why this may be so. After puberty, men have more bone at most sites than women do. So at peak bone mass, men are at an advantage. What's more, while both men and women begin to lose bone mass as they age, this loss becomes accelerated in women at menopause, when estrogen levels drop. Bone loss in women eventually levels off to about one percent per year. In contrast, men lose only about half a percent per year.

AT THE DOCTOR'S

If you suspect that you have osteoporosis, you should make an appointment with your physician. It's best to have the condition diagnosed as soon as possible, before it progresses too far.

If you are diagnosed with osteoporosis, your physician will probably recommend many of the lifestyle changes mentioned in this chapter. For advanced cases, she may prescribe a back brace to help support your body weight while sitting or standing. Crutches, walkers, or a cane may assist walking.

Although the subject of estrogen replacement in menopause has been controversial, most physicians now agree that this bone-saving treatment is safe and beneficial for women without a family history of breast cancer. You can speak with your doctor to find out whether you might be a candidate for this therapy. If your doctor does prescribe hormones for you, you will need to be carefully monitored, since the drugs can cause adverse side effects. You should also have a physical examination and a Pap test (examination of cells scraped from the vagina and cervix to detect cancer) every six months, because of a suspected link between estrogen supplements and uterine and breast cancer.

PREVENTION

The good news is that osteoporosis can usually be prevented with some simple lifestyle changes. It may also be reversed, to some extent, in individuals who are already suffering from the condition. (However, if you have been diagnosed as having osteoporosis, speak with your doctor before beginning any program of home treatment.)

Start exercising. One of the most crucial strategies for preventing osteoporosis is to start a life-long exercise program. The reason is that the skeleton is responsive to mechanical load,

the amount of force you use against your bones. The more mechanical load you apply, the more your bones increase in mass. The best way to "load up" is to engage in activities, such as weight-bearing exercise, that use the body's own weight as a force against gravity. These types of exercise stimulate bone-cell production. Notice the well-developed swinging arm of professional baseball and tennis players (the mechanical load in these sports is the ball striking the racket or bat).

Running is a good bone-building exercise, but some find that their joints take too much of a pounding. Walking may be the better choice for you; it's less strenuous on the joints, and it can be done almost anywhere without expensive equipment. A brisk walk helps the whole body, including the heart. Lower-impact activities, including swimming and bicycling, are helpful, too.

For best results, perform your exercise of choice for at least one hour a day, three days per week. But don't overdo it: Studies show that excessive exercise can deplete fat and calcium stores, which may cause some women to stop menstruating. This exercise-induced amenorrhea, just like menopause, puts overzealous athletes at increased risk for getting osteoporosis.

Avoid being underweight or overweight. You may have dieted and suffered for your slim figure, but being about ten percent or more lighter than the average weight for your age and height puts you at higher risk for developing a deficiency of calcium and other vitamins and minerals important to your bones. Those who are overweight tend to be less active, and exercise is vital to healthy bones.

Lift weights. Weight lifting also prompts the activation of new bone cells. After you've obtained your doctor's OK, start with light weights and very gradually progress to heavier weights as you become stronger.

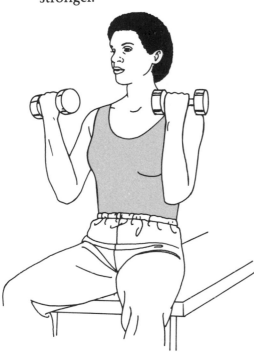

Get more calcium. Since osteoporosis often originates from a calcium deficiency, try to increase your intake of the mineral. The best way to do this is to drink more milk. In addition to its calcium content, milk is fortified with vitamin D, which facilitates the absorption of calcium. The low-fat varieties of milk are healthiest overall.

If you have a hard time consuming enough dairy products to keep up your calcium intake (either because you are dieting, are lactose intolerant, or because you simply don't care for them), there are many other calcium-rich foods that you can—and should—include in your diet. Whenever possible, eat foods raw; cooking foods sometimes robs them of their calcium content. Here are some nondairy, calcium-rich menu suggestions:
• Calcium-fortified orange juice.
• Beans, especially kidney, pinto, and for the adventurous, tofu (soybean curd), which is rich in both calcium and protein.
• Broccoli, preferably raw.
• Nuts, especially hazelnuts, Brazil nuts, and almonds.
• Figs.
• Prunes.
• Leafy greens, especially romaine lettuce, collard greens, and kale. Spinach is not a good choice, since its calcium is not readily absorbed by the body.
• Salmon and sardines, canned, with the bones.

If you are lactose intolerant, you can take the lactase-enzyme tablets available on the market to ease your digestion of dairy products. You can also try eating yogurt and hard cheeses. The lactose, or milk sugar, in yogurt has already been broken down, so your digestive system won't have to do it. However, this holds true only for yogurt containing active cultures (the container will say whether the product contains active cultures). The lactose in hard cheeses breaks down during the aging process. Another tip is to add a small amount of vinegar to leach the calcium out of the bones you use for soup or stew stock. The amount of calcium in a single pint of homemade soup made this way is equal to the calcium found in a quart of milk.

Although increasing your calcium intake is important, it's also crucial not to go overboard, since excess calcium can interfere with the absorption of other nutrients, such as copper and zinc. Stick to the Recommended Daily Allowance (RDA) for calcium, which is 1,200 milligrams for pregnant or lactating women, as well as for women aged 11 through 25. Over age 25, the RDA is 800 milligrams.

Get enough vitamin C. Vitamin C enhances the body's uptake of calcium. Some good sources of vitamin C are orange juice and cantaloupe.

Catch some rays. Women living in colder, more northern climates have a higher incidence of osteoporosis than women living in warmer, sunnier areas. It's not the temperature, but the amount of sunshine, that makes the differ-

ence. The light rays activate the vitamin D in the body. You don't have to roast yourself in the sun for hours at a time to reap the benefits of sunlight. Fifteen minutes of sun exposure each day might do the trick without greatly increasing your risk of skin cancer. Sunscreen blocks out the ultraviolet rays that are needed to activate the vitamin D. So, if you are fair-skinned or have another reason to be very concerned about skin cancer, you may be better off protecting your skin from the sun and trying to make up for the lack of sun exposure with dietary sources of vitamin D, such as fortified, low-fat milk.

Just say no to coffee and tea. And cola, too, because they all contain caffeine. Caffeine promotes the excretion of calcium through the urine. More than two cups of brewed coffee or four cups of brewed tea per day can prompt this increase in calcium loss.

Don't be taken in by a common myth. You might have heard that consuming high levels of phosphorus can influence bone loss and the risk of osteoporosis. However, the Food and Drug Administration has not found any evidence to substantiate this claim.

Consume protein and fiber sensibly. Protein is both friend and foe to healthy bones. In excess, protein in the diet increases the body's excretion of calcium. On the other hand, a proper amount of protein is needed to help maintain collagen, a bone component that is made up of proteins. The problem is not eating too much protein, but rather getting enough calcium to balance out the amount of protein in your diet. If you get enough calcium, don't worry about getting too much protein. However, if you think your calcium intake is substandard, try to avoid going overboard with protein-rich foods.

Fiber can adversely affect calcium absorption in two ways. It combines with calcium in the intestine, and at the same time, increases the rate at which food is passed through the intestinal tract. Don't eliminate fiber, though; it is an important part of a healthful diet. Just try not to eat calcium-rich foods and fiber-rich foods together.

Don't drink alcohol. Alcohol consumption impairs the absorption of calcium.

Quit smoking. Like alcohol, nicotine interferes with calcium absorption. Smoking is associated with lower bone mass.

Consider fluoride. Fluoride is the only known substance that actually increases bone mass. However, experts have not yet come to a conclusion about how much they should prescribe. While the mineral is a bone builder, too much of it can actually make bones brittle. As it stands now, use of fluoride to fight osteoporosis remains controversial. You might want to discuss fluoride with your doctor.

13 Ways to Prevent Osteoporosis

- Start a program of weight-bearing exercise, such as walking or jogging.
- Maintain a healthy body weight.
- Start a program of weight lifting.
- Increase your calcium consumption.
- Make sure that you get enough vitamin C.
- Boost your vitamin D stores.
- Avoid caffeine.
- Don't worry about phosphorus.
- Be careful about your consumption of protein and fiber.
- Avoid alcoholic beverages.
- Don't smoke.
- Get the facts on fluoride.
- Learn about osteoporosis.

Get more info. The more you know about osteoporosis, the more you can do about it. You can get information about osteoporosis from the National Osteoporosis Foundation at 2100 M St. N.W., Suite 602–B, Washington, D.C. 20037. The phone number is 800-223-9994.

Sources: Richard C. Bozian, M.D., Director of Research, Monarch Foundation, Cincinnati, Ohio; Professor of Medicine, Assistant Professor of Biochemistry, Director, Division of Nutrition, University of Cincinnati, Cincinnati, Ohio. Victor G. Ettinger, M.D., Medical Director, Bone Diagnostic Centres, Torrance and Long Beach, California. Robert P. Heaney, M.D., John A. Creighton University Professor, Creighton University, Omaha, Nebraska. Rose Hust, Osteoporosis Coordinator, Knoxville Orthopedic Clinic, Knoxville, Tennessee. Conrad Johnston, M.D., Chief, Division of Endocrinology and Metabolism, Indiana University School of Medicine, Indianapolis, Indiana.

POSTNASAL DRIP

Strategies to

Stem the Flow

YOU KNOW THE FEELING. IT'S THAT annoying sensation that something is in the back of your throat, causing you to hack and cough. You've got postnasal drip.

You probably aren't aware of it, but mucus flows constantly from the back of the nose into the throat and is automatically swallowed. In fact, your sinuses normally produce one to two quarts of the stuff in a day. It's nonirritating and helps keep your nasal tissues and sinuses lubricated. It also helps clean, moisten, and humidify the air you inhale.

CAUSES

The hacking, "gunky" feeling of postnasal drip occurs when your nose produces too much or too little of this mucus. If there's too much mucus, it accumulates behind the nose. If there's not enough, the mucus becomes so thick it can't properly drain down the throat. Often people don't even realize they're suffering from postnasal drip. Instead, they complain of hoarseness, chronic sore throat, and the need to "clear" the throat. When they resolve their postnasal drip problem, the symptoms disappear.

Lots of things cause the sinuses to under- or over-produce mucus:

Allergies. Hay fever–type allergies are one of the most common causes of postnasal drip.

Colds. The common cold (upper respiratory infection) usually produces runny nose symptoms that include postnasal drip.

Nasal or sinus polyps. These are noncancerous growths that can obstruct the passageways of the nose or sinus and block or alter the flow of mucus, affecting air flow. Anatomical abnormalities like a deviated septum (the partition that divides the nose into two sides) can also change mucus production.

Sinus infection. Called "sinusitis," these painful infections of the sinus cavities can occur when the passages become swollen or blocked. Fluid accumulates and microorganisms infect it. If your mucus is yellow or green, you may have a sinus infection. See your doctor for antibiotics.

Dust, smoke, or other irritants. When your nose is exposed to dry, dusty, or smoky conditions, the mucous membranes can become dried out and unable to produce needed mucus. The result is thick mucus and postnasal drip.

Air pollution. Exposure to nitrogen dioxide and sulfur dioxide, the two major components of smog, can cause your sinuses to increase mucus production.

"Drying" medications. Some medications such as antihistamines, diuretics, and certain tranquilizers have a drying effect on mucus production. Any drug that makes your mouth and eyes feel dry probably has the same effect on the sinuses.

Aging. As you age, your sinuses produce less nasal mucus and it is thicker, with a lower water content.

Pregnancy. Some pregnant women complain of postnasal drip. Doctors suspect hormones may be to blame.

"Rebound" nasal sprays. Many people find temporary relief with over-the-counter nasal sprays. These inhalers are "vasoconstrictors" that reduce inflammation and swelling of the nasal passages by reducing blood flow to the area. When they are used for three days or more, products that contain phenylephrine hydrochloride, oxymetazoline hydrochloride, and xylometazoline hydrochloride can have a "rebound" effect and make your postnasal drip worse.

Cold air. Inhaling cold, dry air can promote postnasal drip. This is especially a problem in buildings with air conditioning or forced-air heating. Very dry air, like the air in planes, can also bring on a case of postnasal drip.

Sometimes "gunk" in your throat in the morning isn't from postnasal drip. You may have "esophageal reflux," or heartburn. When you have heartburn, the valve that keeps the stomach contents where they belong doesn't function properly and allows the contents to come back up into the throat during the night. In the morning, you wake up with a bad taste in your mouth, need to clear your throat, and have hoarseness that gets better as the day wears on. If you think heartburn may be the problem, try elevating the head of your bed six to eight inches, avoid overeating and eating within a couple of hours of retiring, and cut back on alcohol and caffeine.

Your throat difficulties may also be due to swallowing problems. As we age, the muscles involved in the complicated process of swallowing weaken and may not function properly. Even stress, and accompanying muscle spasms in the throat, may be your "postnasal" culprit. See your physician for proper diagnosis.

AT-HOME TREATMENT

Here are some home remedy tips to clear out your postnasal problem:

9 WAYS TO RELIEVE THE DRIP

- Irrigate your sinuses.
- Try a saline solution nasal spray.
- Drink plenty of fluids.
- Avoid allergens.
- Humidify your environment.
- Stay inside on smoggy days.
- Avoid cigarette smoke.
- Take a decongestant.
- Try gargling with salt water.

Try irrigation. Clear out nasal mucus by irrigating your nose and sinuses with a saline/baking soda solution. This takes a little practice and an ability to get over your squeamishness, but it works. Mix one cup of warm water, one teaspoon of salt, and a pinch of baking soda. Use a nasal syringe and inject a bulbful of the solution into one nostril while closing off the back of your palate and throat. Tilt your head back, then forward, and then to the sides, eight to ten seconds in each position. The idea is to swish the solution into all eight sinus cavities. Then forcefully blow out the mucus. Inject three or four bulbfuls on each side.

After each use, clean the syringe with alcohol. If you don't have a bulb syringe (they're available at pharmacies), you can cup the salt solution in your hands and inhale through one nostril.

Irrigate your nose and sinuses up to six times a day when postnasal symptoms are present; twice a day for "maintenance."

Go for salt spray. If you're uncomfortable with the syringe method, try an over-the-counter saline nasal spray (NaSal, Ocean, Ayr). Don't use a decongestant nasal spray that can have a rebound effect.

You can also make your own nasal spray. Boil one liter of water and add one tablespoon of salt. Bring the water to a boil again. Let cool. Use the cupped-hand inhalant method or put it in a spray bottle. Keep the solution in a closed container in the refrigerator when you're not using it.

Drink, drink, drink. Don't allow yourself to become dehydrated, especially if you suffer from postnasal drip. Drink at least eight glasses of nonalcoholic, noncaffeinated fluid per day (water is a great choice).

Stay away from allergens. If allergies are responsible for your postnasal drip, try to identify what you're allergic to and avoid it.

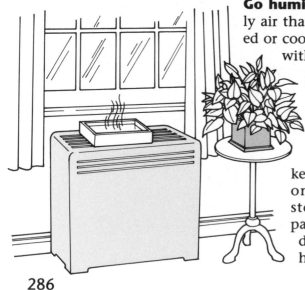

Go humid. Dry air, especially air that is artificially heated or cooled, can play havoc with your sinuses and your nasal passages. Try getting more moisture into the air with a home or room humidifier. You can also keep a kettle of water on low boil on the stove or place open pans of water on radiators. Green, leafy houseplants can also increase indoor humidity. "Perfect" humidity for the human body is about 60 percent.

Avoid smog. Some of us live in areas where the air is less than clean. If your postnasal drip is related to smog exposure, check the newspaper for air quality and limit your outdoor activities on bad days.

Don't smoke. Cigarette smoke—yours or second-hand—irritates the throat, sinuses, and nasal passages. Postnasal drip is a great reason to kick the habit and stay out of smoky environments.

Decongest. You can help drain your sinuses with over-the-counter decongestants like Sudafed. Just don't use decongestant nasal sprays that can rebound and make your postnasal symptoms worse.

Try gargling. If your throat is sore from postnasal drip, you can get some relief from gargling warm salt water. Add a half-teaspoon of salt to a cup of water.

Sources: **Gary Y. Shaw, M.D.,** Associate Professor of Otolaryngology, Head and Neck Surgery, University of Kansas Medical Center, Kansas City, Kansas. **Anne Simons, M.D.,** Coauthor, *Before You Call the Doctor*; Family Practitioner, San Francisco Department of Public Health; Family Practitioner and Assistant Clinical Professor, Family and Community Medicine, University of California San Francisco Medical Center, San Francisco, California. **James A. Stankiewicz, M.D.,** Professor and Vice-Chair, Department of Otolaryngology-Head and Neck Surgery, Loyola University Medical School, Maywood, Illinois. **Sally Wenzel, M.D.,** Assistant Professor of Medicine, National Jewish Center for Immunology and Respiratory Medicine, Denver, Colorado.

•PREGNANCY DISCOMFORTS

How to Make the Miracle of Birth Easier to Live With

MANY WOMEN SAY THAT THEY NEVER felt better in their lives than they did when they were pregnant. And if you are happy about being pregnant and excited about having a baby, you'll probably feel the same way. However, nobody gets through those nine long months without feeling some discomfort. Hormones, the weight of the fetus, and the exertion of carrying on with day-to-day life throughout the whole wonderful process can all add up to a tremendous strain on your body and your spirits.

Fortunately, there are many tried-and-true home remedies for the discomforts of pregnancy. These tips can help make your waiting go a lot more quickly. And, even if they don't eliminate 100 percent of your symptoms, keep one thing in mind. There is one sure cure for every one of pregnancy's discomforts: Giving birth. Then, happily, you'll be on to a whole new set of problems!

AT-HOME TREATMENT

Only a few decades ago, the discomforts of pregnancy were considered unavoidable consequences of childbearing. Today, however, we know that many of them can be minimized and sometimes treated with good prenatal care, allowing you to get that much more pleasure out of your pregnancy. Since pregnancy is customarily divided into three segments, or trimesters, this section is also divided into three parts: first trimester (the first three months), second trimester (the second three months), and third trimester (the final three months). Each section gives information on treating the discomforts commonly associated with the corresponding months of pregnancy.

THE FIRST TRIMESTER

During the first six weeks or so of pregnancy, the physical changes you experience are due primarily to your increasing hormone levels. Sometimes, these early changes are subtle; so subtle, in fact, that if it weren't for your missed menstrual period, you might not even realize that you are pregnant.

After the first six weeks, some of the physical changes you experience will be caused by the growth of the baby. These changes will become more noticeable as the baby gets larger. Although the most obvious changes occur in your uterus and abdomen, pregnancy affects almost every organ of your body.

The following suggestions should help ease the most common discomforts of the first three months of pregnancy. Consult your doctor or midwife if you have any questions.

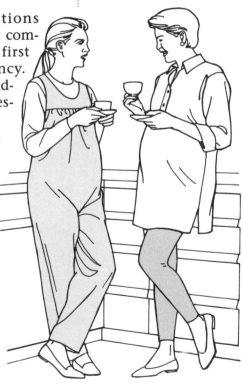

Fatigue. A multitude of changes are taking place in your body at this time. These physical changes, coupled with the mental and emotional adjustments that you are going through, can leave you exhausted. The following tips should help.

Give in to it. Listen to your body. It is telling you that you need extra rest to cope with the changes you are experiencing. Take naps whenever you can. Try to schedule rest periods at regular intervals throughout the day.

287

Reschedule bedtime. If your job makes it impossible for you to take any rest periods, try going to bed a couple of hours earlier than you normally do.

Don't pep yourself up with stimulants. Stimulants, such as over-the-counter caffeine pills, are not appropriate for use during pregnancy. Although drinking one or two cups of coffee or tea a day has not been associated with any adverse effects, taking excessive amounts of caffeine is not recommended. Also, caffeine has a pronounced "rebound" effect, causing you to be more tired after its effects wear off.

Reprioritize. Conserve your energy by being organized about your daily tasks. For example, go out only once to run several errands, instead of making three or four trips. Also, give yourself permission to let the little things go. It's okay to skip the ironing or leave the dishes until tomorrow. Right now, you and your baby come first.

Morning Sickness. The nausea and vomiting of early pregnancy, usually referred to as "morning sickness," are two of the most notable pregnancy symptoms. This condition was written about as early as 2000 B.C. Unfortunately, the ancient Egyptians didn't have a cure for it, either.

Some 50 to 70 percent of American women will suffer from nausea or vomiting, or both, during the first three months of their pregnancies. The severity and occurrence vary not only from woman to woman, but also from pregnancy to pregnancy in the same individual.

Some women never have even the slightest touch of queasiness. Some are ill in the morning and recover by lunch. And some stay sick all day for days on end, wondering why it's called "morning sickness" when it lasts 24 hours.

No one knows what causes morning sickness. It is less common among Eskimos and native African tribes than in Western cultures. But today's physicians emphasize that it's not psychological, as was once believed.

Since hormones are rapidly changing during early pregnancy, researchers theorize that these abnormal hormonal levels contribute somehow to the existence of morning sickness. A suspected culprit is human chorionic gonadotropin (HCG), the hormone tested in home pregnancy kits, which hits an all-time high in those first months. But other hormones may play a role, as well. High levels of progesterone, for example, result in smooth-muscle relaxation, slowing down the digestive process.

The good news about morning sickness? (You doubt that there's anything good to say about this subject?) Studies have shown that women who experience nausea and vomiting early in their pregnancies are more likely to deliver full-term, healthy babies. Researchers in Colorado Springs, Colorado, and Albany, New York, studied 414 pregnant women. Nearly 90 percent said they had some of the symptoms of morning sickness. But these women were more likely to carry their pregnancies to full term and deliver a live baby than the women who had no morning sickness at all. On the other hand, don't panic if you don't experience morning sickness. Plenty of women sail through pregnancy without nausea and end up delivering healthy babies.

If you are suffering from this unpleasant condition, you are probably finding it difficult to see the silver lining; you just want relief. Time will eventually take care of it; the condition usually subsides after the third month. (Scant words of comfort.) While you're waiting for the second trimester to arrive, however, try the suggestions that follow.

If morning sickness persists past the third month, or you find yourself so ill that you're losing weight, see your physician. Watch out, too, for becoming dehydrated; you'll feel dizzy when you stand or your urine output will be scant and dark in color.

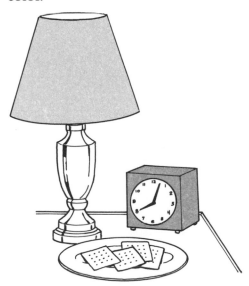

Help your blood-sugar level rise, even before you do. Keep a few low-sodium crackers on a table next to your bed. Eat them immediately upon waking, before you get out of bed. An empty stomach is a common cause of nausea in early pregnancy. That's because acids in the stomach have nothing to digest when there's no food around.

Eat frequent, small meals. If hunger pangs seem to bring on feelings of nausea, you may want to eat five to six small meals a day instead of three large ones. This way, your stomach won't get too empty. Another tip is to eat high-protein foods throughout the day. This prevents a drop in your blood-sugar level, which is also believed to be linked to feelings of nausea.

Don't overload your stomach. Just as an empty stomach can cause nausea, so can a belly that's overly full. One way to avoid having too much bulk in the stomach at once (besides grazing on smaller, more frequent meals) is to drink your fluids between meals, instead of during meals.

Keep up your fluid intake. Dehydration can cause feelings of nausea. You need at least eight glasses of fluid a day, not including coffee or tea, which are diuretics (they pull fluid from your system). Water and diluted noncitrus fruit juices are good choices. Citrus juice and soda may cause heartburn, gas, or indigestion. You may also find that it is easier on your tummy to emphasize liquids over solids. Soups and bouillons are soothing solid-meal alternatives.

Skip the salsa. Common sense dictates that bland foods are less likely to cause problems with your digestion than spicy ones.

Choose easy-to-digest foods. Complex carbohydrates, such as pasta, bread, and potatoes are soothing and easy to digest.

Nix the french fries. Along with the advice to avoid spicy foods, you should also skip fatty foods. Fats are harder to digest than carbohydrates or proteins.

Avoid odors that you know will make you nauseated. Certain odors often trigger feelings of queasiness. Pay attention to what these triggers are and avoid them. For example, if the smell of onions or fish cooking bothers you, let someone else do the cooking.

Take it slow. Quick changes of position can leave you light-headed and nauseated because of a condition known as postural hypotension (temporarily lowered blood pressure due to a change in position). Postural hypotension often strikes when you get up quickly after lying down. So take your time and get up gradually.

Take an anti-morning-sickness vitamin. A number of physicians recommend vitamin B_6 for morning sickness because of the nutrient's ability to fight nausea. Talk to your practitioner before trying a supplement, however, and be sure not to exceed 25 milligrams of the vitamin each day.

Take care of your teeth. If you do fall prey to frequent vomiting, make sure that you brush afterward. Otherwise, the frequent contact with the harsh acids in what you throw up can eat away at tooth enamel.

Breast Tenderness. As the breasts enlarge under the influence of your increasing hormone levels, they will become sensitive and tender. The following tips may help.

Buy a new bra. As soon as you become aware of tenderness in your breasts, begin wearing a well-fitting, supportive bra during the day. All-cotton bras without an underwire tend to be the most comfortable. You may go through a few different sizes, since your breasts may enlarge by as much as three cup sizes by the end of your pregnancy. If you find that you need a new bra during the last several weeks of your pregnancy and you plan to breast-feed your baby, consider purchasing nursing bras. These bras, which are designed to be comfortable and supportive, open to expose the breast for nursing. They can double as maternity bras in the last trimester. Don't buy nursing bras any earlier than your seventh or eighth month, since

6 COMMON DISCOMFORTS OF THE FIRST TRIMESTER

- Fatigue
- Morning sickness
- Breast tenderness
- Constipation
- Vaginal discharge
- Frequent urination

your size may change in the last weeks.

You may wish to wear a bra while sleeping, especially if your breasts have become very large. Some practitioners feel that continuously supporting the breasts may help prevent damage to the tissue that supports the breast, thereby minimizing sagging after the breasts return to their pre-pregnancy size.

Apply cool compresses. Towels soaked in cool water can serve as soothing compresses for tender breasts. Apply the compress for a few minutes, several times a day.

Constipation. Constipation is a common complaint among pregnant women. It is usually the result of the relaxation of the smooth muscle in your digestive tract and the pressure of the enlarging uterus on the rectum. The condition may be further aggravated by iron supplements, lack of adequate fluid intake, and inactivity. The following tips may help get things moving again.

Bulk up. Increase the fiber in your diet by eating more leafy vegetables, whole-grain cereals, and breads. Muffins and cereals containing wheat, oat, or rice bran are ideal choices.

Keep drinking. Drink two to three quarts of liquid each day. This will help keep your stool soft.

Keep moving. Exercise—even if it's only walking—is one of the best ways to prevent constipation from occurring and to set a stubborn digestive system in motion.

Rely on an old standby. One sure cure for constipation is eating prunes. Other fruits that may help include raisins and figs. Integrate these naturally sweet options into your daily diet.

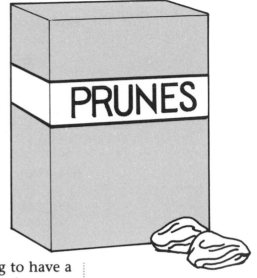

Try to establish a routine. Some people find it helpful to try to "train" the digestive system by attempting to have a bowel movement at the same time every day. After your morning meal is an ideal time.

Vaginal Discharge. A thin, milky-white to yellowish vaginal discharge is normal during pregnancy. Like most other discomforts in the early months of pregnancy, this is caused by your increasing hormone levels. A normal discharge should not cause pain, itching, or burning. It causes no harm and requires no treatment. However, if you find the discharge bothersome, you can try the following tips.

Wash it away. The discharge is not dirty. However, if you find it unpleasant, cleanse the skin outside of your vagina with a mild solution of soap and water two or three times a day.

Go natural. Wearing natural fibers, especially cotton underpants, will allow your vaginal area to breathe, keeping it dry and preventing irritation.

Wear a panty liner. A panty liner or minipad can prevent vaginal discharge from staining your clothing.

Never douche. Douching is not recommended during pregnancy, unless it is specifically recommended by your practitioner for a medical purpose.

Frequent Urination. As the enlarging uterus presses up against the bladder and decreases the bladder's capacity, you will have the urge to urinate more frequently. This is a normal and unavoidable symptom of early pregnancy (it gets a little better in the second trimester and much worse again in the third). However, there are ways to decrease the inconvenience of constantly running to the bathroom.

If your urination is extremely frequent (more than once an hour) or if pain or burning occurs, call your practitioner. These may be signs of a bladder infection.

Drink your fluids during the day. If your sleep is disturbed by your frequent need to urinate, you might try not drinking any liquids within two to three hours before bedtime.

Thoroughly empty your bladder. Making sure that your bladder is completely empty will keep you out of the bathroom for longer intervals. This is especially important before traveling in a car, train, or bus, where facilities may not be available or may be inconvenient to use. You can try this trick: After you have finished urinating, stand up for a second, then sit back down again on the toilet. Lean forward and try to urinate again. Leaning forward compresses the bladder so that it can release every last drop.

THE SECOND TRIMESTER

By the beginning of the second trimester, most of the symptoms and discomforts of early pregnancy will have passed, and you'll probably be experiencing a renewed sense of energy. On the other hand, you'll also begin to develop new symptoms that are related not only to your increasing hormone levels but also to your rapidly growing baby. The suggestions below may ease some of your discomfort.

Back Pain. This nearly universal annoyance of pregnancy occurs when your posture changes to accommodate the increased size and weight of your uterus and baby. Stress is placed on the muscles and ligaments in the lower part of your back, causing an aching sensation in this area.

Of course, there's nothing you can do about the increasing size and weight of your uterus. But the less additional stress you place on your back, the better you will feel. You may find the following tips helpful for minimizing or relieving backache. (For more information on back pain, see the corresponding chapter in this book.)

Back pain, especially if it is constant and severe, may be a symptom of a more serious problem, such as a kidney infection or a slipped disk. If you follow the suggestions below and your back pain does not improve, call your practitioner.

Straighten up. When walking, standing, and sitting, support the weight of the uterus and baby by using good posture. The straighter your body, the less strain is put on your back muscles.

Skip the high heels. Wear comfortable shoes with a slight heel (one to one-and-a-half inches high) and good support. Avoid wearing high-heeled shoes, since they will cause you to arch your back and strain your muscles.

Take a load off. Avoid standing for extended periods of time. Sit down when you can and assume a good sitting posture. Sitting on the floor, Indian-style, will shift the weight of your uterus to the front, taking some of the strain off of your back.

Use your arms and legs. Whenever you are rising from a sitting or lying position, use the muscles of your arms and legs to push yourself up, rather than using your back muscles to assist you in rising.

Take it easy. Avoid heavy lifting or pushing that may strain your back.

Don't get soft. Sleeping on a firm mattress may be best for your back. Placing a board between the mattress and box spring may also help.

Apply heat. A heating pad or warm bath may be helpful in relieving back pain. However, don't allow the pad or bath to become too hot and don't stay in a hot bath too long. Also, never sleep under an electric blanket during pregnancy. Raising your body temperature for extended periods of time has been found to be harmful to a developing fetus.

Get a rubdown. The healing touch of a massage therapist or a loving spouse can do wonders for an aching back.

Squat, don't bend. Whenever you must reach down for anything, bend your knees and squat down, keeping your back straight. Do not bend your back. Pull whatever you are reaching for close to your chest. Then, use your leg muscles to push yourself up to a standing position.

Do back exercises. A program of exercise designed to strengthen your back is probably the best preventive measure against back pain. Ask your practitioner or childbirth educator for recommendations of specific exercises.

Skin Changes. Pregnant women commonly experience a variety of skin changes, including itching, dryness, increased perspiration, oiliness, and increased pigmentation on the face and abdomen.

Apply a lotion to dry, itchy skin. This is most important after bathing, when skin usually feels driest. Some women feel that cocoa-butter-based products are best. Also, try using a mild cleansing bar, such as Dove, Neutrogena, or Aveeno, instead of soap. Use the cleanser only in places that really need it, such as on the face, under the arms, and in the groin area, instead of using it all over your body. You may also choose to skip the cleanser

293

entirely. Lastly, take warm—not hot—baths and showers; hot water is drying to the skin.

Frequently cleanse oily areas. A mild soap or cleansing bar is the best choice. Check with your doctor before using products containing benzoyl peroxide or other over-the-counter skin medications. Also, be aware that overdrying the skin may actually cause a "rebound effect" in some people, causing the skin to produce excess oil to compensate for the dryness.

---

8 Second Trimester Discomforts

- Back pain
- Skin changes
- Stretch marks
- Bleeding gums
- Leg cramps
- Heartburn
- Indigestion
- Gas

Use a sunscreen and avoid direct exposure to sunlight. Increased pigmentation of the skin, especially on the face, is common in pregnancy. Some women experience melasma, which is sometimes called the "mask" of pregnancy. This increased pigmentation usually occurs on the cheeks, nose, and forehead, which makes it resemble a dark mask. Using a sunscreen and staying out of the sun can help lighten the areas of darkened skin. In the meantime, if you find the melasma unsightly, cover it with makeup. Don't worry: Melasma will disappear after you give birth.

Stretch Marks. Contrary to common belief, applying cocoa butter, oil, or any other product to the skin will not prevent stretch marks from developing. In fact, there is no way to prevent these deep, red marks from appearing on the skin of the abdomen, breasts, and thighs (some women even get them under their arms and on the skin on the inside of the knees). The marks appear to run in families, so if your mother had them, you probably will, too.

Sometimes, the stretching skin of the abdomen becomes very itchy and irritated. Applying a heavy moisturizer may help. Although stretch marks will never completely disappear after pregnancy, they will fade to thin, silvery lines that are much less noticeable.

Try thinking of them as a badge of motherhood. Wear them with pride, knowing that they are a sign that you have given birth to another human being. After all, your baby is much more important than looking perfect in a bikini, right?

Bleeding Gums. The increasing volume of blood in your body is responsible for what dentists call "pregnancy gingivitis," or gums that bleed when you brush or floss. Although it may be worrisome, the problem is harmless and will disappear after you give birth. Using a soft-bristled toothbrush and avoiding harsh scrubbing may help. Don't neglect good dental hygiene, however. Regular brushing and flossing will help prevent the buildup of plaque, a sticky substance that can cause dental decay, and will reduce the likelihood that gum disease will develop.

Leg Cramps. The leg cramps that some women experience during pregnancy may be more painful than the contraction pains they go through during their labors. These cramps, which usually occur in the calves, may result from an imbalance of calcium and phosphorous in the body, from tight calf muscles, or from the strain placed on the leg muscles by poor posture.

Up your calcium intake. Drinking more milk and consuming more dairy products and leafy green vegetables can add calcium to your diet. Besides easing leg cramps, an adequate calcium intake is important for your baby's developing bones and teeth. If you don't get the extra calcium from your diet, your growing baby will steal it from your own bones.

Be careful with phosphorus. Phosphorus may contribute to the development of leg cramps. Some calcium supplements contain this element in the form of calcium phosphate. If your practitioner recommends that you take a calcium supplement, stick to preparations containing calcium carbonate.

Keep your calf muscles flexible. Doing calf stretches will help to keep the calf muscles long and flexible, reducing the likelihood that you will experience leg cramps. Try standing a couple of feet away from a wall, with both feet together. Lean into the wall, placing both palms on the wall at about shoulder height. Try to press your heels into the floor and hold the stretch without bouncing.

Stay in alignment. Muscle cramps may also be due to the strain caused by poor posture. Pay close attention to the alignment of your body when you are standing and sitting.

Stretch out the cramp. If you do experience a leg cramp, sit down in a chair and extend your leg with your toes pointed upward. Then have a partner gently push your toes toward you to stretch your calf muscle. If no one is available to help you, reach down and gently pull your toes toward you. This will often relieve the cramp on the spot.

Heartburn, Indigestion, and Gas. There are three reasons why you may experience heartburn, indigestion, or gas during your pregnancy. First, the hormone progesterone, which is produced by the placenta, slows the action of your digestive system and causes the stomach to empty into the intestines more slowly. Second, progesterone relaxes the tight band of muscle between the esophagus and the stomach. Finally, the enlarging uterus pushes up on the stomach and decreases its capacity to hold food. All these factors combine to allow food and acid to back up into your esophagus, producing heartburn or causing indigestion or gas. The following measures may help prevent or relieve these discomforts. Be aware that indigestion may also be associated

295

with more serious conditions, such as gallstones. If simple home treatments do not relieve your digestive discomfort, call your practitioner.

Avoid overloading your stomach. Eat several small meals every day instead of three large ones. Excess food may back up into the esophagus, causing heartburn.

Stay upright. Avoid lying down for two hours after you eat or drink. Lying down may promote the upward flow of stomach acids into the esophagus.

Elevate your head and back. For the same reason that you should stay upright after meals, sleeping with several pillows underneath your head and back can help prevent heartburn.

Stick to bland and mild foods. Spicy foods may promote heartburn.

Avoid gas producers. Beans, onion, and cabbage may cause excess gas and stomach pain.

Take Tums, with your practitioner's approval. Tums antacid tablets are very effective in relieving heartburn and indigestion (they are less helpful for gas). Often, doctors approve their use in pregnancy, since their active ingredient is calcium carbonate, a nutrient that pregnant women need a lot of. As with any medications, check with your doctor before taking Tums.

THE THIRD TRIMESTER

Your time is drawing near; your patience might be wearing thin or running out altogether. As you enter the final three months of pregnancy, your energy may wane, and you may grow weary of carrying around such a heavy load.

Your body, too, is feeling the impact of your growing baby. The result may be a series of discomforts that build to a peak just before the baby is born. It might be encouraging to remember that most of these physical changes (and the emotional ones, too) are quite normal and that they'll be quickly overshadowed by the joy you feel when you give birth.

Shortness of Breath. As the uterus continues to enlarge during the last three months of pregnancy, it will push up on your lungs, and you may experience shortness of breath. If you ever suddenly experience shortness of breath, especially if it is not relieved by standing up or resting, call your practitioner, since this could be a sign of a more serious condition, such as pneumonia.

Stay upright. The best way to relieve the sensation of being out of breath is to maintain an upright position as often as possible.

Never lay flat on your back. The flatter your position, the greater the pressure of the uterus on your lungs. Sleeping on your left side is best for you and the baby during pregnancy. If you absolutely must sleep on your back, place two pillows under your head and one under your back so that your body is at a slight angle, thus helping to relieve the pressure on your lungs while you are in a reclining position.

Hemorrhoids. This problem is also caused by pressure that the enlarging uterus puts on the veins in the abdomen. The following suggestions may help.

Don't strain while trying to move your bowels. Straining may cause hemorrhoids to develop and may make existing ones larger. Follow the tips above for constipation if you have problems moving your bowels.

Stay off your feet. Try to lie down frequently during the day.

Use witch hazel. Witch-hazel pads, which you can purchase at a drugstore, can relieve the pain of hemorrhoids. Apply them directly to the hemorrhoid.

Soak in a warm bath. Make sure the bathwater is not too hot.

Call your practitioner. Your practitioner can recommend safe medications, such as stool softeners and pain-relieving hemorrhoid creams and suppositories, if simple measures do not relieve your discomfort. If extreme pain develops in the rectal area, or if you experience any rectal bleeding, notify your practitioner at once.

Varicose Veins. These are common side effects of pregnancy, and they tend to become more severe with each subsequent pregnancy. Varicose veins are caused by the pressure the enlarging uterus places on abdominal blood vessels that carry blood from the legs back up to the heart. The walls of the veins in the legs weaken as a result of being overfilled with blood. This eventually causes the veins directly below the skin of the legs to bulge and ache.

The following suggestions may be helpful for varicose veins that appear during pregnancy. For more general information, turn to the chapter on varicose veins.

If you ever experience severe pain or tenderness in your legs or notice redness over a leg vein, call your practitioner immediately. This may be a sign of a blood clot.

Rest as often as you can. If it is possible during the day, take frequent rest periods and lie down with your head and shoulders elevated and your feet propped up on a low stool or on several pillows. Avoid laying flat on your back, which could cause shortness of breath.

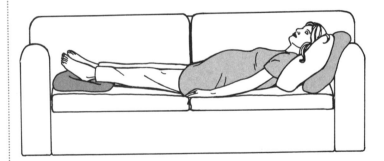

Elevate the foot of your bed. Placing six- to eight-inch blocks under the foot of your bed can raise your legs at night and reduce the pressure on the walls of the leg veins.

Sleep on your left side. Sleeping on your left side will help move the uterus off of the veins in the abdomen and thereby reduce the pressure in the leg veins.

Swelling of the Legs, Feet, and Ankles. This common problem is also caused by the heavy weight of the uterus pressing on blood vessels in the abdomen. It is usually most apparent after you have been standing or sitting for a long period of time. The following tips may help.

While swelling of the legs is common during pregnancy, swelling of the hands or face may be a sign of preeclampsia. If you ever experience swelling of the hands or face, or if your feet, ankles, or legs swell suddenly, notify your doctor immediately.

Elevate your feet. Lying down or sitting with your feet elevated as often as possible can help relieve swelling.

Wear loose clothing. Do not wear constricting panties, stockings, or girdles during pregnancy.

Sleep on your left side with your feet elevated on pillows. Lying on your left side, besides being useful for varicose veins and shortness of breath, can also help prevent fluid retention and swelling in the legs. It also allows for freer blood circulation, which is important for the baby.

6 COMMON DISCOMFORTS OF THE THIRD TRIMESTER

- Varicose veins
- Shortness of breath
- Hemorrhoids
- Swelling of the legs, feet, or ankles
- Pelvic pain
- Vision problems

Use salt in moderation. Excess salt in your diet may cause you to retain excess fluid, causing swelling. However, some salt is important during pregnancy. It's best just to avoid heavily salted foods, such as pickles, and hold back on the salt shaker at the table.

Pelvic Pain. Aches in the vagina, groin, and hips are caused by the pressure of the enlarging uterus and by the loosening of the joints and ligaments in the pelvis that results from your changing hormonal levels. There is no treatment for this pain. However, you should avoid activities that may strain these joints and ligaments. Move carefully and avoid sudden twisting or bending. Also, turn over slowly when you are in bed or getting up.

Vision Problems. Women who wear glasses or contact lenses may find that their vision during pregnancy is not as good as it was prior to pregnancy. Vision changes may occur if the shape of the eyeball alters slightly due to increased fluid in the tissues. If you do have this problem, you may need to have your lens prescription changed during pregnancy. See your eye doctor if you think you should have your eyes retested.

Call your practitioner immediately if you ever experience blurred or double vision during pregnancy. These may be signs of preeclampsia.

AT THE DOCTOR'S

This chapter is not intended to be a substitute for medical treatment. Good prenatal care is associated with babies of higher birth weight, fewer stillbirths, and healthier children. You should see an obstetrician or family physician immediately upon learning that you are pregnant. Thereafter, monthly visits are customary until the ninth month of pregnancy, when you will probably see your practitioner weekly.

If you experience any vaginal bleeding; severe abdominal pain; swelling of the hands or face; a burning sensation while urinating; vaginal discharge that is heavy or causes itching or burning; severe, frequent vomiting; a sudden overnight weight gain; or feelings of no longer being pregnant, contact your physician immediately. You should also call your practitioner if you have any other symptoms that cause you severe discomfort or that worry you. Of course, if you feel that you are going into labor (especially if your due date is more than a month away) or if you see anything protruding from your vagina, call your practitioner at once. Lastly, never take any medication, herb, or remedy during pregnancy without contacting your physician. Many substances can travel through the placenta and harm your growing baby.

Sources: Cheryl Coleman, R.N., B.S.N., I.C.C.E., Director, Public Relations, International Childbirth Education Association; Childbirth Educator, Hillcrest Medical Center, Tulsa, Oklahoma. Donald R. Coustan, M.D., Professor and Chair, Obstetrics and Gynecology, Brown University School of Medicine; Chief, Obstetrics and Gynecology, Women and Infants Hospital of Rhode Island, Providence, Rhode Island. Kermit E. Krantz, M.D., University Distinguished Professor, Professor of Gynecology and Obstetrics, Professor of Anatomy, University of Kansas Medical Center, Kansas City, Kansas.

11 SYMPTOMS THAT WARRANT MEDICAL ATTENTION

Call your doctor if you experience:
- Vaginal bleeding.
- Severe abdominal pain.
- Swelling of the hands or face.
- A burning sensation while urinating.
- Vaginal discharge that is heavy or causes itching or burning.
- Severe, frequent vomiting.
- A sudden overnight weight gain.
- Feelings of no longer being pregnant.
- Signs of labor, especially if your due date is more than a month away.
- Anything protruding from the vagina.
- Any symptom that you find worrisome.

PREMENSTRUAL SYNDROME

Easing Before-

Period

Symptoms

YOU FEEL BLOATED; YOUR BREASTS ARE sore and tender. Your back and head hurt and you feel exhausted. You've eaten every sweet treat in the refrigerator and if your kids don't leave you alone, you know you're going to kill them. Sound familiar? Then you, like most women of reproductive age, know about premenstrual syndrome, or "PMS."

Have you seen the bumper sticker that reads, "I have PMS and I carry a gun"? With all the jokes about women and "that time of the month," sometimes it's hard to sift through what's fact and what's fantasy. For years, the male-dominated medical profession told women that their mood swings, weight gain, bloating, breast tenderness, and other symptoms during the week before their period were just "all in their heads." However, in the last 20 years, doctors have realized that premenstrual syndrome symptoms do, in fact, have a physiological basis.

SYMPTOMS

Premenstrual syndrome isn't a disease, but a complex set of physical and emotional symptoms many women experience during the week before the menstrual period begins. These symptoms include bloating, breast swelling and tenderness, fatigue, weight gain, headaches, food cravings, back and muscle aches, diarrhea and/or constipation, dizziness, shakiness, acne, lack of coordination, and emotional upsets, including depression, anger, irritability, and "spaciness." Some women experience many of these symptoms; others just one or two. The symptoms may be mild or debilitating. Usually the severity of symptoms is the same month after

month, but some women experience changes in their symptoms due to other illnesses or increased stress.

CAUSES

Researchers aren't sure exactly what causes PMS, but they suspect it's related to the cyclic changes in the levels of sex hormones, particularly estrogen, that occur around the menstrual period. One theory suggests PMS symptoms may be due to an ovarian hormone imbalance of either estrogen or progesterone. Another theory says symptoms are due to a brain hormone change or deficiency. Some researchers believe that PMS mood swings may be related to deficiencies in vitamin B_6 and magnesium.

Symptoms appear five to 14 days before menstruation. Usually, they disappear with the onset of the menstrual period. Doctors generally diagnose PMS symptoms by their cyclic regularity—beginning before the period and disappearing when the menstrual flow begins.

How do you know if your symptoms are caused by PMS? Ask yourself these questions:

• Do you have the same or similar symptoms every month?

• Do you suffer from symptoms such as headaches, backaches, muscle aches, etc., right before your period?

• Do your symptoms disappear when your period starts?

• Do you have at least two symptom-free weeks every month? (If you answer no to this question, see your physician. You may have a more serious health condition such as endometriosis, a vaginal or pelvic infection, fibroids, or you may have depression or anxiety disorder.)

If you answered "yes" to all or most of these questions, you probably have PMS. If you're still not sure whether you have premenstrual syndrome, keep a PMS diary. You can use a regular calendar. Or, on one side of a piece of paper list symptoms (headache, water retention, breast swelling/tenderness, weight gain, etc.); across the top of the page, write categories for the date these symptoms start, the date the symptoms end, their severity (1=mild, 2=moderate, 3=severe), and the date your period begins. By tracking your symptoms for two or three months, you should be able to tell if your symptoms are due to premenstrual syndrome.

AT-HOME TREATMENT

Unfortunately, just as doctors aren't sure what causes PMS, neither do they have a definitive cure. However, there is plenty you can do to ease your PMS discomforts.

Check your diet. Eat from a well-balanced menu that includes fresh fruits and vegetables, starches, whole grains, fish, and lean poultry.

Talk to others. Some women say their PMS symptoms make them feel isolated and "crazy." It helps to talk with other PMS sufferers. Many communities offer PMS support groups. Talk with your friends and family, too. Many women say one of their biggest stressors during PMS is family. Often family members don't understand the tension and mood swings. By talking with them about your symptoms and the causes of PMS, you can help them under-stand your condition and enable them to take your situation seriously and give you support. If your PMS symptoms are causing serious problems in your relationships, see a mental health professional.

Omit the sugar. Many women have food cravings before their periods, particularly a craving for sweets. Eating too much sugar can actually make you feel worse by intensifying your anger and irritability. Try cutting out all sweets, all month long. Instead of sugary snacks or junk foods, stave off your sweet tooth by keeping healthy finger foods (unbuttered popcorn, cut-up vegetables with low-fat yogurt dip, etc.) close at hand. Choose foods with natural sugars, like fresh fruits that can satisfy your need for sweet while also providing nutrients. Apples, pears, and berries are all relatively low in sugar and taste terrific. Tropical fruits (pineapples, bananas, mangos, etc.) contain more sugar and should be on the "omit" list. Skip artificial sweeteners, too. They may have the same effects as sugar.

Nix the booze. Right before your period isn't the time to drink alcohol. It's metabolized like sugar so it can contribute to mood swings and can leave you dehydrated and even more

301

11 STRATEGIES FOR BEATING THE PMS BLUES

- Eat a well-balanced diet.
- Get support from friends, family, and other PMS sufferers.
- Cut out sugar.
- Don't drink alcoholic beverages.
- Cut out caffeine completely.
- Lower your intake of dietary fat.
- Use less salt.
- Effectively manage your stress.
- Plan ahead for PMS.
- Treat yourself kindly.
- Exercise regularly.

fatigued. Alcohol also depletes your stores of B vitamins (believed to be related to PMS mood swings) and interferes with carbohydrate and hormone metabolism, which can result in excessively high estrogen levels. If you're in a social situation where alcohol is served, opt for soda water with a twist of lime or some other nonalcoholic beverage.

Eat a little, often. A good way to keep your blood sugar from fluctuating wildly and keep your moods on a more even keel is to eat small, frequent meals. Eat every three to four hours.

Cut out caf. Some studies have shown that even a small amount of caffeine can trigger PMS symptoms in some women, especially mood swings and breast tenderness. Eliminate it completely for a few months and see if your symptoms lessen. Don't forget that caffeine isn't just found in coffee and tea, but also in cocoa, chocolate, colas and other sodas, and many over-the-counter medications. Try substituting herbal teas or grain-based coffee substitutes such as Pero, Postum, and Caffix.

Go easy on dietary fat. Cutting the fat in your diet is a good idea for everyone, but it's especially important for PMS sufferers. Eating too much fat can interfere with liver function and some beef also contains small amounts of synthetic estrogens. Substitute fish and skinless poultry for higher-fat cuts of red meat, and eat plenty of beans, peas, seeds, nuts, whole grains, rice, vegetables, and fresh fruits.

Cut the salt. Too much sodium can increase fluid retention and contribute to breast swelling and tenderness. Don't salt your food while cooking. Taste your food before salting and then use the salt shaker only sparingly, if at all. Cut down on high-sodium foods like bouillon, salad dressings, ketchup, and sausage.

Manage your stress. By learning to effectively manage your stress throughout the month, you can lessen your PMS symptoms. Try biofeedback, progressive relaxation, yoga, deep breathing, meditation, or any number of stress reduction techniques. Often local hospitals or community colleges offer stress reduction classes.

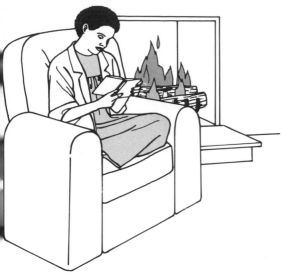

Treat yourself with TLC. In some ancient cultures, women went away to special lodges right before and during their menstrual periods. You can take a clue from the ancients and learn to take special care of yourself right before your period. Do things that make you feel comforted and taken care of, such as reading a book by the fire, walking in the woods, going to a movie, listening to music you love, or taking a warm bubble bath.

Plan accordingly. Use your calendar and your head. Don't plan major social events or other demanding occasions right before your period if you can help it. The added stress will only make your PMS symptoms worse. Whenever possible, put off stressful events until another time. Reduce your stress as much as possible during this touchy period.

Get out and move. Okay, you feel achy, bloated, and depressed. You don't want to get out and exercise, but this is exactly what can make you feel better. Aerobic exercise is the body's own "feel-good elixir." It trig- gers the release of endorphins, natural brain opiates that make you feel good. It also increases pelvic circulation, which can help reduce some of the bloating associated with PMS. Good choices for aerobic exercise include jogging, brisk walking, stair-stepping, low-impact aerobics, and bicycling. A workout of 20 to 30 minutes is enough to bring on the PMS-reducing benefits. If you simply feel too fatigued to exercise right before your period, don't force yourself. Just make sure you exercise regularly throughout the rest of the month.

AT THE DOCTOR'S

The vast majority of women can effectively reduce their PMS discomfort with the home remedies discussed in this chapter. However, some women have PMS symptoms that are so severe they require medical intervention.

Just as doctors don't have one explanation for PMS, neither do they have a single treatment. Most offer a variety of medications. Talk to your physician about finding the combination of treatments that is right for you.

Sources: Phyllis Frey, A.R.N.P., Nurse Practitioner, Bellegrove GYN, Inc., Bellevue, Washington. Sadja Greenwood, M.D., Assistant Clinical Professor, Department of Obstetrics, Gynecology, and Reproductive Services, University of California at San Francisco, San Francisco, California; Coauthor *The Medical Self-Care Book of Women's Health.* Anne Simons, M.D., Coauthor, *Before You Call the Doctor*; Family Practitioner, San Francisco Department of Public Health; Family Practitioner and Assistant Clinical Professor, Family and Community Medicine, University of California San Francisco Medical Center, San Francisco, California. Harold Zimmer, M.D., Obstetrician and Gynecologist, Bellevue, Washington.

Strategies to

Cope with

Scaly Skin

IF YOU HAVE PSORIASIS, CHANCES ARE you're feeling pretty frustrated. Psoriasis is a chronic, incurable skin problem in which the skin produces round, dry, scaly patches of different sizes with white, grey, or silvery scales. Although an estimated three to four million people have psoriasis, doctors don't know what causes it or how to cure it. A particular medication or treatment works for some, but it may not work for you. A treatment that seemed to help yesterday will mysteriously stop working. One day the disease will show only a few patches; the next, huge scales will cover large portions of your body.

SYMPTOMS

Psoriasis is a rashlike skin condition that commonly occurs on the scalp, lower back, and over the elbows, knees, and knuckles. When it occurs on the toenails and fingernails, it can cause pitting and brownish discoloration. Sometimes, it causes the nail to lift and crack. When the thick scale appears on the scalp at the hairline, it resembles severe dandruff. Psoriasis lesions leave no scars, but they can itch, especially when they appear in body creases.

In some people, psoriasis is mild and causes only a few tiny patches. In others, it covers large areas of the body with thick scales, cracks, and blisters and causes pitted, deformed nails, a rash in the genitals, profuse shedding of dead skin flakes, and a form of arthritis that involves the spine and large joints. In a few people, the disease becomes so severe that it causes chills, painful reddening of the skin, and shedding of large areas of scaled skin ("exfolia-

tive psoriasis") and requires hospitalization.

CAUSES

No one knows what causes psoriasis. The National Psoriasis Foundation says that 150,000 new cases of psoriasis are diagnosed every year. It appears to run in some families (about 30 percent of sufferers report having a relative with the condition), but many people who have psoriasis have no family history of the disease. It can appear at any age, although it typically first appears in teens and young adults. It has been diagnosed in children and even in infants.

Doctors can't even agree on exactly what psoriasis is. They know it isn't an infection or an allergic reaction. It doesn't appear to be caused by foods or by a vitamin or mineral deficiency. Psoriasis somehow makes the mechanism of skin cell production shift into overdrive. It causes the normal growth and replacement cycle to go haywire and makes the upper layer of skin overgrow. Normally, skin cells are replaced every 28 to 30 days. Old cells are continuously shed from the skin's surface and replaced by new cells formed in the deeper layers. It takes the new cells about 30 days to migrate up to the skin's surface where they live for about a month before they die, flake off, and are replaced by new cells. In psoriasis, the process is shortened to three or four days. Cells rapidly move to the surface and die. The results are the dry, irritating, scaly cell patches called plaques.

Once you have psoriasis, a variety of factors can cause it to flare up. While stress isn't the cause, it can worsen an already existing condition. Skin injuries like bruises, cuts, or burns can cause an outbreak, usually eight to 18 days after the injury occurs. Infections, especially upper respiratory infections like the common cold, can aggravate the problem. Psoriasis is even sensitive to the weather. Many psoriasis sufferers say their skin condition worsens during dry, cold winter months.

Psoriasis is a disease of flare-ups and remissions. Sometimes the patches disappear for months or even years. Some people report their psoriasis improves with age. For others, it worsens.

AT-HOME TREATMENT

There may not be a cure for psoriasis yet, but until then, there is plenty you can do to make living with psoriasis easier.

Stay upbeat. It's tough to keep a positive mental attitude with such a mysterious ailment. However, psoriasis isn't life-threatening and a positive attitude can help you find relief. Doctors are developing new treatments every day, and treatments that may have once worked for you may work again. Don't give up trying to treat your condition. Instead of focusing on the fact that you have a chronic skin condition, put your energy into learning more about managing it.

Keep it moist. When skin, any skin, becomes dry, it can itch and crack. Skin that has psoriasis is very dry, which can lead to more psoriasis, itching, and more flaking. Very dry skin can also crack and bleed, making it

susceptible to secondary infection. It's vital to keep your skin moist with emollients. Moisturizing your skin will reduce inflammation, help maintain flexibility (dried plaques can make moving certain parts of the body difficult), keep the condition from getting worse, and make the plaque scales less noticeable.

Use thick moisturizers. The thicker and greasier the moisturizer, the more it's able to "lock in" skin moisture. You can use something inexpensive like Vaseline, cooking oils, or even vegetable shortening. Or you can opt for thick commercial moisturizers such as Eucerin, Aquaphor, and Neutrogena Norwegian Formula Hand Cream. Apply the moisturizer right after bathing and throughout the day.

Go for water. Since psoriasis skin tends to be dry, one solution is to rehydrate it with showering, swimming, soaking in a tub, or applying wet compresses. The water not only adds moisture to the skin, but also removes the thick, scaly patches without damaging the skin underneath. Since thick patches can act as a barrier to both medications and ultraviolet light, it's important to gently remove as much scale as possible.

A regular soak also helps reduce the itching and redness

of the lesions. However, don't opt for a steamy soak. Water that is too hot can make you itch even more. Instead, use tepid water and add a little mineral oil to the bath to help seal in the water.

Soaking can remove scales, but it can also remove your skin's natural oils, which hold in moisture. To prevent over-drying your skin, pat (don't rub) it moist-dry after bathing and immediately after the soak (within three minutes) apply a heavy emollient.

Bring on the sun. You've probably heard health authorities warn about protecting your skin from excessive exposure to sunlight. They have a point, of course, but sunlight is good for psoriasis. Many people are actually able to clear their lesions with exposure to sunlight.

Doctors don't know exactly why ultraviolet light works, but it appears to slow skin cell replication. For years, psoriasis sufferers have flocked to the Dead Sea for relief from psoriasis plaques. Authorities first thought it might be something in the sea's water, but now they believe it's the unique properties of sunlight at 1,300 feet below sea level that's the key.

You don't have to travel to the Dead Sea to get relief for your skin condition. Sunlight right in your backyard will help your psoriasis. Just be sure not to damage your skin further by burning it. Before going out into the sun, grease your scaly patches with Vaseline or miner-

al oil and don't overdo it. To reduce your risk of sunburn and skin cancer, apply sunscreen to areas where you don't have scale.

Try UVB. According to the National Psoriasis Foundation, 80 percent of psoriasis sufferers find they get significant relief with ultraviolet B light (UVB) therapy. Home models of UVB lamps are now available, but never use a home UVB unit without first talking with your physician and getting clear instructions. Also, be careful to avoid burning your skin, and have your doctor check your skin regularly to ensure you aren't developing cancerous skin lesions (malignant melanoma).

Ask these questions from the National Psoriasis Foundation when choosing your home UVB unit:
• Does the unit have safety features like key switches or disabling switches that keep the machine from being used when you're not around?
• Does it have a reliable and accurate timer?
• Are there safety guards or grids over the lamps?
• Is the equipment stable and durable?
• Are replacement bulbs readily available? How much do they cost?

Tar it. Tar-containing products such as shampoos, creams, and bath additives (e.g., Baker's PNS) have been effective psoriasis remedies for years. They're designed to loosen and remove scale. Tar-containing bath oils are particularly good for psoriasis that is widespread on the body.

Tar does tend to increase the skin's sensitivity to sunlight (photosensitivity). Some tar products can be used in combination with sunlight or with UVB treatments. Just be careful not to overdo it. Discontinue any tar product (or other product) that causes your skin to burn or become irritated.

Try salicylic acid. Another effective psoriasis treatment is salicylic acid. Added to shampoos and creams, it "eats" scale.

Go for the cortisone. Mild cases of psoriasis often respond well to over-the-counter 0.5-percent cortisone creams. They're especially effective for psoriasis that occurs in the folds and creases of the skin and on the face. These products are too mild to have much effect on thick plaques, but stronger, one-percent cortisone creams are now available in pharmacies and may be more effective.

Wrap it up. Doctors have known for years that "occlusive therapy," or covering up psoriasis lesions, helps them go away. Covering the lesions forces medications into the skin and helps it retain moisture.

Inexpensive plastic wrap is perfect for occlusive therapy. Or you can buy over-the-counter patches (Actiderm). Apply the medication or moisturizer; then cover the area. Many psoriasis sufferers use this technique overnight. Be careful, however, that the skin doesn't become too soggy or it may become vulnerable to secondary infection.

Watch those soaps. The wrong kind of soap can make your psoriasis even more irritated and itchy. Forego harsh, detergent-type soaps. Instead choose mild, unscented ones (fragrances often contain chemicals that can irritate the skin). Some mild, "superfatted" soaps such as Basis, Purpose, Oilatum, Alpha Keri, and Nivea Cream Bar contain moisturizing ingredients that help the skin retain moisture. If your skin is really dry and irritated, you can use a nonsoap cleanser such as Lowilla Cake, Aveeno Cleansing Bar, or pHisoDerm Dry Skin Formula.

Rinse, rinse, rinse. It doesn't matter what kind of soap you use if you don't wash it off thoroughly. Any kind of soap residue can cause drying, itching, and irritation. Rinse and then rinse again to make sure you get it all off.

A little olive oil, please. Psoriasis scales can be a real problem on the scalp. To help soften and remove them, warm a little olive oil and massage it onto the scalp.

Try antihistamines. Any psoriasis sufferer can tell you that flaky plaques can itch like crazy. The natural response, of course, is to scratch, but scratching can damage the skin, which can be serious with psoriasis. When the itch becomes more than you can handle, use over-the-counter antihistamines. Follow package instructions.

Pass the fish oil. Studies from the University of Michigan at Ann Arbor and from the University of California at Davis suggest that large oral doses of fish oil may be a psoriasis remedy. Greenland Eskimos rarely suffer from psoriasis, and some researchers believe that their diet, which is rich in cold-water fish, may be the reason. Since

you probably don't want to switch to an Eskimo diet and the participants in the fish-oil studies had to take unusually large quantities of fish oil supplements to achieve results, you should talk with your doctor before trying fish oil yourself.

Bring up the humidity. Whenever the humidity drops below 60 percent, the dry air can pull moisture from the skin. That's bad enough when you have normal skin, but when you have psoriasis, it can be an itchy, scaly disaster. Consider using a room humidifier. You can also keep a kettle of water on low boil, set a pan of water on the radiator, or buy lots of green, leafy plants to increase the humidity in your home or office.

Be careful of injuries. When you have psoriasis, even mild injuries like sunburn, scratches, or sore areas caused by rubbing, tight clothing can cause a dramatic flare-up of the disease. Called "Koebner's phenomenon," an outbreak of psoriasis often occurs at the site of the injury. Be extra careful and avoid injuring your skin.

Watch the irritants. Many commonly used products like solvents, cleaners, hair dyes, and hair straighteners can irritate the skin. People with psoriasis are more susceptible to such irritation. Avoid these types of substances whenever possible, and when you can't, always wear cotton-lined vinyl gloves. If you opt for hair-care prod-

---

23 TIPS FOR TREATING YOUR PSORIASIS

- Maintain a positive attitude.
- Moisturize your skin.
- Use thick moisturizers.
- Soak in tepid water.
- Expose your skin to sunlight.
- Try UVB therapy.
- Go for tar-containing products.
- Try salicylic acid.
- Apply cortisone.
- Try occlusive therapy.
- Use mild soaps or soap alternatives.
- Rinse soap off thoroughly.
- Try olive oil for scalp scale.
- Take over-the-counter antihistamines for the itch.
- Consider fish oil.
- Increase the humidity in your environment.
- Avoid injuries.
- Be careful with irritants.
- Treat infections promptly.
- Stay trim.
- Be careful with medications.
- Manage your stress.
- Try kitchen solutions.

ucts like dyes, make sure your skin is in excellent shape before using them. Never use these products if your skin is broken or irritated.

Pay attention to infections. Another cause of psoriasis flare-ups is systemic infections like strep throat. If you suspect that you have such an infection, have it treated right away by your doctor.

Stay trim. Doctors don't know why, but if you're overweight, your psoriasis will likely be harder to control. Lose excess pounds with a low-fat diet and regular aerobic exercise.

Easy on the drugs. In some people, drugs like antimalarials, beta blockers, and lithium, among others, can cause psoriasis to flare up. Be sure your doctor knows about your psoriasis, and talk with him or her about reduced dosages or, when possible, alternative drugs or other therapies.

Take it easy. While stress doesn't cause psoriasis, doctors know it can certainly make it worse. You can't escape stress, but you can learn to manage it. Try meditation, biofeedback, yoga, progressive relaxation, deep "belly" breathing, or other stress management techniques.

Head for the kitchen. Try these home remedies from the National Psoriasis Foundation: For an anti-itch compress, dissolve 1½ cups of baking soda in three gallons of water or add three tablespoons of boric acid (available in pharmacies) to 16

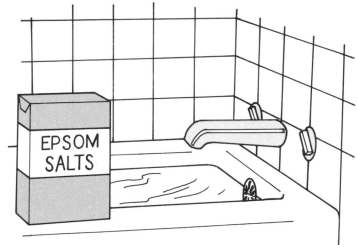

ounces of water. For itch relief, try adding a handful of Epsom salts, Dead Sea salts, or a cup of white vinegar to your bath. To soothe irritated skin, add two tablespoons of olive oil and eight ounces of milk to your bath.

Sources: Diane Baker, M.D., Clinical Professor of Dermatology, Oregon Health Sciences University, Portland, Oregon; Advisor, National Psoriasis Foundation. **Jon M. Hanifin, M.D.,** Professor of Dermatology, Oregon Health Sciences University; Board Member, Eczema Association for Science and Education, Portland, Oregon. **Mark Lebwohl, M.D.,** Medical Advisor, National Psoriasis Foundation; Director of Clinical Dermatology, Mt. Sinai School of Medicine, New York, New York. **Robert Matheson, M.D.,** Dermatologist, Portland, Oregon. **Frank Parker, M.D.,** Professor and Chair, Department of Dermatology, Oregon Health Sciences University, Portland, Oregon.

How to Beat

Winter

Depression

"THE SUN WILL COME OUT TOMORrow." It's an expression that means that things are looking up. Something about the sun just beams cheerfulness. It's no surprise that people who live in dreary northern climes have higher rates of depression, suicide, and alcoholism than everyone else.

SYMPTOMS

For most people, winter means nothing more than a time to pull the sweaters out of the cedar chest. However, for some of us, the increasing darkness and cold signal a Jekyll-and-Hyde change in personality—from happy and relaxed to depressed and tense. As winter progresses, concentration becomes difficult, irritability begins to rise, urges to munch (especially on carbohydrates) strike frequently, and just getting out of bed becomes a real challenge. Then spring comes along and Dr. Jekyll returns.

Seasonal Affective Disorder (SAD) can hit in varying degrees. Some patients may require hospitalization every winter. Others say that they don't feel all that depressed; they simply have such low energy that they aren't able to accomplish the things they would like to accomplish.

For most people with SAD, it takes two or three days of bright sunshine to elicit a reversal of symptoms. Consequently, a tipoff that you may have SAD is that you find relief from your symptoms when you spend some time closer to the equator.

SAD doesn't discriminate. It is found in men and women of all ages and races and in all parts of the country. However, it does seem to occur in women more often than in men, and specifically in women who are in their reproductive years.

CAUSES

Until about ten years ago, people suffering from this seasonal change in personality could only wonder what on earth was happening to them. Norman E. Rosenthal, M.D., author of *Seasons of the Mind,* was the first to make the connection between the shorter, darker days of winter and the onset of seasonal depression. He and his colleagues began studying this phenomenon and gave it the name "seasonal affective disorder."

Experts are not sure about the exact cause of this seasonal problem. They have proposed several theories. One theory suggests that a delay in the timing of the body clock in SAD patients causes their temperature minimum to occur at 6:00 A.M. rather than at the normal time of 3:00 A.M. As a result, they are attempting to wake up in what, for them, is physiologically the middle of the night. When these people are treated with bright light between 6:00 A.M. to 8:00 A.M., their mood improves. Their temperature minimum also shifts to an earlier time.

Another theory is that the secretion of the hormone melatonin is responsible for the low mood and lack of energy. The secretion of this hormone regulates the hibernation and reproductive cycles of animals. Melatonin is only secreted in the dark and is very light-sensitive. During the long summer days, melatonin secretion is markedly reduced because the nights are shorter. But during the long winter nights, melatonin secretion increases. Human melatonin production is also responsive to light, but it takes much more light to stop that production than it does in animals.

When melatonin is administered to normal individuals, it tends to lower their body temperature and cause drowsiness. This suggests the possibility that people with winter depression are secreting a lot of melatonin during the winter and not much during the summer. Following this theory, light therapy is thought to work because it shuts off the melatonin production.

AT-HOME TREATMENT

Taking a warm-weather vacation every few weeks is impractical for most of us, so what can you do about SAD right here at home? According to the experts, the following may help:

Avoid chemical stimulants. Your reduced energy level and depression may prompt you to turn to coffee or alcohol for a boost. However, the very brief lift you experience from caffeine can be accompanied by anxiety, muscle tension, and gastrointestinal problems. Alcohol is even worse; its depressive effects can further darken your mood.

Get moving. Exercising, especially outside in the morning light, may give you a feeling of control and lift your spirits. It is known that aerobic exercise boosts the body's production of natural painkillers, called endorphins. However, if you have been sedentary or if you suffer from any special medical conditions, consult your physician before beginning any program of exercise.

Get up with the birds. You may think that your home and office are lit well enough, but even brightly lit interiors are only one-tenth as intense as outdoor natural light, even on a cloudy day. Get out and see the light, especially early in the morning between 6:00 A.M. and 8:00 A.M. Take a morning walk or sit by a large window.

Get outside—whenever you can. Although the morning light seems to be the most helpful, any daylight is better than nothing. If you can't get outside first thing in the morning, at least get out on your lunch break.

Same time to bed, same time to rise. Retiring and rising at the same time every day will help synchronize your body's clock.

Increase your home's natural light. Make an effort to keep the blinds or curtains open as much as possible during the daylight hours. Some patients also report that moving from a room that faces north to a room that faces east, so the morning sun can wake them, makes a tremendous difference.

Enjoy an artificial dawn. Low-level light boxes can simulate dawn in your bedroom. They switch themselves on early and slowly get brighter and brighter as the morning wears on. In fact, even people without SAD say that these simulators make them feel more energetic. However, dawn simulators produce the best results when they are used under the supervision of a qualified professional.

Go south for the winter. It's an extreme solution, but moving to an area with a sunnier climate may lessen the severity of your symptoms. However, this treatment is impractical for most people.

---

8 WAYS TO KEEP SADNESS AT BAY

- Get as much natural light as possible between 6:00 A.M. and 8:00 A.M.
- Stay away from caffeine and alcohol.
- Start a program of mild aerobic exercise.
- Use every opportunity you have to spend time outside.
- Go to bed and get up at the same time every day.
- Let as much light into your home as possible.
- Move to an eastward-facing bedroom, if possible.
- Invest in a dawn simulator.

AT THE DOCTOR'S

If the suggestions in this chapter do not help your depression, it's time to seek the help of a licensed health professional who has experience in the use of light therapy. This could be a psychiatrist, psychologist, social worker, doctor, or nurse. However, it's best to see your personal physician first to rule out any physiologic cause for your depression, such as a thyroid disorder.

In addition to asking your doctor for a referral to a specialist in SAD, you can check the following sources to find a health practitioner in your area who has worked with patients who suffer from SAD.

- Your local medical school's department of psychiatry. Call and ask if there is any research program in your area for this disorder.
- Your local branch of the American Psychiatric Association. It may have a list of people who specialize in light therapy.
- The book *Seasons of the Mind* by Norman E. Rosenthal, M.D. In addition to giving you a wealth of information about SAD, the book contains a listing of health professionals from all over the country who specialize in this field.
- The Society for Light Treatment and Biological Rhythms (SLTBR). While this is a nationwide professional society for experts in the field, its membership roster includes health professionals who are qualified to do light therapy. You can write to SLTBR at P.O. Box 478, Wilsonville, Oregon 97070, or call 503-694-2404.
- The National Organization for Seasonal Affective Disorder. This national support group can help in both seeking treatment for and coping with the condition. You can write to the organization for information at P.O. Box 451, Vienna, Virginia 22180.

The treatments you would most likely receive from a professional include light-box therapy, dawn-simulator therapy, or tricyclic anti-depressants.

Sources: David H. Avery, M.D., Associate Professor of Psychiatry and Behavioral Sciences, University of Washington School of Medicine, Harborview Medical Center, Seattle, Washington. **Raymond Lam, M.D., F.R.C.P.** Assistant Professor, Department of Psychiatry, Psychiatrist, Mood Disorders Program, University of British Columbia, Vancouver, British Columbia, Canada. **Dan Oren, M.D.,** Senior Clinical Investigator, National Institute of Mental Health, National Institutes of Health, Bethesda, Maryland.

Tips to Take

the Tenderness

out of Teeth

Do COLD BEVERAGES MAKE YOU wince? Do hot coffee and soup give your teeth a painful message? When you eat or drink something very sugary or sour, do you feel an ache that goes all the way down into your gums? If you bite down on something hard, do you wish you could trade in your painful teeth? Welcome to the Sensitive Teeth Club. While it doesn't mean your teeth are going to fall out overnight, having sensitive teeth can certainly make you very uncomfortable.

Sensitivity to temperature, pressure, or sweet or sour means your teeth have been compromised in some way. It's a signal from your mouth that something is wrong. It might be as simple as a minor trauma from biting down too hard. Or it might be a sign that your tooth pulp is dead (necrotic) and you need root-canal work.

CAUSES

"Sensitive teeth" is a catchall term for a wide range of things than can make your teeth go "ouch." Most often, it's a simple case of exposed dentin, the material underneath the enamel. Dentin is also the substance that forms the teeth's roots. It contains microscopic nerve fibers that, when exposed, feel pain, especially in response to temperature and sweet and sour. Plenty of things can cause dentin to become exposed and sensitive. The gums may recede slightly due to gum disease or natural age-related changes. Or, if you're an enthusiastic toothbrusher, which many of us are, you may have caused a minor abrasion by brushing with too much pressure or using a toothbrush that's too stiff.

Sometimes teeth are sensitive because they are bruised. Think of that sensitive feeling in your tooth after you've had it drilled and filled at the dentist's office. It's probably a little bruised from the dental work. Depending on the extent of the trauma, this kind of sensitivity can take weeks or even months to go away. A tooth bruise can also be caused by an action as simple as biting down on something hard. Or it may be that you're a grinder or clencher, and you habitually grind your teeth or clamp your jaws down tightly. Usually this type of sensitivity isn't a problem, especially if it happens only once or twice and disappears within a day or two.

Sometimes sensitive teeth mean that your bite, the way the teeth fit together, is off. One or more teeth may be hitting too soon or too hard, causing uncomfortable pressure on certain teeth. While we think of teeth as being hard and stationary,

---

8 TIPS FOR BRUSHING CORRECTLY

Using a soft toothbrush and light pressure, follow these tips for correct brushing:

- **Vibrate or jiggle the brush head gently, letting the brush bristles stay in the same place. Avoid using a scrubbing action.**
- **Spend about ten seconds on each tooth.**
- **Place the brush at a 45-degree angle, aiming the brush into the margin between the teeth and gums.**
- **Use a back-and-forth stroke to clean the upper and lower teeth.**
- **For the inside of the front teeth, tilt the brush vertically and use an up-and-down motion.**
- **For the inside and outside of the back teeth, use short, angled strokes.**
- **Be sure to clean the outer surfaces, inner surfaces, and biting surfaces of both the upper and lower teeth.**
- **Gently brush your tongue (it can harbor bacteria).**

they really aren't. They move around slightly. As we age, bone is reabsorbed, or sometimes, childhood habits like thumb sucking can move teeth around and change how they come together.

AT-HOME TREATMENT

If your tooth sensitivity is caused by simple enamel abrasion or normal gum recession, home remedies can help relieve your discomfort. However, anytime you experience sensitivity in one or more teeth, you should see your dentist to determine the cause before trying self-care.

Desensitize it. You can't just fill enamel abrasion or gum-line recession like you can a dental cavity. But you can desensitize your teeth by brushing with one of the many over-the-counter desensitizing toothpastes available. The tooth's dentin contains minute tubules that lead to the tooth's blood and nerve supply (the pulp). These tiny tubules and the dentin's nerve endings can become exposed and sensitive. Desensitizing toothpastes contain chemicals that help seal up the tubules, thus decreasing sensitivity. Try putting some of the toothpaste on your finger or on a cotton swab and spreading it on sensitive spots before you go to bed. Spit, but don't rinse afterward. In most cases, you should see considerable improvement within two or three weeks.

Rinse it. Another way to desensitize your teeth is to use fluoride rinses, available over the counter at pharmacies or in the dental section at grocery stores. Once a day, swish it around in your mouth, then spit. Don't rinse. In addition to decreasing sensitivity, the fluoride acts as a cavity inhibitor.

Some people with sensitive teeth need fluoride rinses that are stronger than what's available over the counter. This may be true for you, especially if you've had extensive gum (periodontal) work like root planing to get rid of plaque. Your dentist can prescribe a stronger fluoride rinse.

Stay clean. If you have sensitive teeth, it's especially important to keep them free of plaque, the white sticky substance that forms on teeth. As the plaque metabolizes, it forms acid that can further irritate the sensitive teeth and make them even more reactive. Brush at least twice a day (plaque develops roughly every 12 hours), particularly after eating, and floss at least once a day. Have your teeth professionally cleaned once a year, preferably twice a year.

Use a softie. Toothbrushes come in soft, medium, and hard bristles. For sensitive teeth, you need to use the softest bristles you can find.

Lighten up. Even if you use a soft-bristled toothbrush, you probably need to lighten up on your brush stroke. Most people brush their teeth too hard, using too much pressure. Not only does this make it difficult for the bristles to move around and clean the teeth, it can damage the enamel and particularly the much-softer dentin. Avoid using a scrubbing action when you brush and apply as little pressure as possible.

Nix the snuff. "Snuff," "dip," "chew"—they all mean chewing tobacco and they're all bad for your teeth and gums. In the past, chewing tobacco was the domain of men and boys, but lately many young women, especially teenagers, have taken up the habit. They mistakenly believe that chewing tobacco is less harmful than smoking cigarettes. In reality, snuff causes gums to recede, a major cause of tooth sensitivity and decay. Tongue and throat cancer are two more dire consequences of chewing tobacco.

Skip the chewable vitamin C. You might wonder how vitamin C could be bad for you. Actually, chewable vitamin C tablets are hard on your teeth. The vitamin eats away at tooth enamel, exposing the sensitive material underneath. If you need vitamin C supplements, take them in pill form.

Use caution with candy. Hard candies that you suck on can also cause abrasion and tooth sensitivity. This is especially true of candies that you "pack" into your cheek against the gumline.

Call the dentist. In most cases, you can handle your sensitive teeth with home remedies. However, you should call the dentist if:

---

9 STRATEGIES TO SOOTHE YOUR SENSITIVE TEETH

- **Brush with desensitizing toothpaste.**
- **Rinse with fluoride.**
- **Keep your teeth clean.**
- **Use a soft-bristle brush.**
- **Brush with light pressure.**
- **Never use snuff.**
- **Be careful sucking on hard candies.**
- **Avoid chewable vitamin C tablets.**
- **If your symptoms warrant it, call your dentist.**

- Pressure consistently causes you discomfort.
- A single tooth is sensitive.
- Teeth don't respond to desensitizing toothpastes.
- You have pain that lasts longer than one hour.
- Your gums change color, especially around sensitive teeth.
- You have obvious dental decay.

Sources: Jack W. Clinton, D.M.D., Associate Dean of Patient Services, Oregon Health Sciences University School of Dentistry, Portland, Oregon. **Sandra Hazard**, D.M.D., Managing Dentist, Willamette Dental Group, Inc., Portland, Oregon. **Ken Waddell**, D.M.D., Dentist, Tigard, Oregon. **Ronald Wismer**, D.M.D., Past President, Washington County Dental Society; Dentist, Beaverton, Oregon.

●SEXUAL DIFFICULTIES

Ways to Get

More Pleasure

THIS IS HOW A ROMANTIC SEXUAL interlude goes, according to Hollywood: He sweeps her into his arms, crushing her lips with a passionate kiss. He deftly slips off her clothing and lifts her onto the bed. Within 30 seconds or so, she's writhing in orgasmic pleasure. Again and again, he brings her to a passionate orgasm until she's exhausted and falls asleep in her lover's arms.

Does that sound like what goes on in your bedroom? Not likely. Sexual desire and sexual pleasure can play a major role in a relationship. It can increase communication, solidify commitment, and deepen intimacy. However, for many women, sex can be a cause of tension, disagreement, and even physical pain.

Sex and sexuality are full of myths. It's time to correct a few of the more common misconceptions:

- Sexual pleasure is not solely a physical response. There's no denying the physical element of sex, but sexual desire and the ability to achieve sexual satisfaction are as much in one's head as they are in one's body, particularly for women. Many things—tension, worry, past sexual abuse, ambivalence about one's partner—can get in the way of sexual pleasure.
- Sexual pleasuring does not necessarily come naturally. Many women assume enjoying sexual relations is innate and being able to pleasure one's partner is just something we're born knowing about. However, like many other human activities, becoming "sexually successful" is learned. It takes practice and good communication.
- Successful sex partners do not have to have equal sexual desire.

It's rare that two people have identical desires for sexual frequency. Wanting more or less sex is often a source of tension and disagreement in relationships.

- Intercourse is not the only kind of "real" sex. There are many ways to sexually pleasure one another. In fact, many women aren't able to orgasm during intercourse. Most women require direct stimulation of the clitoris for orgasm.
- Good lovers do not always have multiple orgasms. It's a common misconception that a woman should always have multiple orgasms. After orgasm, some women do retain a high level of arousal and can achieve another orgasm shortly after the first. However, few of us have multiple orgasms and women shouldn't feel inadequate if they don't have them. After orgasm, most men cannot immediately get an erection (a few younger men are able to become erect shortly after orgasm) or attain orgasm. Women shouldn't expect a male lover to be "ready and able" with rapid re-erection.

CAUSES

With so many misconceptions and expectations about sex, it's no wonder many women have sexual difficulties. The most common causes of sexual difficulties in women include:

- Orgasm problems. Up to 50 percent of all women have difficulties achieving orgasm from vaginal intercourse, and many never achieve orgasm regardless of the type of sexual stimulation.
- Pain with intercourse. Called "dyspareunia," painful intercourse can

make this form of lovemaking a real turnoff for many women. Painful intercourse can be caused by vaginal or urinary tract infections, estrogen deficiency (due to breastfeeding, birth control pills, or age-related changes), endometriosis, scarring from surgery, or vaginismus, involuntary contraction of the vaginal muscles. However, by far the most common cause of painful intercourse for women is lack of lubrication due to not taking enough time for arousal.

- Loss of sexual interest. Some authorities believe that Americans are undergoing an "epidemic" of loss of sexual interest due to career commitments, aging, hormonal changes associated with pregnancy, alcohol and drug abuse, illness, fear of AIDS, and other problems.
- Desire differences. When one partner consistently wants to make love and the other doesn't, it can cause tension and other relationship difficulties. In heterosexual relationships, men are stereotypically viewed as "sex fiends" and women as "frigid" when there are desire differences.

AT-HOME TREATMENT

Sexual difficulties often respond to self-care. However, if your sexual problems persist, see a professional for assistance.

Take extra time. We live in a "hurry up" society. But as women, we typically need more time than men do to become aroused. Don't schedule lovemaking when you don't really have time for it. Although a "quickie" once in a while can

be fun, for satisfying lovemaking, most women need sufficient time to become aroused and achieve orgasm. If your partner wants to have intercourse too soon for you, ask him to slow down and take enough time so that you can enjoy each another's entire body—not just the genitals.

Try nonintercourse pleasuring. For both women and men, an orgasm is the same regardless of whether it is achieved through intercourse, mutual masturbation, oral sex, anal sex, a vibrator, or other stimulation. Many women cannot achieve orgasm through intercourse no matter how long it lasts. It simply doesn't provide enough stimulation to the clitoris. Experiment with forms of lovemaking other than intercourse and tell your partner what feels good.

Use a lubricant. If more foreplay and nonintercourse lovemaking aren't enough to provide sufficient lubrication for intercourse, you may need to use a lubricant. You can purchase commercial products like K-Y Jelly, Astroglide, or Surgilube at the pharmacy. However, keep in mind that a lubricant isn't a substitution for arousal.

Use less alcohol. We've long known that alcohol may increase sexual desire and decrease caution, but it also decreases the ability to satisfy that desire. In men, alcohol makes erections more difficult. In women (and men), too much alcohol can numb the senses, interfere with good communication, and make orgasms difficult to achieve.

Don't abuse drugs. Many prescription medications and street drugs can make it difficult if not impossible to get sexual satisfaction. Drugs that work on the central nervous system such as narcotics, barbiturates, hypnotics, and sleeping aids impair sexual responsiveness. So-called "recreational" drugs like crack, cocaine, and amphetamines increase desire, but impair orgasms. If you're taking prescription medications and are having sexual difficulties, talk with your physician about alternative medications.

Talk about it. Some couples have been together for years and never talk about their sexual relationship. To be mutually satisfying, a sexual relationship must be based on open communication. Women are often afraid to talk directly about what they want and need from their sexual partners. No one can read your mind. Ask for what you want. Tell your partner what feels good and what doesn't.

If you have desire differences, set aside some time to discuss them. Take a walk or drive together and talk about how you can come to satisfying compromises.

Make a "turn-on" list. We often assume our lovers know exactly what we like. No one can read your mind. Have each of you make a list of what arouses you. Then share your lists. You may be surprised at how stimulating and enlightening this exercise can be.

Engage in nonsexual play. We often become so engrossed in living—responsibilities at work, volunteer duties, demands from children—that we get out of touch with our partners. Take time to be together in pleasurable, nonsexual ways. Make "dates" to rediscover having fun together. If you can't enjoy spending time out of the bedroom together, it's unlikely you'll enjoy one another in the bedroom.

Don't fall for "getting old" myths. OK, you may not be a hot-blooded teenager anymore, but sexual activity can be a lifelong source of pleasure and intimacy. Desire may change after about age 40, but you can still have an active and enjoyable sex life. Remember, you're never too old for sex.

Exercise regularly. You probably won't feel like having sex if you're not feeling good about yourself or if you feel rundown. Regular moderate exercise can lift your spirits, increase your energy, make you feel healthier, boost your self-esteem, and increase your sexual desire.

Manage your stress. Worries, tension, and anxieties can all impair your ability to enjoy sex and achieve orgasm. Take time to look at your commitments and priorities. Are there ways you could manage your time more effectively? Make a list of your priorities. What's really important in your life? What things could you let drop? Experiment with different stress management techniques such as biofeedback, meditation, progressive relaxation, deep breathing, visualization, or other techniques, and see which ones work for you.

Avoid "faking" it. Many women have "faked" their orgasms, fearing their partners would think they were cold or unresponsive if they didn't achieve orgasm. You'll never be able to break the cycle of miscommunication if you don't stop faking. Talk with your partner and tell him what works for you and what doesn't work. If that kind of direct communication feels too scary, try being more responsive and making pleasurable noises when your partner does something you enjoy.

Try self-pleasuring. Some women have been raised to believe that there's something "wrong" or "dirty" about masturbation. However, sex experts say that masturbating can make a woman more responsive with a sex partner. It can also be very helpful for women who have never had an orgasm or who aren't sure what they need to achieve one.

Vary your lovemaking routine. Couples who have been together for a number of years often become bored with one anoth-

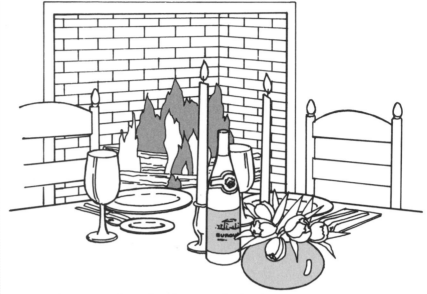

er because they don't vary their sexual routine. They make love on the same day of the week, at the same time, in the same way. You don't have to get out the whipped cream or engage in exotic sexual practices to escape your sexual rut. Simply changing your lovemaking location (you don't have to always make love in the bedroom), timing (nighttime isn't the only time to make love), or ambiance can help. Add music. Lower the lighting. Use massage oil. Spread a blanket and make love in front of the fireplace.

Don't make love when you're tired. Many busy couples try to squeeze lovemaking into a narrow slice of time right before going to sleep. This may be the worst time to make love. Both of you are probably exhausted from the day's challenges. Instead, try to find other times—perhaps early morning, during weekends, or earlier in the evening—when you're more rested and responsive.

Ask for what you want. If you want to make love, say so to your partner through words and/or actions. Don't take the attitude that "If you really loved me, you'd just know." Some women are afraid to take the lead and show any assertiveness in lovemaking, but men enjoy feeling desired, too, and most men really enjoy when a woman takes initiative in lovemaking.

Schedule "child-free" time. New parents often experience sexual difficulties. Demanding newborns and young children can leave parents exhausted and in no mood for lovemaking. It's vital to your relationship that you schedule some "child-free" time into your life. Work your sexual schedule around your child's nap schedule. Hire a baby-sitter to enable you to get away and have some privacy.

Get away from it all. Sometimes a change of scenery is just what the doctor ordered for an ailing sex life. Taking a brief vacation, even if it's just for the weekend, can help you get away from your daily cares and free you up for reigniting romance.

Stop smoking. Cigarette smoking increases fatigue and decreases energy, including the energy needed for sex. Also, if you smoke and your lover doesn't, the taste and smell can be a real turnoff.

Get professional help. If you feel you've tried your best to work out problems in your relationship and your sex life and you still have difficulties, consider talking with a mental health professional, particularly one who specializes in relationships and sexuality.

Problems like the involuntary muscle contractions of vaginismus can stem from deep psychological trauma like sexual abuse. These kinds of issues require professional assistance. Other mental health problems like depression, eating disorders, or severe anxiety, among others, can contribute to loss of sexual desire and other sexual difficulties. Problems with self-esteem or body image can also

---

21 TIPS FOR INCREASING YOUR SEXUAL PLEASURE

- Take enough time to become aroused.
- Try nonintercourse pleasuring.
- Use a lubricant.
- Talk about it with your partner.
- Drink less alcohol.
- Don't abuse drugs.
- Share "turn-on" lists.
- Engage in nonsexual play.
- Don't fall for "getting old" myths.
- Exercise regularly.
- Vary your lovemaking routine.
- Manage your stress.
- Avoid faking it.
- Try self-pleasuring.
- Don't make love when you're tired.
- Ask for what you want.
- Get away for a little vacation.
- Schedule "child-free" time.
- Don't smoke.
- Seek professional help.
- Call the doctor.

create problems in a sexual relationship. A mental health professional can often help.

Call the doctor. Some sexual difficulties in women are caused by medical problems like endometriosis, vaginal infections, urinary tract infections, vaginal irritation that is due to lack of estrogen, or scarring from past surgical procedures. These are conditions that require a doctor's help. If you've tried the home remedies listed here without success or if you suspect your difficulties are related to another health condition, call your physician.

Sources: **Michael Castleman,** Former Editor, *Medical SelfCare* Magazine; Author *Sexual Solutions,* San Francisco, California. **Sadja Greenwood, M.D.,** Assistant Clinical Professor, Department of Gynecology, Obstetrics, and Reproductive Services, University of California at San Francisco, San Francisco, California; Author, *Menopause Naturally;* Coauthor, *The Medical SelfCare Book of Women's Health.* **Anne Simons, M.D.,** Coauthor, *Before You Call the Doctor;* Family Practitioner, San Francisco Department of Public Health; Family Practitioner and Assistant Clinical Professor, Family and Community Medicine, University of California San Francisco Medical Center, San Francisco, California.

●SEXUALLY TRANSMITTED DISEASES

Strategies for

Staying Safe

NOT SO LONG AGO, THE STEREOTYPE was that only "those" kinds of girls and women contracted sexually transmitted diseases, also called "STDs," "venereal disease," or "VD." Today, we know that any woman (or man) can contract a wide range of infections passed through sexual contact. Some, like trichomonas, are highly treatable. However, for women, even many treatable STDs carry the risk of developing into potentially fatal pelvic inflammatory disease (PID). Others, like acquired immune deficiency syndrome, or AIDS, are themselves fatal.

Many of us will have more than one sexual partner in our lifetimes. The reality is that you're having sexual contact with every other person your partner has had sex with. Even if your sexual partner hasn't had intercourse with anyone else for months or even years, some STDs like AIDS or syphilis persist for years and can be readily transmitted to new sexual partners. Some people think they're safe as long as they always use condoms during intercourse. However, some STDs like genital herpes and syphilis (at certain stages) can be passed through skin-to-skin contact or kissing.

TYPES OF STDs

There are many sexually transmitted diseases. Each has its own set of symptoms and its own treatment. The only thing they have in common is that they are spread primarily through sexual contact. Let's look at the types of STDs: AIDS, chlamydia, genital warts, genital herpes, gonorrhea, syphilis, and trichomonas.

AIDS. Short for "acquired immune deficiency syndrome," AIDS is due to a viral infection that attacks the body's immune system. It usually begins with loss of weight, fevers, night sweats, infections, and/or a type of pneumonia. The human immunodeficiency virus (HIV) that causes AIDS attacks and destroys the type of white blood cells called "T cells." It turns these cells into tiny factories that replicate more and more of the virus. Without the T cells as the body's first line of defense against a wide range of infectious agents, the body becomes highly vulnerable. As the disease progresses, the body's entire immune system collapses and organisms that are normally fought off become deadly. AIDS can also kill by causing a form of cancer or by attacking the brain.

The recent epidemic of AIDS worldwide has created many misconceptions and myths about the disease. Here we'll tell you the facts:

• Anyone can get AIDS, not just gay men and intravenous drug users. In fact, AIDS is spread much more easily from men to women than from women to men. Anal intercourse is especially dangerous. When professional basketball player Earvin "Magic" Johnson announced he was HIV positive (meaning he's been exposed to the HIV virus, but has not yet developed full-blown AIDS), he underscored the reality that anyone who has unprotected sex can contract HIV.

• You can't get AIDS from casual contact. You can't get AIDS from shaking hands or touching someone who is HIV positive or who has AIDS. You can't get it from living with an HIV-positive person, breathing the same air, or sharing utensils. And you can't get it from telephones, toilet seats, water fountains, showers, or other inanimate objects. AIDS can be transmitted only through blood, saliva, or sexual contact, or from mother to fetus.

- Donating blood doesn't give you AIDS. The equipment used to extract donated blood has been sterilized and is used only once before it is disposed of.
- A negative AIDS test does not mean that you're completely safe. It depends on when the test was performed and when you were exposed. It takes a few months after exposure for the HIV antibodies to show up in blood tests. People who have been infected since testing or who were tested right after exposure may test negative and still be HIV positive.

At this time, there is no cure for AIDS. Prevention is the only protection you have. We'll talk about prevention later in this chapter.

Chlamydia. This is one of the most deadly STDs for women, yet it's been so poorly publicized that many women have never even heard of it. Caused by a virus-like bacterium, *Chlamydia trachomatis,* it affects both men and women, but in women it can cause a potentially deadly pelvic infection, pelvic inflammatory disease (PID), that affects the fallopian tubes. It's also a major cause of fertility problems in women.

Chlamydia is passed during vaginal or anal intercourse. Doctors still aren't sure whether chlamydia can be transmitted through oral sex. It can also be passed from mother to child during birth, resulting in ear

---

5 IMPORTANT AIDS FACTS

Because AIDS is still a new and very frightening idea to many people, the rumors about the disease seem to get more publicity than the cold, hard facts. These are some of the truths about how the AIDS virus is transmitted:

- If you're a straight female, this doesn't mean you're safe from AIDS. Anyone can get the disease, not just gay males.
- You can't get AIDS from touching an infected person or from inanimate objects that have been touched by an infected person.
- AIDS can be transmitted through blood, saliva, sexual contact, or from mother to fetus.
- It's safe to donate blood. The equipment used won't give you AIDS.
- One negative test is not a guarantee that you don't have the HIV virus. It takes a few months for HIV to show up in tests.

---

infections and pneumonia in the newborn. In addition, chlamydia has been linked to an increased risk of stillbirths and to sudden infant death syndrome (SIDS).

Unfortunately, the majority of women exhibit no symptoms with chlamydia until they have a pelvic inflammatory infection. Some women do have early symptoms, including: vaginal discharge and sometimes painful urination, vaginal bleeding, bleeding after sex, and lower abdominal pain. In men, symptoms include penile discharge and sometimes painful urination.

Chlamydia is effectively treated with antibiotics (doxycycline, tetracycline, erythromycin). It does not respond to penicillin.

Herpes. These are feverlike blisters in the genital area caused by either of two viruses, herpesvirus type 1 or type 2. Usually, type 1 is the kind that causes fever blisters (cold sores) on the mouth, face, and lips. Type 2 involves sores in the genital area. Either type may infect the genitals.

Herpes is a "contact" virus, which means you can get it from skin-to-skin contact with someone who is infected. It's passed from partner to partner through oral or genital sex. It can be passed when an infected person has active sores or is in the pre-active state when the sore areas feel itchy or tingly but have not produced blisters yet.

Once you have herpes you have it for life. The virus enters the body through mucous membranes and travels to the base of the spine where it lies dormant, feeding off cell nutrients. An outbreak can recur at any time.

Herpes can't be cured, but prescription medications can sometimes shorten outbreaks and relieve symptoms.

Genital warts. Also called "venereal warts," these are just what they sound like, warts in the genital area. They are soft, moist, and pink and may be flat, raised, single, or multiple viral growths. They are painless and may go unnoticed. In women, they often occur on the outer part of the vagina, in the vagina, on the cervix, or on or near the anus. When they occur inside, some women have burning or vaginal discharge.

Caused by the human papilloma virus (HPV), genital warts can grow to be quite large when they are left untreated, causing discomfort during intercourse, urination, or bowel movements. Some medical authorities believe that genital warts increase a woman's risk of developing cancer of the cervix.

If you have genital warts and become pregnant, the pregnancy may make the warts grow faster. Usually they shrink after birth. The wart virus can be transmitted from mother to baby, sometimes causing warts in the baby's throat.

Warts are spread through sexual contact with an infected person. They usually develop six to eight weeks after exposure. They're often treated with caustic chemicals or are burned off (cauterized) or frozen off (cryosurgery). Unfortunately, despite treatments, warts often recur.

Gonorrhea. This is a highly contagious bacterial infection spread through direct sexual contact. Also called "GC" or "the clap," gonorrhea is a major cause of fertility problems and the potentially fatal pelvic inflammatory disease in women. In men, gonorrhea primarily affects the penis. In women, it can infect the throat, the anus, and the vagina. It can also infect the eyes if genital secretions come in contact with them (e.g., a person rubs their eyes after touching infected genitals). Left untreated, gonorrhea can infect the blood and become a serious systemic infection, which can cause sterility, arthritis, and even heart trouble. A gonorrhea-infected woman can pass on the infection to her newborn.

Unfortunately, in women, gonorrhea may exhibit no symptoms. Women who exhibit symptoms have vaginal discharge and frequent, painful urination. When the throat is infected, a woman may not notice any symptoms or she may have a scratchy or inflamed sore throat. When gonorrhea leads to pelvic inflammatory disease, symptoms include fever, chills, vaginal discharge, vomiting, and lower abdominal pain.

It's easier to spot gonorrhea in men. They display thick, yellowish penile discharge, inflamed urethra, and pain or burning on urination.

Gonorrhea responds to injections or oral treatments of penicillin or tetracycline.

Syphilis. This serious and highly contagious STD is one of the oldest in the world. It is caused by spiral-shaped bacteria called spirochetes, which, over time, can affect the brain, bones, spinal cord, heart, and reproductive organs. Left untreated, syphilis can cause blindness, brain damage, heart disease, and death. It can be passed from mother to fetus and cause blindness, deafness, and other serious health problems.

Syphilis has three distinctive phases: primary, secondary, and tertiary. Sometimes in women, syphilis does not cause symptoms, which can make it particularly dangerous. Usually, however, the first stage is characterized by the appearance of a tiny, open sore called a chancre 10 to 90 days after exposure. This lesion is painless and usually occurs on the genitals. It can also appear on the rectum, cervix, lips, tongue, fingers, or anywhere direct contact with the bacteria was made. After a few weeks, the sore disappears without treatment.

A body-wide rash appears in the second stage of syphilis, usually within six weeks to six months of exposure. Other symptoms may include flulike symptoms—fever, sore throat, headache, fatigue, aching joints, and enlarged lymph nodes—and red or reddish brown erosions on the lining of the mouth, external sex organs, the anus, and warm, moist areas like under the arms. Often, these symptoms are ignored or confused with other conditions. Usually, these symptoms pass without treatment within three to six weeks, although in some cases, they come and go sporadically for years. At this stage a person infected with syphilis can pass on the disease through casual contact like kissing or skin contact with an open sore.

In the third stage of syphilis, all symptoms disappear and the disease appears to be dormant. During this period, the infected person isn't contagious except to unborn offspring. This final stage can last indefinitely and cause body-wide destruction and possibly death.

Syphilis is treated with penicillin (or other antibiotics if you're allergic to penicillin). In very advanced cases, syphilis cannot be treated.

Trichomonas. Also called "tric," it is caused by a single-celled protozoan (the trichomonad). It is sexually passed from one partner to another, but may develop or recur several years after exposure.

In some women, trichomonas causes no symptoms. In most, however, it causes a frothy, yellowish, smelly vaginal discharge. When the infection spreads to the bladder, women may need to urinate frequently. In many men, trichomonas doesn't cause symptoms. Other men will develop painful urination, a watery discharge, and penile itching if they are infected.

Trichomonas is treated by doctors with a single dose of metronidazole (Flagyl). If you're taking metronidazole, don't drink alcohol, which can cause nausea, abdominal cramping, numbness in the arms and legs, and even seizures.

AT-HOME TREATMENT

All sexually transmitted diseases require a doctor's care. If you think you have an STD, see your doctor immediately. If you do have one of these diseases, the following strategies can help.

Get tested. If there's even the slightest possibility that you might have been exposed to a sexually transmitted disease, get tested, especially if you begin to exhibit any symptoms. Prompt diagnosis and treatment are important in preventing complications and the spread of STDs. Be sure to tell your doctor about all the areas where you may be infected (e.g., mouth, throat, rectum, anus, genitals).

Let all sex partners know. One way to stop the chain of transmission of STDs is to let any sexual partner know if you contract a sexually transmitted disease. Your physician or county health department can assist you in notifying past and present sex partners.

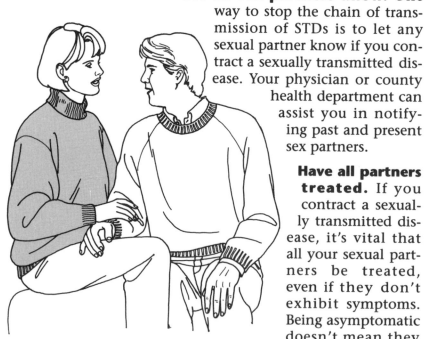

Have all partners treated. If you contract a sexually transmitted disease, it's vital that all your sexual partners be treated, even if they don't exhibit symptoms. Being asymptomatic doesn't mean they aren't infected. Often men don't exhibit noticeable symptoms for many STDs, and they pass them on or reinfect their partners.

Take ALL your medication. Many STDs are treated with a course of antibiotics. Often, symptoms will subside within a few days after starting the medication. This does not mean that you are free of the infection. Be sure both you and your partner take the entire course of medication.

Ask for other tests. If you've been diagnosed with gonorrhea, ask to be tested for chlamydia and syphilis. Women should also insist on a Pap smear for genital wart (HPV) infection.

Go for a follow-up visit. While medical treatment for most STDs (other than AIDS or herpes) is usually effective, you may be infected with an antibiotic-resistant strain. For women, this can mean you think you're cured and then you develop a potentially fatal pelvic infection. At your first doctor visit ask, "When should I return for a follow-up?" Then make sure you and your partner(s) keep the appointment.

Request a retest. Insist that your doctor retest you for the STD after you've taken all the medication to ensure that you're infection-free. If you're not, get treated again.

Abstain from sex while infected. It's a good idea to avoid sexual contact altogether while you're being treated for an STD. If you must engage in sex during this time, be sure to use a latex condom and don't have unprotected oral sex.

Tell your OB. If you have an STD and become pregnant, be sure to let your obstetrician know immediately. Many STDs can harm the fetus.

Herpes. Use these herpes home remedies. Genital herpes isn't curable, but you can get some welcome relief using these at-home treatment strategies:

Manage your stress. Often emotional and physical stress trigger outbreaks of herpes. Learn some strategies to keep stress under control.

Use ice. At the first sign of a herpes outbreak, apply ice to reduce pain and swelling. Cover an ice pack with a thin cloth and apply it directly to sores for ten to 15 minutes at a time. Reapply several times throughout the day.

Use drying remedies. Drying remedies like baking soda and corn starch can reduce itching and help dry sores. You can also try a hand-held hair dryer on the low setting.

Avoid tight-fitting clothing. Don't wear tight-fitting underwear, nylons, or pants that can irritate the genital area and stimulate an outbreak of genital herpes.

Apply black tea bags. Placing cold, wet tea bags on the sores can soothe irritated tissues.

Use Burow's solution. Apply cool compresses of Burow's solution (ask your pharmacist) four to six times a day.

---

10 WAYS TO TREAT YOUR STD

- **Get tested early.**
- **If you're infected, inform all your sexual partners.**
- **Have all your sexual partners treated.**
- **Take all your medication.**
- **Request other tests.**
- **Go for a follow-up visit.**
- **Get retested.**
- **Abstain from sex while you're infected. (See this chapter for more detailed information on when to abstain from sex if you have herpes.)**
- **Let your obstetrician know if you're pregnant and contract an STD.**
- **Use herpes home remedies.**

Take pain relievers. Aspirin, acetaminophen, or ibuprofen can help relieve pain.

Keep your genital area dry. After showering or bathing, pat (don't rub) your genital area dry or use a hand-held dryer on the cool setting. Use a separate towel for your genital area to prevent spreading the virus to other parts of your body. Don't share your towels with anyone.

PREVENTION

As you can see, many sexually transmitted diseases are deadly serious. None of them can be treated with self-care. They all require professional diagnosis and treatment. Prompt diagnosis and treatment can, in many cases, prevent complications and spread of the STD. You can use the strategies below to keep yourself safe and reduce your risk of contracting a sexually transmitted disease.

Forget "casual" sex. Having sex with strangers or casual acquaintances may have been in during the 1970s and early 80s, but such contact is too dangerous today. Don't simply ask whether your potential partner has ever contracted an STD. Really get to know a person before having sex with them. Careful partner selection may be the single most important thing you can do to prevent contracting an STD.

Always use a latex condom. OK, some men don't like wearing them, but insisting your male partner(s) use latex condoms may save your life. (AIDS has become increasingly widespread among the heterosexual population in the U.S. and many other countries.) Make sure your partner uses latex condoms, not animal membrane "skin" types, which provide less effective protection. Using condoms doesn't have to break up the flow of your lovemaking if you make putting them on part of your sexual play.

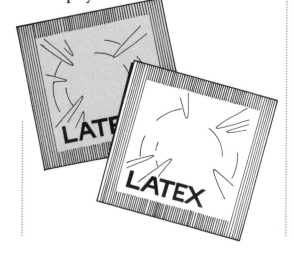

Limit the number of your sex partners. The more sex partners you have, the greater your risk of contracting a potentially deadly STD.

Avoid oil-based lubricants. Some women, particularly postmenopausal women, need additional lubrication for intercourse to be comfortable. Oil-based lubricants like Vaseline or mineral oil can cause condoms to break down. (They're also not good for a woman's genital health.) Opt for water-based commercial lubricants like K-Y Jelly or Astroglide.

Use spermicidal jellies or creams. Spermicidal products that contain nonoxynol-9 can provide extra protection against infection from STDs like AIDS in case of condom breakage. (It can also provide additional contraceptive protection.) Using a spermicidal jelly alone will not provide adequate protection against STDs or pregnancy.

Don't have unprotected oral sex. It used to be that young women worried only about becoming pregnant. Oral sex was a pregnancy-free alternative to intercourse. Now, however, we know that unprotected mouth contact with the penis, vagina, or anus can spread STD organisms.

Avoid sexual acrobatics. Some sexual practices are more likely to cause tears in the anus, vagina, or penis. Such tears make you and your partner much more susceptible to transmission of STD organisms. Take it easy and prevent these kinds of injuries.

Never use intravenous drugs. STDs like AIDS are readily passed from person to person through intravenous drug use. If you do use intravenous drugs, never share needles with anyone, even people you know very well.

Examine your partner before having sex. It may not sound too romantic, but it's important to examine your partner carefully for bumps, sores, tears, and so on in the genital area before engaging in any sexual activity. Also, pay attention to any changes such as different smells, tastes, or discharges. Often STDs are passed between partners before either one is aware that one partner has been infected.

Pay attention to your body. If you're sexually active, tune into your own body and watch for any symptoms or changes. Look for symptoms like discharge, burning with urination, sores, lumps and bumps, and itching. Never ignore symptoms, even mild ones. Serious sexually transmitted diseases like syphilis and gonorrhea may exhibit only mild symptoms.

Have regular exams. A regular Pap smear and pelvic examination is a must for gynecologic health. Yearly exams can help you spot problems before they become too great. If you experience symptoms, don't wait

---

12 STRATEGIES FOR PREVENTING STDs

- Know your sex partners well.
- Use latex condoms.
- Limit the number of sex partners you have.
- Don't use oil-based lubricants.
- Use spermicides that contain nonoxynol-9.
- Don't have unprotected oral sex.
- Be gentle in lovemaking.
- Don't use intravenous drugs.
- Examine your partner for symptoms before having sex.
- Watch your body for symptoms.
- Have regular gynecologic exams.
- Inform your OB–GYN about your STD history.

---

for your regular exam to have them checked out.

Let your OB–GYN know. If you're pregnant or considering becoming pregnant and have a history of STD, be sure your gynecologist and/or obstetrician has the complete story. Untreated STDs or "lifelong" STDs like genital herpes or genital warts can harm the fetus.

Sources: **Michael Castleman,** Former Editor, *Medical SelfCare* Magazine; Author *Sexual Solutions,* San Francisco, California. **Amanda Clark, M.D.,** Assistant Professor, Department of Obstetrics and Gynecology, Oregon Health Sciences University, Portland, Oregon. **Sadja Greenwood, M.D.,** Assistant Clinical Professor, Department of Gynecology, Obstetrics, and Reproductive Services, University of California at San Francisco, San Francisco, California; Author, *Menopause Naturally;* Coauthor, *The Medical SelfCare Book of Women's Health.* **Anne Simons, M.D.,** Coauthor, *Before You Call the Doctor;* Family Practitioner, San Francisco Department of Public Health; Family Practitioner and Assistant Clinical Professor, Family and Community Medicine, University of California San Francisco Medical Center, San Francisco, California. **Sue Woodruff, R.N.,** Childbirth and Parenting Education Coordinator, Tuality Community Hospital, Hillsboro, Oregon.

•SHINGLES

Ways to

Relieve the

Pain

IT STARTS WITH A TINGLING OR PRICKLING of the skin. Then burning or shooting pain begins. Within a couple of days, a rash of small, red spots has developed. It itches like crazy and the pain gets worse as the spots enlarge and blister. Eventually, they fill with pus, burst, and crust over. Welcome to one of life's déjà vu experiences—you have shingles, otherwise known as "adult chicken pox."

SYMPTOMS

Shingles may sound funny, but when you've got them, it's no laughing matter. The rash is itchy and painful, and the pain increases as the rash becomes more swollen. The blisters that follow may last five days to three or four weeks before they crust over and disappear. The agony of shingles may not end with the rash either. Even after the rash and blisters have disappeared, you may experience sharp, shooting, piercing pain that can last for months or perhaps years. Doctors call it "postherpetic neuralgia." The older you are, the more you're at risk for this lingering pain. Fortunately, only about one in ten people who suffer from shingles have postherpetic neuralgia, and prompt medical attention can often reduce your risk.

Shingles commonly attack the nerves of the chest, back, neck, buttocks, arms, legs, or face. The painful rash usually occurs as a band or strip along the nerve, hence the name "shingles" from the Latin and French words for belt or girdle. One important clue in distinguishing shingles from the myriad of other skin rashes: Shingles occur only on one side of the body.

CAUSES

Medical experts disagree about the causes of shingles. Some say that when you were younger and contracted the varicella zoster virus that causes chicken pox, the virus never really went away. Instead, it lay dormant in your body for years. Then, for some reason such as an injury to the skin or an emotional or physical upset that temporarily weakens the immune system, the virus is reactivated and these "adult chicken pox" develop.

Others contend that the antibodies produced by the body after the initial attack of chicken pox decrease in number and strength over the years and leave us again susceptible to the zoster virus. However, because some of the antibodies from the original chicken pox exposure endure in the body, shingles develop rather than full-blown chicken pox. Of course, if you've never been exposed to chicken pox, you'll get pox rather than shingles, no matter what your age.

The risk of developing shingles increases as you age. It rarely develops in anyone under 15 and is fairly common in people over 50 (more than half of all people who contract shingles are over 50). The good news is that most people only have shingles once in a lifetime.

In a few cases, shingles can spread over the entire body. Usually, this only happens in people who have an underlying disease such as certain forms of cancer. In people whose immune systems are already compromised by a serious illness such as cancer or AIDS, shingles can, in rare instances, be fatal.

The most common complication is the rash becoming infected with bacteria. Not only can this prolong the rash, but it can also cause skin scarring.

AT-HOME TREATMENT

Call the doctor. If you think you might have shingles, the first thing you need to do is see a doctor immediately for proper diagnosis. Prompt medical attention can often reduce your chances of experiencing prolonged pain from shingles and can reduce your risk of complications. Medical attention is particularly important if:

• You're older.

• You have some other serious illness.

• You have shingles on your face, especially near your eyes (it can lead to vision problems).

• You have shingles on your leg, hand, or genital areas.

Once you've seen your doctor, there are plenty of home remedies you can use to help you cope with the pain and itching, blisters, and any lingering discomfort.

Cool it. Ice water can cool the pain and reduce inflammation. Place a cold cloth on the blisters or wrap a towel around the lesion and pour ice water on it. Use the cold packs for 20 minutes, then leave them off for 20 minutes. Repeat until you have relief from the pain.

You can also use cold milk compresses for soothing relief. Or try wrapping a bag of frozen peas or frozen unpopped popcorn in a thin towel and placing it on the hot, rashy area.

---

13 WAYS TO EASE SHINGLES DISCOMFORT

• Call the doctor.
• Use cool compresses.
• Get plenty of rest.
• Try over-the-counter anti-inflammatories.
• Rub on topical anesthetics.
• Don't pop your blisters.
• Wear cotton gloves at night to prevent scratching.
• Avoid infecting others.
• Take warm baths.
• Try capsaicin.
• Use mental strategies.
• Try a TENS unit.
• Consider antidepressants.

Rest, rest, rest. When you've got shingles, your immune system is under attack. The best thing you can do is to rest and let your immune system have the extra energy it needs to fight this virus.

Try anti-inflammatories. Over-the-counter anti-inflammatories like aspirin and ibuprofen can relieve pain and reduce inflammation and swelling. If you can't take aspirin or ibuprofen, try acetaminophen (it will help the pain, but is much less effective as an anti-inflammatory). If the pain is too great to be relieved by over-the-counter pain relievers, ask your doctor to prescribe codeine or another painkilling narcotic.

Get the rub. Ask your doctor to recommend or prescribe a topical anesthetic cream to reduce your pain. Watch out for over-the-counter products that contain any ingredient that ends in "-caine." These can cause allergic reactions that may make your shingles worse.

Hands off. As blisters form, there's a great temptation to pop them. Resist! It will just make matters worse and may put you at risk for a secondary bacterial infection.

Wear nighttime gloves. Try cutting your fingernails short and wearing soft cotton gloves at night to control unconscious scratching.

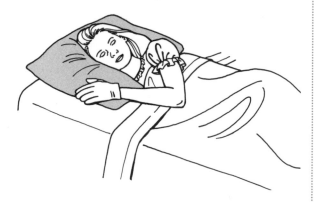

Avoid contact. Once you have shingles, avoid passing it on. It's particularly important not to infect people who have any sort of immune problem and children who haven't yet been exposed to the chicken pox virus.

Take warm baths. It's important to avoid infecting the shingles rash. Taking warm (not hot) baths will soothe and clean your skin. Don't take hot baths, as they can increase itching.

Go for the heat. If your blisters have finally disappeared but you still feel pain, what can

you do? One option is Zostrix, an over-the-counter cream that contains capsaicin, the "hot" ingredient in peppers. Be forewarned: Capsaicin can make you feel worse before it makes you feel better. Many people say that with Zostrix, the pain increases for two or three days before they feel relief.

Use your mind. Using your mind to overcome your pain may be an effective strategy. Guided imagery, meditation, biofeedback, and self-hypnosis can all be used to combat pain. Many books are available to help you learn various techniques, or ask your doctor to refer you to a pain center for instruction.

TENS it. Some people have had excellent pain relief using a TENS unit, a device that delivers a weak electrical current that blocks pain. These units can often be purchased for home use for less than $100. Talk with your physician.

Try antidepressants. Research shows that low doses of antidepressants can help relieve post-shingles pain. Talk with your doctor.

Sources: Philip C. Anderson, **M.D.**, Chairman of Dermatology, University of Missouri-Columbia School of Medicine, Columbia, Missouri. **Judy Jordan, M.D.**, Spokesperson, American Academy of Dermatology; Dermatologist, San Antonio, Texas. **Mitchell Max, M.D.**, Chief, Clinical Trials Unit, Pain Research Clinic, National Institute of Dental Research, National Institutes of Health, Bethesda, Maryland.

Ease the Pain

YOU FELT FINE LAST NIGHT, BUT WHEN you woke up this morning and tried to swallow, you felt as if your throat were coated with sandpaper. When you tried to talk, you croaked. On examining your throat in the mirror, your throat tissues looked swollen and flaming red.

It's easy to pass off a sore throat as a minor inconvenience. After all, most sore throats are just that. However, a sore throat shouldn't just be ignored. It can be a symptom of strep throat, which, left untreated, can cause rheumatic heart disease or kidney damage.

CAUSES

Plenty of things can cause your throat to swell and hurt. The most common causes include:

Bacterial infections. It's the bacteria *Streptococcus* that causes strep throat, which can lead to heart and kidney damage. "Classic" strep throat symptoms include fever, body aches and pains, general malaise (feeling ill), swollen lymph nodes, whitish pus spots on the tonsils, and a severe sore throat.

Viral infections. More than 200 rhinoviruses can cause the common cold, which is usually accompanied by a raw, scratchy throat.

Allergies. Sore throats related to allergies usually are accompanied by a runny nose and watery, itchy eyes. Chronic allergies or sinus infections can cause throat irritation due to the constant flow of nasal mucus dripping down the throat (postnasal drip).

Irritants. Inhaling irritants like cigarette smoke can make your throat feel sore.

When bacteria or viruses attack your system, your body fights back. It's the body's response to the invasion, not the bacteria or viruses themselves, that cause the redness, irritation, swollen tissues, and hoarseness, among other symptoms. When the viruses or bacteria attack, blood vessels in the throat open up to carry more blood and blood-borne invader fighters like white blood cells to the area. It's the extra blood and its infection-fighting substances that cause the throat to become red, swollen, and painful.

AT-HOME TREATMENT

Most sore throats can be effectively self-treated with home remedies. Try the tips below for sore-throat relief.

Pass the salt, please. A mild saline solution (one-half teaspoon of salt to eight ounces of water) used as a gargle can help kill organisms in the throat and will soothe irritated tissues. Gargle every few hours.

Try Listerine. Another soothing gargle is Listerine. Use it straight from the bottle (don't dilute) and gargle every few hours. Be sure not to share your bottle with anyone else if you have a cold.

Go for OTC pain relievers. Aspirin and ibuprofen are both excellent for relieving pain and inflammation. Acetaminophen will relieve pain, but not inflammation. Adults can take any of these over-the-counter analgesics to relieve sore-throat pain. Anyone younger than 21 should only take acetaminophen (children who take aspirin may be at risk for Reye's syndrome, a rare but potentially fatal condition). Pregnant and nursing women should check with a physician before they take any drugs, even over-the-counter medications. Women with a history of ulcers should not take ibuprofen without a doctor's recommendation.

Take a break. Many women's lives are filled with so many demands that sometimes it's difficult to find time to take care of ourselves. A sore throat is a great reason to take a break. Head for bed and read a good book. The extra rest will help your body heal faster.

Make it hot. Drinking hot liquids is like applying moist heat packs inside your throat. Most experts believe that swallowing hot liquids bathes the throat in moist heat, which many microorganisms find noxious. Try drinking warm herbal teas or chicken soup, which is especially good for sore throats due to colds. Stay away from icy drinks. Cold liquids lower the temperature of the throat tissues, which contributes to the replication of viruses.

Try a golden oldie. Some home remedies are so good, they stick around for years. Try this tried-and-true sore throat remedy published more than 130 years ago: Mix one tablespoon of honey (any kind), one table-

spoon of vinegar (preferably apple-cider), and eight ounces of hot water. Sip slowly. Reheat if necessary. Use as often as desired.

Say "yes" to candy. How often have you heard medical authorities advise you to eat candy? This is one of those rare times. Hard candy, cough drops, and lozenges help lubricate the throat and ease pain. The sugar in the candy soothes irritated tissues and helps calm tickly coughs.

Halt the postnasal drip. Postnasal drip is one of the most common causes of sore throat. When mucus accumulates behind the nose (postnasally) and drips into the throat, it can cause irritation and soreness to the throat tissues. Sleeping with your mouth open can also cause your throat tissues to dry out and become sore. To clear out your sinus passages and stop the drip, try taking an over-the-counter decongestant that contains pseudoephedrine (read labels). Or try using a nasal saline spray (available at pharmacies) several times a day. (Stay away from nasal sprays that contain phenylephrine hydrochloride, oxymetazoline hydrochloride, or xylometazoline hydrochloride. Use of these products for longer than two or three days can cause a "rebound" effect that makes postnasal drip worse.) You can also decrease postnasal drip and dry throat problems by using a room humidifier at night.

Try analgesic sprays. They only provide temporary relief, but throat sprays such as Chloraseptic can bring some much-needed respite and can take the edge off extremely sore throats. However, the effects last only a short time. You'll have to respray several times an hour.

Get into a steam tent. "Steaming"—sitting with your face over a steaming bowl of hot water with a towel draped over your head to hold in some of the heat—is one of the oldest and most effective treatments for a sore throat. Modern scientific studies have proven that this remedy may actually shorten the time it takes for the infection to go away.

Drink, drink, drink. When you've got a sore throat, it's a good idea to keep the fluids flowing. The fluids keep the tissues bathed and lubricated and prevent the throat from drying out. They soothe and help prevent irritation and may even shorten the course of your sore throat. Stay with warm or tepid fluids rather than ice-cold ones.

Nix the cigs. Cigarette smoke is an irritant to swollen, sore throat tissues.

See your doctor. Not all cases of strep throat exhibit the "classic" strep symptoms—fever, body aches and pains, pus-filled tonsils, and swollen nodes. Also, some infections can mimic strep throat symptoms. It's important to determine whether your sore throat swelling, redness, and pain are

---

13 WAYS TO EASE YOUR SORE THROAT

- Gargle with salt water.
- Gargle with Listerine.
- Drink hot liquids.
- Sip a honey/vinegar remedy.
- Take over-the-counter analgesics.
- Get some rest.
- Suck on hard candy.
- Treat your postnasal drip.
- Try analgesic sprays.
- Steam it away in a steam tent.
- Drink plenty of fluids.
- Stop smoking.
- See the doctor.

---

caused by the *Streptococcus* organism. The only way to determine this is with a throat culture performed by your doctor. See your doctor if:

- You have the "classic" strep throat symptoms.
- Your sore throat lasts longer than two or three days.
- You have a fever (101 degrees or higher) with no other symptoms.
- You have a rash.
- You experience hoarseness or enlarged lymph nodes that last three weeks or longer.

Sources: Alvin J. Ciccone, M.D., F.A.A.F.P., Associate Professor, Department of Family Medicine, Eastern Virginia Medical School, Norfolk, Virginia. **Stephen Kriebel, M.D.,** Family Physician, Forks, Washington. **V.E. Mikkelson, M.D.,** Retired General Practitioner, Hayward, California. **Robert S. Robinson, M.D.,** General Practitioner, Metter, Georgia. **Anne Simons, M.D.,** Coauthor, *Before You Call the Doctor;* Family Practitioner, San Francisco Department of Public Health; Family Practitioner and Assistant Clinical Professor, Family and Community Medicine, University of California San Francisco Medical Center, San Francisco, California.

●STOMACH UPSET

Ways to Soothe

an Unhappy

Tummy

"I CAN'T BELIEVE I ATE THE WHOLE thing." Sometimes you wonder what possessed you to take that one last bite that seems to have sent you over the edge. When you eat too much or the wrong foods, your stomach may complain loudly with stomach upset. The trick in dealing with an upset tummy is to determine whether it's a temporary problem, such as discomfort from eating too much, or if it's something more serious.

CAUSES

Lots of factors can make your stomach go "tilt." Overeating, eating too fast, excessive drinking, or eating foods that don't agree with you, such as fatty, sugary, or "gassy" foods, can cause bloating, cramping, and gas. The flu can also make your stomach temporarily feel upset. However, abdominal distress may also be caused by problems such as gastritis, ulcer, acid reflux (heartburn), or irritable bowel syndrome, among others.

Without thinking, point to your stomach. If you're like most people, you're pointing to your navel. That's not where the stomach is located. You're pointing at your intestine. The stomach is located beneath the rib cage slightly to the left of the sternum. Because people are unclear where their stomach is, they often complain of an "upset stomach" when the problem has nothing to do with the stomach at all.

To help you determine whether or not your problem is in the stomach—and if it's temporary or something you should discuss with your doctor—answer these questions:

- How long have you had your symptoms? If your distress lasts longer than a few days, see your doctor.
- Where is the distress located? Is it located in the upper area where the stomach is located? If so, the problem may be simple stomach upset or heartburn, or something more serious like gastritis, gallstones, or an ulcer. Is it in the middle abdominal area? Distress in this area indicates the problem may be with the small and/or large intestine. It may mean you have appendicitis, colitis, gas, gastroenteritis, or irritable bowel syndrome. Is the problem in the lower abdominal area? The lower colon and pelvic organs are located in this area. Problems here may indicate "late" appendicitis, colitis, gas, irritable bowel syndrome, or problems with the bladder. In women, it may also indicate problems with the uterus, fallopian tubes, or ovaries.
- What happened before the distress began? If your temperamental tummy hit right after a big meal or party, chances are good that it's temporary discomfort from overdoing it. If your upset began right after emotional stress, the problem is probably what doctors call "psychogenic," or emotionally caused.
- Is your abdominal distress accompanied by any other symptoms?

AT-HOME TREATMENT

You can get relief from temporary stomach upset due to indigestion or the flu from these home remedies:

Nix the milk. Many people mistakenly believe that milk is soothing to the stomach. In some cases, it can be just the opposite. Many adults can't digest milk (lactose intolerance), and it causes bloating, gas, and cramping. If you think you may be lactose intolerant, lay off dairy products.

Forget that morning cup of java. Doctors aren't sure whether it's the acid or the caffeine in coffee that causes the problem, but they do know that coffee can irritate your stomach.

Don't drink. If your stomach is bothering you, the last thing you need is an alcoholic beverage. Alcohol is a known stomach irritant.

Back off on pepper. Some people love red and black pepper, but it doesn't love their stomach. Pepper is a known gastrointestinal irritant. If you love to pile on the pepper, back off for a while and see if your symptoms improve.

Stop smoking. You can put stomach upset on your list of "101 Reasons to Quit Smoking." Cigarette smoking is associated with ulcers and it irritates the stomach.

Check out your diet. Think about what you ate yesterday or the day before. Were your meals full of fried and high-fat foods? Do your stomach a favor and fill your diet with easy-to-digest foods. A high-carbohydrate, low-fat, high-fiber diet is the healthiest and the easiest on your digestive system.

Go for the fiber—slowly. A high-fiber diet can do wonders for your digestive system, but you need to introduce fibrous foods gradually into your diet, especially if you've been eating lots of highly processed foods. Slowly substitute low-fiber foods (such as fast-food apple pie) with high-fiber foods (such as raw apples).

Watch those veggies. Vegetables are an important part of any healthy diet. However, "cole" vegetables like broccoli, cabbage, and brussels sprouts are notorious gas producers.

Skip troublesome fruits. Some people find that certain fruits like apples and melons cause abdominal distress. Pay attention and see if specific fruits cause you problems. If so, avoid them.

Go for the soda. Sipping soda pop, particularly 7-Up or other decaffeinated varieties, helps settle an upset stomach.

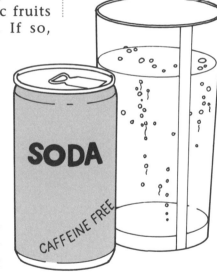

Don't pig out. One of the most common causes of stomach upset is simply eating too much at one time. It's easier on your digestion to eat smaller, more frequent meals.

Take the "music" out of beans. Beans have been known as the "musical" food, but they don't have to be. If you soak the beans, then throw out the water and replace it with fresh water before cooking them, it'll reduce the gas-producing compounds significantly.

Exercise. Every part of your body benefits from a program of regular exercise, even your digestive system. Instead of sitting down in front of the television after a meal, take a short walk.

Drink, drink, drink. Plenty of water helps move the food and waste materials through your digestive tract. Be sure to increase the water you drink as you increase your dietary fiber to prevent a painful back-up in the system. Drink at least six to eight eight-ounce glasses of water daily.

---

18 TIPS FOR TREATING YOUR ACHING TUMMY

- Drink caffeine-free soda pop.
- Don't drink milk.
- Cut out coffee.
- Don't drink alcohol.
- Cut back on pepper.
- Stop smoking.
- Eat a healthy diet.
- Gradually increase your fiber intake.
- Cut back on gassy vegetables.
- Skip problematic fruits.
- Eat smaller, more frequent meals.
- De-gas your beans.
- Exercise regularly.
- Drink plenty of water.
- Don't use laxatives.
- Try aspirin substitutes.
- Use antacids sparingly.
- Learn to relax.

Say no to laxatives. Relying on laxatives to move your bowels can create all kinds of intestinal problems. It's better to increase the fiber in your diet, or use bran or a commercial bulking agent such as Metamucil. If you chronically use laxatives to maintain your weight, see a health professional for assistance immediately.

Skip the aspirin. Many people find that aspirin upsets their stomach. Aspirin and nonsteroidal anti-inflammatory drugs like ibuprofen can actually cause ulcers. If your stomach is aspirin sensitive and you need pain relief, try acetaminophen or ask your pharmacist for enteric-coated aspirin.

Try antacids. Taking antacids can bring your stomach temporary relief. If one brand doesn't work, try switching to another. However, be aware that antacids can also cause side effects if used for more than a couple days.

Take it easy. The cause of stomach upset for a vast majority of people is stress. Stress-related gastrointestinal problems often include indigestion, irritable bowel syndrome, constipation, and diarrhea. The solution? Relax. Take it easy. Get out of your rut and have some fun. For a more permanent solution to your stress, try taking a stress management class.

Sources: Sherman Hess, B.S., R.Ph., Registered Pharmacist and Manager, Hillsdale Pharmacy, Portland, Oregon. **Anne Simons, M.D.,** Coauthor, *Before You Call the Doctor;* Family Practitioner, San Francisco Department of Public Health; Family Practitioner and Assistant Clinical Professor, Family and Community Medicine, University of California San Francisco Medical Center, San Francisco, California. **David M. Taylor, M.D.,** Author, *Gut Reactions: How to Handle Stress and Your Stomach;* Assistant Professor of Medicine, Emory University, Atlanta, Georgia; Assistant Professor of Medicine, Medical College of Georgia, Augusta, Georgia. **Douglas C. Walta, M.D.,** Gastroenterologist, Portland, Oregon.

D O YOU FEEL LIKE YOU'RE LIVING YOUR life in fast-forward? If so, it's not surprising that you've turned to this page. You, like hundreds of thousands of other American women, are probably living a triple life. Most likely, you have a career, a family, and a husband (or maybe you're single and have to do all the work by yourself). You spend all your time juggling the different demands that have been placed on you. It's no surprise that your needs have somehow been left by the wayside.

We all know stress when we see it (or feel it), but it's hard to define. One expert interviewed for this chapter described it as "the individual's perception of losing control of his or her life—a mismatch between expectations and reality."

It's not just the negative events in life that cause stress. Positive happenings such as getting married, starting a new job, being pregnant, or winning an election, while they can make us feel great, can also cause us to tense up.

Stress is not necessarily an evil, either. It arises from the fight-or-flight reaction that helped keep humans alive in the past. By priming the body to react quickly to adverse situations, stress helped people react to physical threats from the environment.

Nowadays, however, we rarely encounter life-threatening situations of this nature. The physiologic reactions of stress go into overdrive, even when we don't need them, causing wear and tear on the body and making us feel "stressed out."

SYMPTOMS

How stress will affect you depends on the chink in your body's particu-

lar armor of resistance. Everything from headaches, upset stomach, skin rashes, hair loss, racing heartbeat, back pain, and muscle aches can be stress-related. Stress can affect every organ in your system—from the skin to the gut to the heart.

AT-HOME TREATMENT

Perception of stress is highly individualized. Something that seems to turn your friend into a nervous wreck may not disturb you at all, and vice versa. Think of the audience at a horror movie, with some relishing every gory thrill, others covering their eyes and wishing they were anywhere but here, and the rest falling somewhere in between. In short, it's not external events that are stressful, but your perception of them. This gives you the power to change the things you perceive as stressful.

Just as the things that cause tension vary from person to person, so do effective techniques for stress management. Some people find meditation dull and annoying; others find it enjoyable and refreshing. Still others find a half-hour jog or a half-hour in front of the television a great way to combat stress. You will have to find out what works for you. The best advice is to develop a "smorgasbord" of stress-busters.

Here is a menu of practical techniques you can choose from to alleviate some of the stress in your life:

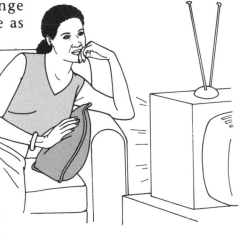

Seek out a caring network. A feeling of connection, of caring attachments to other people, will help you deal with stress more effectively. These connections can be with friends, relatives, or both. One illustration of the power of a support system is that across both sexes of all races and all age groups in all countries, married people have better health than single people. If your busy life has prevented you from forming attachments where you live, consider joining a support group through a local hospital, church, or synagogue.

Have the serenity to accept what you cannot change. The world is full of things that we as individuals don't have the power to alter. Sometimes we can't avoid heavy traffic, irrational bosses, natural disasters, or the death of a loved one. Ask yourself if you are attempting to shoulder the burden of unpleasant situations that you cannot change. Are you a perfectionist who tenses up when the littlest things get off track? Are you a "fixer" who makes it your business to get involved with the problems of everyone around you? Are you a compulsive overachiever? If you fit one of these descriptions, try separating out the things that you cannot change from those you can. Wisdom comes in the form of accepting and letting go of the problems that you are not able to solve. Then you can direct your energy and time toward things you can influ-

ence; you'll be achieving more, and you'll be feeling better about it.

Have the courage to change the things you can—especially at work. Having said that you can't control everything around you, it is also true that if you have some power over certain key areas of your life—particularly your job—you may be better able to deal with stress. In fact, studies have shown that people who have some sort of autonomy in the workplace tend to feel less stress than those who have no control over their work.

What can you do if you're in a line of work that leaves you completely out of the loop? Well, first off, know that you're not alone. We all feel overburdened by the pressures of our jobs at times, and often the worst part about it is that it seems we have no authority to change the situation. One study of stress in the workplace recommended several ways that employers can reduce on-the-job stress. Giving employees more control over their own jobs can ease the pressure. So can improving communications between management and employees and allowing flexible scheduling of work hours. Instituting progressive policies that support the worker on the job and at home can make a difference also.

If you're in a position to make any of the above changes in your workplace or department, by all means, do so. If your position is too low on the totem pole for you to make any major changes, perhaps you could make some suggestions to your supervisor on how to change little things that you know would help.

Develop a sense of why your life holds meaning. Having a clear understanding of what you can and do accomplish in your life can help you manage your stress. Experts say that you can see the glass as half-full or jog until your heart gives out, but if you're not in touch with your life's purpose, you may still have big problems coping with stress. So, how exactly does one develop a sense of purpose? A good place to start is to sit down and write a list of all the reasons that your world needs you. This may consist of the obvious, such as your children needing you to care for them. It may also range to the more obscure, such as people with HIV needing you to help garner support for better health insurance. Whatever it is, get in touch with the ways you are needed and the ways you plan to make a difference. Hold onto these goals and think of them often, especially when you begin to feel overwhelmed.

Run away. Three 20-minute sessions of aerobic exercise a week can help keep your mind and body healthy and energetic. This kind of exercise can soften your body's response to stressful situations, and it can put you in a good mood. So take a break to run, walk, swim, bike,

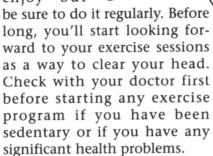

row, or aerobicize. And remember, you don't have to be a prime jock to reap exercise's benefits. Just do something to increase your heart rate, something you can also enjoy—but be sure to do it regularly. Before long, you'll start looking forward to your exercise sessions as a way to clear your head. Check with your doctor first before starting any exercise program if you have been sedentary or if you have any significant health problems.

Don't take a coffee break. Don't take a cigarette break, either. Instead, take breaks to enjoy a few calming deep breaths. Caffeine and nicotine can add to stress and can make you feel nervous even when you're not stressed out.

Turn the devil on your shoulder into an angel. The things we say to ourselves can either heighten or lessen the tension of a situation. If we focus on life's challenges in a negative way, the challenges will be more stressful; if we look at things in a positive, confident way, life will seem less stressful. It can be likened to a miniature devil sitting on one shoulder, giving us negative messages, versus a little angel on the other shoulder, telling us that everything is going to be OK.

Pessimistic or self-critical thoughts might be habitual for you. If they are, don't beat yourself up if you're unable to change the habit in a day. Instead, try to slowly modify the messages you give yourself, a little at a time. As Mark Twain once said, "Habit is habit, and not to be flung out of the window by any man, but coaxed downstairs a step at a time."

Laugh it off. Humor helps us keep things in perspective and avoid the stress we feel when we blow problems out of proportion. In a 12-year study of 1,200 people who claimed to be resistant to stress, researchers found that one of the things these people had in common was a good sense of humor or exposure to others with a good sense of humor. Laughing also initiates physiologic changes that can put you in a better mood. So, just for a moment, put your troubles aside and laugh your stress away.

Make your mental health a top priority. In the same study of stress-resistant people, all said that they set aside 10 or 15 minutes each day to do something relaxing. For example, some participants used relaxation techniques on a regular schedule or when they were feeling stressed out. One such relaxation exercise focuses on the muscles: Starting at your toes and working up to your face, tighten the various groups of muscles in your body as you inhale and then relax them as you exhale.

Visualization is another technique. Close your eyes for five minutes and breathe slowly and deeply as you imagine you are in a calm, relaxing place, such as an open meadow or perhaps your favorite comfortable chair. Imagine what all of your senses would experience there—what you'd smell, taste, feel, see, and hear. Another option is to look for the things in your life you find relaxing and rely on them—chatting with a special friend, painting or drawing, listening to jazz music, or pursuing some hobby such as photography or pottery.

Clean up your finances. Financial problems are a common source of stress. For example, many people get in over their heads using credit cards. In fact, credit-card debt may be one of the leading causes of divorce. Try to avoid the temptation to overspend with plastic; it will help you ward off lots of problems and keep your stress level from skyrocketing. You can also take advantage of credit-counseling services that can help you get your debts under control.

Reprioritize. In our society, we often feel pressured to attain wealth, power, and success, along with a great personal and family life. This striving to have it all may be one of our most stressful dilemmas. If you feel you might be trying to do too much, review your current goals and consider eliminating a few of the less important ones.

Ask for help. When things get out of control, seek good advice from the best sources you can. Often, self-help will go far, but when you have major problems with your job, marriage, spiritual beliefs, friends, or children, don't be afraid to ask the people around you to lend a helping hand. You may also wish to seek counseling. A little outside help can do a lot to get things under control, and that's what stress management is all about.

Use your breath to help you control stress. When a stressful situation arises, try taking steady, slow abdominal breaths to cool off so that you can think more clearly. The following breathing technique is based on five-second intervals: Inhale deeply and slowly for five seconds. Then hold your breath for five seconds, and finally exhale slowly for five seconds. Wait five seconds without taking a breath, and then repeat the exercise. Don't repeat it a third time; you could hyperventilate.

Don't turn allies into scapegoats. If you're having trouble at work, taking it out on your family and friends won't solve anything. Focus your energy on understanding the problem areas in your life and working to improve them.

AT THE DOCTOR'S

If you feel that your life is truly out of control, if you feel hopeless, depressed, or suicidal, it's a good idea to seek help from a psychologist, pastoral counselor, or psychiatrist. These professionals will be able

---

14 WAYS TO GET A HANDLE ON STRESS

- **Form a caring network of friends and family.**
- **Learn to accept the things you cannot change.**
- **Work to gain more autonomy at your place of employment.**
- **Develop a sense of purpose.**
- **Start a program of regular aerobic exercise.**
- **Avoid coffee and nicotine.**
- **Develop more positive dialogues with yourself.**
- **Hold on to your sense of humor.**
- **Take time for relaxation.**
- **Get your finances under control.**
- **Focus on what's important to you.**
- **Ask for help.**
- **Learn the art of deep breathing.**
- **Don't take your frustrations out on people who don't deserve it.**

---

to give you the counseling you need to get your life back on track again. Your family doctor may be able to give you a referral to a competent professional in your area. Some of the cost of therapy may be covered by your medical insurance (check your policy to be sure). If you're on a tight budget or are uninsured, there are sliding-scale therapists who may be able to help.

Sources: **Robert Eliot, M.D.**, Director, Institute of Stress Medicine, Jackson Hole, Wyoming; Professor of Cardiology, University of Nebraska Medical Center, Omaha, Nebraska. **Raymond Flannery, Jr., Ph.D., F.A.P.M.**, Author, *Becoming Stress Resistant*; Assistant Professor of Psychology, Department of Psychiatry, Harvard Medical School at the Cambridge Hospital, Cambridge, Massachusetts. **Paul Rosch, M.D.**, President, The American Institute of Stress, Yonkers, New York.

● STY

Strategies to

Ease the Eye

Pain

YOU JUST RECEIVED A PROMOTION AND you're planning on having your photograph taken today for the corporate newsletter. But what's this? There's a red, unsightly bump on your eyelid. You've got a sty.

CAUSES

A sty, or what doctors call a "hordeolum," occurs on the inner or outer surface of the eyelid when an oil or sebaceous gland at the root of an eyelash becomes blocked due to an infection. The infecting agent is commonly the *Staphylococcus* bacteria. The gland swells, turns red, and can hurt like the devil. After a few days, the swollen boil forms a "head"—a pimple-like white point. (A sty on the inside of the lid shows only as a protrusion on the lid.) The head eventually bursts, the pus and cell debris from inside discharges, and the pain subsides. At that point, the affected eyelash also falls out. Unfortunately, sometimes more sties develop when the bacteria from the original sty spread and infect other eyelash follicles.

When you get a sty, it feels like you've got something in your eye. The eye may tear up and feel tender. It may also become very sensitive to the touch and to light.

9 WAYS TO TREAT YOUR STY

- Use warm compresses.
- Don't squeeze, poke, or prick your sty.
- Gently pull out the affected eyelash to drain the pus.
- Apply a thin line of antibacterial ointment.
- When you have a sty, don't use eye makeup.
- Wash your eyelashes with a mild cleanser.
- Remove your eye makeup daily.
- Never share your makeup or applicators with others.
- Call the doctor if symptoms persist.

AT-HOME TREATMENT

Most sties can be effectively treated at home. In fact, if you're prompt and consistent in your use of home treatments, you can speed healing and keep a sty from coming back to pester you again.

Bring on the heat. Warm compresses applied to the sty stimulate circulation to the area, bringing more white blood cells—an important part of the body's immune system—to clean up the problem. Wring out a clean washcloth in warm water. Make the water as hot as you can tolerate, but not so hot that you burn your skin. Place the compress on the eyelid for five minutes at a time. Rewet the washcloth as needed to keep it hot.

Hands off. Don't squeeze, poke, or prick the sty. If you prematurely burst the pus sack, you risk spreading the infection deeper into the eyelid tissue. Let the sty drain on its own.

Try the eyelash pull. If you absolutely can't stand to leave the sty alone and the pain is too much to bear, you can try to gently pull out the affected eyelash. This releases the pus. Immediately wash the eyelid and surrounding area carefully with warm soap and water to remove all the pus.

Use antibacterial ointment. After the pus drains and you've cleaned the area with soap and water, apply a thin layer of antibacterial ointment containing bacitracin like Neosporin to the eyelid.

Nix the makeup. You can do it. You don't need eye makeup when you have a sty. If you use your eye makeup when you have this highly contagious infection, you risk contaminating your makeup and contracting more sties.

Keep it clean. To prevent sties from returning, always practice good hygiene. Wash the roots of your lashes each day with diluted baby shampoo or mild soap on a cotton ball or washcloth. Better yet, use Cetaphil (available over the counter at pharmacies), which won't sting or dry out the skin on your eyelids too much.

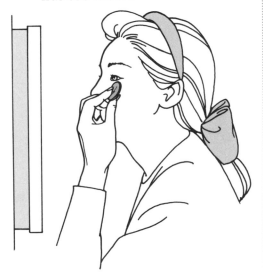

Take off your P.M. makeup. One of the major causes of blockage and subsequent infection of the sebaceous glands of the eyelashes is eye makeup. Once your sty is healed and you begin wearing eye makeup again, be sure you thoroughly remove it every day. If you're wearing eye makeup on Friday night, don't wait until Saturday morning to remove it. Take it off before you go to bed. Use a cold cream or other cleansing agent to make it easier to remove. Wash your lids again before reapplying makeup.

Be stingy. "Oh, let me just borrow a little mascara." Don't do it! Sharing your eye makeup or applicators is one of the fastest ways to spread infection.

Call the doctor. Most sties can be effectively treated at home. However, you need to see a doctor if:

• A sty or any eye swelling develops in a child for more than 24 hours. In children, problems can progress more quickly. Don't risk later vision difficulties by delaying medical attention.

• You've been applying warm compresses and you fail to see any improvement within 48 to 72 hours.

• You have recurring sties or any bump on the lid that remains for weeks. You may have a chalazion, a different type of blocked gland. Warm compresses are also the first line of defense for a chalazion, but if it doesn't clear up or is unsightly, ask your doctor to drain it.

Sources: **Barbara J. Arnold, M.D.,** Associate Clinical Professor, University of California Davis, Davis, California. **Monica L. Monica, M.D., Ph.D.,** Ophthalmologist, New Orleans, Louisiana. **Anne Simons, M.D.,** Coauthor, *Before You Call the Doctor;* Family Practitioner, San Francisco Department of Public Health; Family Practitioner and Assistant Clinical Professor, Family and Community Medicine, University of California San Francisco Medical Center, San Francisco, California.

TARTAR AND PLAQUE

Steps to a

Brighter Smile

WHEN YOU DON'T BRUSH YOUR TEETH, a sticky white film forms on them. That's called plaque. When you go to the dentist to have your teeth professionally cleaned, the hygienist has to chip and scrape off a hard, white substance. That's the calcified form of plaque and debris, called tartar. Together, these two dental villains are responsible for gum (periodontal) disease—the major cause of tooth loss for adults over age 35—and for dental decay, including serious problems like root damage.

CAUSES

Plaque, the soft, sticky stuff, is actually an organized mass of oral bacteria. These bacteria cause gum disease and tooth decay. Nearly invisible, this pervasive substance accumulates on teeth, fillings, crowns, and dentures. It's ever-present, beginning within the first ten hours of a baby's life and continuing until the end of life.

Plaque's cousin, tartar, or calculus, is a white, chalky substance that's a form of mineralized plaque and bacterial debris. Tartar enables plaque to stick better to the teeth, but it's less harmful than plaque and is largely a cosmetic problem.

Plaque is the big gun in dental troubles. As plaque sticks around and gets older, it changes chemically and becomes even more dangerous. Bacteria in the plaque feed off fermentable carbohydrates, such as sugars in fruit and milk and starches such as breads, pastas, and crackers. In the process, they produce an acid that literally eats away tooth enamel, causing cavities. Other bacteria in the plaque can attack the gums and cause redness, inflammation, and bleeding—the first stages of gingivitis. If left untreated, gingivitis, the earliest stage of gum disease, can advance to the point where the bone that anchors the teeth is destroyed.

Part of the difficulty with plaque and tartar is that they form both above and below the gum line. While you can often remove much of the plaque from above the gum line with a program of good oral hygiene, it takes a professional hygienist or dentist to remove plaque below the gum line. Only professional cleaning can remove hardened tartar. Regular professional dental care and cleaning—as often as your dentist recommends—will make your own home care more effective. Regular dental checkups with gentle periodontal probing can also help stop gum disease before it progresses too far.

AT-HOME TREATMENT

There's plenty you can do to control tartar and plaque and brighten your smile. Try these strategies:

Check your brushing technique. If you brush incorrectly ten times a day, you won't get the benefits of one or two correct brushings. Dental experts say that regular brushing is important, but how you brush is even more important than how often. Use this technique:

1) Go for the gum line. When we brush, most of us are worried about getting corn flakes or spinach out from between our teeth and we completely miss the gum line. But this is where most of the plaque and tartar destruction goes on. Hold the brush at a 45-degree angle

against the gum line. When you're cleaning the upper teeth, point the brush upward, toward your nose; for the lower teeth, point the brush downward, toward your chin.

2) Use the right stroke. Use a short, back-and-forth motion to clean the outer surfaces of the teeth. Focus only on one or two teeth at a time. Don't use a "traveling" stroke that covers five or six teeth at once. Also, don't use too much force. Most people act as if they are scrubbing the bathtub instead of their teeth and use too much pressure, which can result in gum injuries, enamel abrasions, and sensitive teeth.

Use the same stroke on the inner surfaces of the teeth, except the front ones. Keep the brush angled at a 45-degree angle toward the gum line.

3) Don't miss the chewing surfaces. Gently scrub the chewing surfaces of your back teeth with the same back-and-forth motion, holding the brush flat.

4) Go up and down for front teeth. Many people forget to brush the back sides of their front teeth. Tilt the brush vertically and use the front part of the brush in short up-and-down strokes to clean the inside surfaces of the teeth.

5) Brush your tongue. The tongue can harbor disease-causing bacteria. Give it a gentle brushing.

Be picky about your brush. Toothbrushes come in soft, medium, and hard bristles.

Hard bristles can actually wear away the enamel that protects your teeth and can cause grooves in the teeth where bacteria can multiply. Your tooth enamel may be hard, but it isn't that hard. You don't need the Brillo-Pad approach to teeth cleaning. Using brush bristles that are too hard or brushing with too much force can also damage your gums, causing them to recede or pull away from the teeth.

Choose a soft nylon brush with rounded-end, polished bristles. Buy a brush that's small enough to reach all the teeth, even the ones way back in your mouth. Some adults have better results using a child-size toothbrush. And replace your toothbrush often, at least every three months. Don't wait until the bristles become worn or frayed. Some brushes now come with a col-

---

14 WAYS TO TREAT YOUR TEETH RIGHT

- Use correct brushing technique.
- Choose a soft, round-bristle brush.
- Try an electric toothbrush.
- Use fluoride-containing products.
- Choose tartar-control toothpaste.
- Floss regularly.
- Use waxed or unwaxed floss.
- Try Interproximal cleaners or oral irrigators.
- Stick to an oral hygiene routine.
- Use disclosing tablets or solutions.
- Keep the saliva flowing.
- Don't rely on plaque rinses.
- Eat a tooth-healthy diet.
- See your dentist.

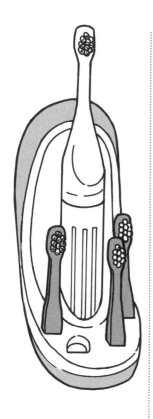

ored strip that changes over time and tells you when to replace them.

Try electric. You certainly don't have to go high-tech to get a good toothbrushing. Your plain, old-fashioned tooth-brush will do just fine. But if you have dexterity problems or if you just like electric gadgets, you might find that one of the new electric toothbrushes can help you do a better job of keeping your teeth clean.

Fluoride it. The American Dental Association (ADA) puts its seal of approval on dental products like toothpastes that have met rigorous testing guidelines and actually do what they advertise. Look for a fluoride toothpaste with the ADA's seal of approval. Fluoride "remineralizes" and strengthens teeth by binding with the minerals in saliva, which helps prevent cavities. Many adults mistakenly believe that as they get older their teeth stop getting cavities, so the type of toothpaste they choose isn't important. Nothing could be further from the truth. As you age, your gums recede, exposing tooth roots, which lack the protective enamel coating and are more prone to a type of dental decay called root caries.

Get that tartar control. If your dental hygienist looks exhaust-ed after your cleaning, your teeth probably accumulate a lot of tartar. Give your dental hygienist, and your teeth, a break by using a tartar-control

toothpaste. These products contain chemicals, such as pyrophosphate, that interfere with deposits of calcium salt, an element in tartar. If you use a tartar-control toothpaste on a regular basis, you can reduce your tartar deposits by more than one-third.

Floss, floss, floss. Your dentist or hygienist probably asks, "Do you floss your teeth every day?" If you're like most of us, you can't say yes and be com-pletely honest. Flossing isn't just to remove celery strings or popcorn kernels that are stuck in your teeth. It's the only way to clean plaque and food debris from between the teeth and under the gums.

Flossing correctly is easy once you get the hang of it. Try this technique:

1) Use plenty of floss. Wrap most of 18 to 24 inches of floss around the middle or index finger of one hand.

2) Wrap the remaining floss around the same finger on the opposite hand. Use this finger as the take-up spool for the used floss. Don't be stingy. Floss is inexpensive and if you don't use enough floss, or if you don't use a clean piece of floss on each tooth, you're sim-ply re-introducing bacteria to another tooth.

3) Be taut. Hold the floss tightly with your thumbs and forefingers, leaving about an inch of floss between your two hands. Keep the floss taut.

4) Use a sawing action. Pull the floss between the teeth,

using a gentle "sawing" action. Don't snap the floss into your tender gums.

5) "C" the gums. At the gum line, gently curve the floss into a "C" shape, fitting it snugly around the tooth and slide it into the space between the gum and the tooth. Be careful not to injure your gums.

6) Side scrape. Bring the floss out from under the gum and scrape the side of the tooth to remove the plaque. After you pull out the floss, use a clean section of floss to clean the tooth on the other side.

7) Last, but not least, don't forget to clean the back side of the last tooth on each side.

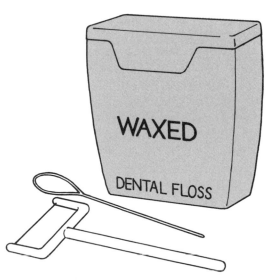

Wax it or unwax it. Dental floss comes waxed, unwaxed, and even in different flavors. The kind of dental floss you use isn't important; however, the waxed variety may be a little easier to get between your teeth. The flavored brands simply taste better. If you have trouble handling the floss or if you have a lot of complicated bridgework that makes flossing a real challenge, try using floss threaders or floss holders, which are available over the counter at pharmacies. Your dentist can help you with instructions on how to use these devices properly.

Try other tooth toys. There's no substitute for flossing, but you might enhance your dental hygiene program with items like interproximal cleaners (Stim-u-Dents), which look like tiny bottle brushes. Oral irrigators are also good for getting out large pieces of debris from tricky spaces. However, don't use interproximal cleaners or oral irrigators until after you've flossed or you risk pushing the debris or bacteria deeper into crevices or pockets.

Be routine. It's great to be creative about some things, but flossing and brushing are best done in a routine manner, the same way every time. Start at the same spot in your mouth each time and work your way around. Using a routine will help keep you from missing spots as you brush and floss.

Check yourself. Just how well do you clean your teeth? If you really want to know, you can buy "disclosing" tablets or solution at the drug store. These products stick to plaque, revealing the presence of plaque after cleaning. The results can be startling. They can help you learn where you need to clean more thoroughly.

Stay wet. Saliva keeps the mouth clean and helps fight bacteria. Sometimes, however, the mouth doesn't have enough saliva to do its job. Many drugs, such as antidepressants, antihistamines, and high blood pressure medications, can cause dry mouth. Diseases like Sjögren's syndrome can also slow the flow of saliva and cause dry mouth and dry eyes. Even radiation therapy for cancer of the head and neck can damage the salivary glands.

If you suffer from dry mouth, try chewing sugarless gum, sucking on hard candy, or using artificial saliva (available over the counter at pharmacies). Or keep your mouth moist by taking frequent sips of water, rinsing with a mixture of one teaspoon of glycerine in a glass of water, or coating your lips, mouth, and tongue with mineral oil (spit it out), especially before bed at night, when dry mouth tends to worsen.

Don't rely on plaque rinses. Only two products have received the ADA's seal of approval for fighting bacteria: prescription Peridex and Listerine, an over-the-counter mouthwash. Even these products don't replace regular flossing and brushing.

Consume a tooth-healthy diet. The foods and beverages you consume can have a big impact on your dental health. Follow these guidelines from dental experts:
• Limit how often you eat sugar-containing foods. Eat your dessert with your meals. Don't suck on sugary hard candies all day.
• Don't sip sweet drinks all day.
• Chew sugarless gum. Gum stimulates the flow of saliva, which cleanses your mouth and protects your teeth.
• Munch on tooth-healthy foods. Certain foods can actually help prevent cavities. Snack on raw vegetables, crunchy fruits, plain peanuts, and cheeses. Drink plain club soda, or unsweetened or artificially sweetened tea, coffee, or soda instead of sweetened drinks.

Call the dentist. You need to see your dentist if:
• You have persistent bad breath.
• You have pus between the teeth and gums.
• Your "bite" (how your teeth fit together) feels off.
• You have loose or separating teeth.
• Your gums consistently bleed.
• The gums at the gumline look "rolled" rather than flat.
• Your partial dentures fit differently than they used to.

Sources: Erwin Barrington, D.D.S., Professor of Periodontics, University of Illinois in Chicago, Chicago, Illinois. **Sabastian G. Ciancio, D.D.S.,** Past President, American Academy of Periodontology; Professor and Chairman, Department of Periodontology, Clinical Professor of Pharmacology, Director, Center for Clinical Dental Studies, School of Dental Medicine, State University of New York at Buffalo, Buffalo, New York. **Christine Dumas, D.D.S.,** Consumer Advisor/Spokesperson, American Dental Association; Assistant Professor of Clinical Dentistry, University of Southern California, Los Angeles, California. **Michael G. Newman, D.D.S.,** President of the American Academy of Periodontology; Adjunct Professor of Periodontology, University of California at Los Angeles School of Dentistry, Los Angeles, California.

Temporomandibular Joint Syndrome

Ways to Ease

Your Pain

Sometimes it causes only a bothersome "clicking" or "popping" sensation in the jaw. Other times, it causes wracking pain in the head, neck, and shoulders. Most of the time, it's a mysterious condition that goes undiagnosed, misdiagnosed, or untreated. We're talking about temporomandibular joint syndrome, or TMJ syndrome for short, which causes a number of symptoms due to the misalignment of the temporomandibular joint, or lower jaw joint, just below the ear. This is the joint that allows your mouth to open, close, and move sideways.

TMJ is a controversial disorder. Some medical authorities doubt that it even exists, adding that many dentists, chiropractors, and physicians are profiting handsomely from this "non-disorder." Others suggest TMJ is a psychogenic problem that originates in the mind. However, most experts, and certainly the people who suffer from it, know it's a real problem with physiologic origins.

Symptoms

If you suffer from headaches, bothersome clicking and popping in the jaw, dizziness, ear aches, ear ringing, muscular tension, or pain in the face, neck, shoulders, limbs, or back, you may have TMJ syndrome. The American Dental Association estimates that as many as ten million Americans suffer from TMJ dysfunction. As a woman, you're nine times more likely to seek treatment for this problem than a man. No one knows if this means women have more TMJ problems or if they just recognize the problem and seek professional help more often.

Causes

Two of the reasons that TMJ disorder is controversial are that its symptoms often mimic other health conditions, and it has no single cause. The underlying problem is a misalignment of the temporomandibular joint, but it can also involve the nerves and muscles of the head, neck, and shoulders.

Understanding the physiology of the jaw may shed some light on why this syndrome is so widespread. The temporomandibular joint is attached by a complex system of five pairs of muscles and ligaments that allow you to open and close your mouth and enable you to move your jaw up, down, and side-to-side. Any problem that prevents this system of joints, muscles, ligaments, and nerves from working together can cause pain and the other symptoms associated with temporomandibular joint syndrome.

Some of the more common causes of TMJ misalignment include the following:

- Incorrect "bite." When the teeth of the upper and lower jaw don't fit together properly, the bite is off and it causes undue pressure and stress on certain teeth and on the temporomandibular joint.
- Tooth grinding. Habitual grinding of teeth (bruxism) or clenching the jaw can create tremendous pressures on the jaw.
- Postural problems. The head and neck are delicately aligned with the spine. Postural problems can throw off this balance and cause undue stresses.
- Bad habits. Unconscious habits like cradling the phone between the ear and shoulder can cause TMJ problems.

351

- Injuries. Whiplash or a blow to the chin or jaw can misalign the joint.
- Diseases. Health problems like arthritis can contribute to TMJ symptoms.

In addition, stress plays a role in TMJ disorder. Many people experience their first TMJ symptoms during stressful times.

Is It TMJ Syndrome?

TMJ can be very tough to diagnose. Many people suffer needlessly for years because of misdiagnosis. If you answer yes to one or more of these questions, you may have TMJ syndrome.

- Do you have frequent headaches, especially in the morning?
- Do you clench or grind your teeth?
- Have you noticed any teeth, especially the eye teeth, becoming worn down?
- Do your jaw muscles feel tender?
- Does your jaw make popping, grating, or clicking sounds?
- Do you have difficulty opening or closing your mouth?
- Do you have pain in your face, teeth, neck, or shoulders?
- Is it painful to chew, yawn, or open your mouth widely?
- Do you feel pain in or around your ears?
- Do your ears feel stuffy or itchy?
- Do you have ear noises (ringing, roaring, hissing, or buzzing)?
- Do you feel dizzy?

At-Home Treatment

Pain and discomfort from mild misalignments of the TMJ can often be handled with home treatment. Here are some ways to ease your distress:

Massage 'em. When muscles go into spasm, the blood supply is temporarily cut off. The muscles complain loudly by sending out pain messages via the nerves. To ease the pain, you have to relax the spasm. Try massaging the jaw joint just in front of your ears and your neck and shoulders.

Try heat. Heat brings blood to the area and helps relax tight muscles. Place a heating pad or hot-water bottle on painful areas. Keep the heat low enough so that you don't cause skin burns.

Ice it. Applying ice packs to your sore jaw, neck, and shoulders is also an excellent pain reliever.

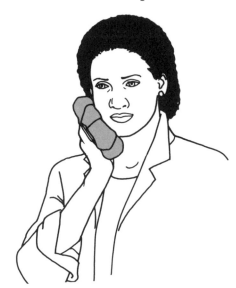

Take aspirin, ibuprofen, or acetaminophen. These over-the-counter pain relievers can ease pain and reduce inflammation.

Change your habits. Start to become aware of habits that may contribute to your TMJ problems. Do you cradle the phone between your cheek and shoulder? Do you habitually clench or grind your teeth? Consciously work to replace these habits with less stressful ones.

Learn to relax. Stress can create a cycle of muscle tension and pain that is self-perpetuating. When you feel stressed, you tense the muscles of the jaw, neck, and shoulders, which cuts the blood supply and causes the muscles to spasm. This, in turn, causes pain, which creates even more tension and spasm. The tension-pain-tension cycle must be broken to achieve relief from TMJ symptoms. Learning and using stress management techniques can help.

You can also use techniques like progressive relaxation. Sit in a quiet place where you won't be disturbed. Take a few deep breaths. Then, starting with your head and neck, tighten the muscles and then relax them. Work down your entire body, alternating tensing and relaxing each muscle group until you're completely relaxed.

Taking a "mental vacation" with visualization can help to relax you, too. In a quiet place, close your eyes and take a few deep breaths. Now imagine you're in a restful, beautiful place. Perhaps you're in a lush meadow, beside a lake, or on the beach. Really engage all your senses. Imagine what the breezes smell like and how they feel on your skin. Feel yourself relaxing in this special place. There is no place you have to go, nothing you have to do. Just relax. After several minutes

---

7 TIPS FOR TREATING YOUR TMJ

- **Massage your tense muscles.**
- **Try heat.**
- **Apply ice.**
- **Take over-the-counter pain relievers.**
- **Correct your bad habits.**
- **Learn to relax.**
- **Get professional help when needed.**

---

of enjoying your mental vacation, take another couple of deep breaths, and slowly open your eyes.

There are a number of other effective stress management techniques you can learn, including meditation, yoga, and deep breathing. Check with the community college in your area for classes or ask your dentist for a referral. If you can't get your stress under control with stress management techniques on your own, a mental health professional can often help.

Hello doctor? Conservative treatments like ice, heat, massage, and pain relievers work in mild cases of TMJ syndrome. However, for permanent relief, many people need help from TMJ specialists. Sometimes successful treatment for severe TMJ disorders requires a team approach, including help from a dentist who specializes in TMJ; an orthopedist; a neurologist; an ear, nose, and throat specialist; and a physical therapist.

Sources: **Gregg R. Morris**, D.C., Chiropractor, Beaverton, Oregon. **Ken Waddell**, D.M.D., Dentist, Tigard, Oregon. **Ronald Wismer**, **D.M.D.**, Past President, Washington County Dental Society; Dentist, Beaverton, Oregon.

•Toothache

Easing the

Pain

I T'S IMPOSSIBLE TO IGNORE. IT STARTS OUT as a tiny twinge. Then it escalates to a dull ache that comes and goes. Before long, it's a sharp pain that won't stop. Head for the nearest dentist; you've got a toothache.

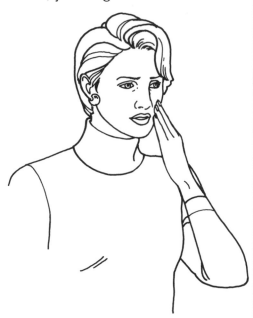

Any time your body gives you a pain message, it's trying to tell you that something is wrong. This goes for your teeth, too. Pain from your mouth may be referred to other areas such as your ears, neck, or even shoulders. Pain in or around your mouth or jaw may not even be related to your teeth, but may indicate some other health problem. For example, coronary problems can appear as pain in the jaw. Tooth pain may not be related to dental disease, but to a misalignment of the jaw joint (temporomandibular joint syndrome). This misalignment can cause pain in the teeth, neck, face, head, and shoulders. Never ignore pain in the head or neck. Even minor dental discomfort should be checked out by a dentist to ensure that it's nothing serious.

CAUSES

Tooth pain isn't something you can ignore for long. Sometimes it's just a temporary minor pain caused by sensitive teeth. You eat or drink something sugary, hot, or cold, and you feel a momentary "ouch." This kind of pain may be caused by trauma to the teeth such as biting down too hard on something, or from recent dental work. Discomfort of this type usually goes away within a few days to a few weeks. Your sensitivity may also be caused by exposed dentin, the sensitive material beneath the gums. If your discomfort is limited to the upper teeth and several teeth are affected at once ("generalized sensitivity"), chances are your tooth pain is related to sinus problems.

A sharp pain when you bite down may indicate a cavity, a loose filling, a cracked tooth, or damage to the pulp, the inner core of the tooth that contains the nerves and blood vessels. If pain lasts for more than half an hour after you eat hot or cold foods, it may also indicate pulp damage from a deep cavity or from a blow to the tooth. Pain that is severe and constant, with swelling and sensitivity, is a sure sign that something is wrong with your tooth and that you need to see a dentist immediately. Any time dental pain wakes you up during the night, it's an indication that something serious is wrong, such as an abscess in which the pulp of the tooth has died and become infected. Left untreated, these infections can spread to the gum and even into the bone itself.

Don't think a problem has gone away just because the pain has disappeared. For example, if the pulp is damaged it can cause the tooth's nerves—and the tooth's ability to send pain signals—to die. So the pain disappears, but not the problem. The tooth can then become infected, or abscessed.

AT-HOME TREATMENT

Much tooth pain can be prevented by a combination of regular home dental hygiene (flossing and brushing), professional care, and eating a diet low in sugar. If the area where you live doesn't have fluoridated water, use fluoride rinses and toothpastes, and ask your dentist about having fluoride professionally applied to your teeth to minimize tooth decay.

When you do have dental pain, see your dentist. No dental pain should be handled with home remedies alone. Some people try to self-treat tooth pain because they're afraid that a toothache means they'll lose a tooth. With the advances in dental technology, a bad toothache doesn't mean the tooth will have to be extracted. Even when a tooth's pulp has been damaged severely enough to cause its roots to die, the tooth can often be saved with root canal therapy. This involves making a small opening in the tooth, removing the diseased pulp, and then filling the canal with an inert material. Sometimes tiny metal rods are inserted into the tooth's root canals to help strengthen and anchor it. The tooth is then capped with a crown and will likely last for many years.

If your toothache occurs in the middle of the night or at some other time when you can't get to your dentist immediately, here are some home remedies to help:

Take OTC pain relievers. Over-the-counter pain relievers like aspirin, acetaminophen, and ibuprofen can go a long way toward relieving mild tooth pain. If you have inflammation as well as pain, your best choice is ibuprofen, for its anti-inflammatory action. Pregnant women and those with a history of ulcers should not take aspirin or ibuprofen without a doctor's recommendation.

Clove it. An ancient and effective home remedy for toothaches, oil of cloves applied to an aching tooth, can immediately numb the pain. Oil of cloves is available over the counter in pharmacies and health-food stores. Follow the directions on the package and apply the oil directly to the tooth, not on the gums (it can burn tender gum tissue).

Compress the swelling. Many times toothaches, especially those caused by abscesses, are accompanied by swelling. You can decrease the swelling by placing a cold compress on the outside of your cheek near the painful tooth.

Cool it. Ice is excellent for calming pain-excited nerve endings. For a painful tooth, try holding an ice cube or cold water in your mouth. If it aggravates the pain, discontinue it.

Elevate it. When the pain in your teeth is pounding, keep your head upright to decrease the pressure in the area.

Nix the aspirin. Placing an aspirin directly on an achy tooth is an

12 WAYS TO STOP THE TOOTH PAIN

- Take over-the-counter pain relievers.
- Apply oil of cloves to the tooth.
- Decrease swelling with cold compresses.
- Stop the pain with ice or cold water.
- Keep your head elevated.
- Don't put aspirin directly on your teeth or gums.
- Rinse with warm water or warm salt water.
- Floss to remove food debris.
- Avoid hot, cold, or sweet foods or beverages.
- Cover the painful tooth.
- Use an over-the-counter anesthetic.
- Call for an emergency appointment.

old home remedy that can make your situation worse. Aspirin doesn't work topically and can burn your gums or cheek tissue. If you want an aspirin remedy, swallow it with a glass of water.

Try warm water. You can never rinse away a dental problem, but rinsing with warm water can help remove any food particles that may be trapped and causing problems. To soothe inflamed tissues, try rinsing with a mild saline solution (one teaspoon of salt in eight ounces of water).

Floss it. When food particles become lodged in the gums or between teeth, they sometimes cause pain that mimics pulp problems. Remove trapped food particles with flossing. Or use the rubber tip on the end of your toothbrush. If you don't have anything else, you can use a toothpick (very carefully).

Don't aggravate it. When your teeth are feeling sensitive and painful, the last thing you need to do is irritate them. Stay away from hot, cold, or excessively sweet foods or beverages.

Keep the air out. Sometimes when a tooth aches, it's sensitive to air. Cover it with gauze or even sugarless gum until you can get to your dentist.

Use OTC anesthetic. You can temporarily numb your tooth pain with over-the-counter topical anesthetic products like Anbesol. Remember that these numbing agents don't solve the problem, they just temporarily mask the pain.

Call the dentist—quickly! You need an emergency dental appointment if your tooth:
- Causes you constant pain.
- Wakes you up at night.
- Is accompanied by facial or gum swelling or any fever.

Sources: Roland C. Duell, D.D.S., M.S., Professor of Endodontics, Department of Oral Health Practice, University of Kentucky College of Dentistry, Lexington, Kentucky. Alan H. Gluskin, D.D.S., Associate Professor and Chair, Department of Endodontics, University of the Pacific School of Dentistry, San Francisco, California. Joseph Tenca, D.D.S., M.A., Past President, American Association of Endodontists; Professor and Chairman, Department of Endodontics, Tufts University School of Dental Medicine, Boston, Massachusetts.

AT FIRST, YOU THOUGHT IT WAS HEART-burn or indigestion from something you ate. It started as a burning sensation in the middle abdominal area near your navel. Even though you'd eaten only an hour or so ago, the sensation felt like hunger pangs. So you ate a little something and the discomfort went away. Was it just heartburn, indigestion, or hunger? Nope. You've got the classic signs of an ulcer.

The word "ulcer" means "open wound." When you have an open wound in your digestive system—esophagus, stomach, or first section of the small intestine (duodenum)—you have a peptic ulcer. When you eat, the strong hydrochloric acid in the stomach breaks down and digests the food. The lining of the stomach is made of tissues that are able to withstand exposure to this strong digestive acid. However, sometimes an eruption occurs on the surface of the stomach or other digestive organs. When the hydrochloric acid comes into contact with this ulcer, it causes a burning pain.

CAUSES

Thirty years ago, men had ulcers 20 times more often than women. Today, if you're a woman, you've got the same chance as a man for getting an ulcer. Why the increase? Doctors aren't sure, but they suspect increases in levels of stress in women's lives might be one reason. Another possible reason is that larger numbers of women are drinking and smoking these days.

Ulcers were one of the first diseases the medical community recognized as stress-related. The theory says that hard-driving, ambitious individuals who are under a great deal of stress are more likely to have ulcers. The idea is that too much stress causes the body to produce excess stomach acid, which produces ulcers. Population studies, however, have shown that ulcers don't just occur in hard-driving, type "A" personalities. In fact, ulcers cut across all racial, ethnic, and occupational groups. They can occur in young children and in elderly people.

It is true that the body produces more hydrochloric acid under stress. However, not everyone who is under stress gets ulcers, and doctors are still at a loss to explain exactly why. Some researchers say that certain individuals simply produce more stomach acid than others. While this may be true, it doesn't explain why some people with ulcers produce less stomach acid than normal.

Other authorities suggest that some people may have "weaker" stomachs than others. The lining of the stomach in these vulnerable individuals may be less able to withstand the onslaught of gastric acids. The same lifestyle factors that aggravate ulcers may cause this stomach-lining weakness.

Some experts believe that certain lifestyle factors may increase the risk of ulcers developing. Drinking large amounts of alcohol or coffee and smoking cigarettes all increase acidic stomach secretions. Some medications, such as aspirin or aspirinlike products, also increase stomach acids.

A newer ulcer theory that's getting a lot of attention focuses on a bacterial infection by an organism called *Helicobacter pylori*. Proponents of the bacteria-ulcer theory say that this particular microorganism has been found in large numbers of people with ulcers and that eliminating the organisms cures the ulcers. Opponents of the *H. pylori* theory point out that many people are infected with this organism and don't have ulcers.

AT-HOME TREATMENT

While doctors argue over the exact causes of ulcers, you can use these home remedies to cope with your ulcer.

10 WAYS TO TREAT YOUR ULCER

- Identify and avoid your "trigger" foods.
- Eat small, frequent meals.
- Avoid drinking milk.
- Manage your stress.
- Don't smoke.
- Avoid aspirin.
- Cut out or cut down on coffee.
- Limit your alcohol intake.
- Take antacids with caution.
- Call the doctor.

Check your diet. When you think of an "ulcer diet," you probably think of bland, boring, tasteless foods prepared without spices. Doctors used to recommend such foods for people with ulcers, believing that spicy foods caused or aggravated ulcers. Today, gastrointestinal specialists tell us that individual tolerances to different types of foods vary. Pay attention to how your ulcer reacts to particular foods. If you feel pain after eating a highly spiced meal, chances are good that the spices are aggravating your condition. The same goes for other foods. Avoid those foods that cause you discomfort.

Eat less, more often. Most ulcer sufferers say that the pain is worse when their stomach is empty. That's because the excess hydrochloric acid has nothing to work on. Keep some food present in the digestive tract by eating small, frequent meals. A word of caution: Be careful not to overeat on this frequent-meal regimen. Eating too much causes the formation of more gastric juices and, of course, can also cause you to gain weight.

Skip the milk. Drinking milk is a time-honored tradition among people with ulcers, but it may actually make your condition worse. Calcium increases the production of stomach acids. While the protein in the milk may feel soothing, the calcium can make your stomach even more acidic.

Manage your stress. Even if stress doesn't cause ulcers, it can certainly aggravate existing conditions. Work on ways to cope with your stress more effectively. Take a stress management class, learn to meditate, exercise regularly, or do whatever helps you cope.

Stop smoking. If you've been waiting for a really good reason to stop smoking, this is it: Cigarette smoking is a known stomach irritant. It inhibits the secretion of prostaglandins, which normally act against an attack of hydrochloric acid and pepsin.

Avoid aspirin. Aspirin inhibits prostaglandins and reduces the digestive system's defenses.

Watch the alcohol. If your family has a history of ulcers, the last thing you need is an alcoholic beverage. Doctors aren't sure why, but people who drink heavily have a higher risk of getting ulcers than those who drink little or not at all.

Reach for the antacids. Antacids can be effective in relieving the discomfort of a peptic ulcer attack. They not only neutralize stomach acid, they may also help the ulcer heal. However, they can cause problems if you overuse them. Keep these caveats in mind:

• Overuse of antacids that contain aluminum can cause constipation and interfere with the absorption of phosphorus, which can lead to bone weakness and damage.

• Taking too much magnesium-containing antacid can cause diarrhea. If you have impaired kidney function, using magnesium-based antacids can cause the blood levels of magnesium to rise and lead to weakness and fatigue.

• When you use antacids over a long period of time and suddenly stop, it can cause an increase in stomach acid.

• All antacids can interfere with the absorption and metabolism of other drugs. Talk with your doctor or pharmacist about possible drug interactions.

• By using antacids, you may be masking symptoms of a more serious health problem.

• Consistently using over-the-counter antacids in lieu of stronger prescription medications can end up costing you more money in the long run.

• If you need to use antacids constantly, or if you need more and more antacid to get relief, talk with your doctor.

Cut the coffee. The caffeine and acids in coffee and in tea can irritate your stomach. Substitute herbal teas or cereal-based coffee beverages like Pero.

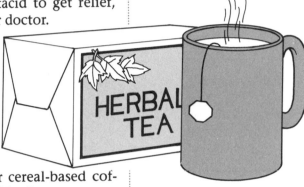

Call the doctor. Consult a doctor immediately if you have any of these symptoms:

• Vomiting blood. This is a sign of gastrointestinal bleeding.

• Black, red, or bloody stools. This is also a sign of gastrointestinal bleeding.

• Sudden, severe abdominal pain. This may indicate a perforation in which the stomach contents spill into the abdominal cavity. This is a medical emergency. Get help immediately.

Sources: Lawrence S. Friedman, M.D., Associate Professor of Medicine, Jefferson Medical College, Thomas Jefferson University, Philadelphia, Pennsylvania. **Gayle Randall, M.D.,** Assistant Professor of Medicine, Department of Medicine, University of California, Los Angeles, School of Medicine, Los Angeles, California. **Norton Rosensweig, M.D.,** Associate Clinical Professor of Medicine, Columbia University College of Physicians and Surgeons, New York, New York. **Anne Simons, M.D.,** Coauthor, *Before You Call the Doctor*; Family Practitioner, San Francisco Department of Public Health; Family Practitioner and Assistant Clinical Professor, Family and Community Medicine, University of California San Francisco Medical Center, San Francisco, California.

●VARICOSE VEINS

What to Do

About

Unsightly

Veins

I N A PERFECT WORLD, NO ONE WOULD ever get stretch marks. Our hair would retain its original color until the day we died. And no one would get varicose veins.

Varicose veins are swollen, stretched veins in the legs that develop close to the surface of the skin. By themselves, they are not much to worry about, but they may lead to a more serious condition, such as a skin ulcer, phlebitis (inflammation of a vein), or thrombosis (formation of a blood clot).

SYMPTOMS

How do you know if you have varicose veins? They are usually noticeable, since they form close to the surface of the skin. They appear as bulging, bluish, cordlike lines running down the legs. They may be accompanied by feelings of achiness, heaviness, and fatigue in the legs, especially at the end of the day; itchy, scaly skin covering the affected areas; and, in advanced cases, swollen ankles, pain shooting down the leg, and leg cramps at night.

Eighty percent of varicose-vein sufferers will also get spider veins. And half of all spider-vein sufferers also have varicose veins. Unlike knotty varicose veins, spider veins are thin and weblike in appearance (hence the name) and show up most often on the legs, neck, and face. These veins are actually dilated blood vessels that appear no thicker than a thread or hair. Besides a link to pregnancy and hormones, no one knows for sure why they crop up. But on the plus side, they rarely cause problems.

CAUSES

Blood from the legs must return to the heart uphill, against the force of gravity. The leg veins have one-way valves to prevent blood from flowing back down toward the feet. When pressure on the veins stretches them or when the valves are injured in some way, the valves cannot close properly and some blood travels back down. This blood accumulates in pools, which stretch the veins even more. These stretched, bulging veins are called "varicose veins."

It's estimated that 25 percent of all women and ten percent of all men are affected by varicose veins. Women seem to be more susceptible, largely due to hormonal factors, especially during pregnancy. Surging hormones during pregnancy weaken collagen and connective tissues in the pelvis in preparation for giving birth. Unfortunately, as a side effect, the hormones may also weaken the collagen found in the veins and valves of the body. These weakened tissues have more difficulty standing up to the increased blood volume that comes with carrying a baby. In addition, the weight of the fetus itself may play a role in the development of varicose veins and spider veins in the legs. These veins may recede, however, after you give birth.

AT-HOME TREATMENT

Although you probably cannot completely cure an existing case of varicose veins, there are ways to prevent or, at the very least, postpone their development and decrease their severity. Follow these tips to help your varicose veins:

Do a family leg check. A tendency toward varicose veins can be inherited. If, for example, a person has an abnormality in a gene involved in vein development, that abnormal gene can be passed on to some or all of that person's descendents. Family members may also have a flaw in the design of their valves or veins that would predispose them to varicose veins. Talk to your doctor about taking preventative steps if you have a family history of this condition.

Stay active. Exercise can help prevent or postpone varicose veins by keeping blood from pooling in the veins. When you use your legs, you improve the circulation. Running, weight training, calisthenics—anything that gets your legs moving will also get your blood moving.

Shed extra pounds. If you are overweight, your body is probably less able to pump blood back to the heart, and your blood vessels will be forced to carry more blood. Both these things increase your risk of varicose veins developing.

Take a load off. When you're standing up, the blood in your legs has to fight gravity to get back to your heart. Therefore, it is more likely to pool in your legs. If you find yourself standing for long periods of time, make a point of taking a break to sit down from time to time.

Don't become a couch potato. While resting occasionally is important, sitting for too long can also contribute to varicose veins. When your knees and hips are bent, your veins have

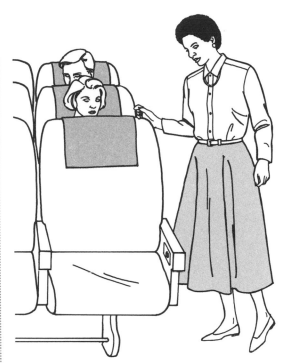

to push harder to get the blood around the corners. Get up and stretch your legs once in a while during a long plane trip or during a day of sitting at the office. Another circulation booster is to stand on your toes and flex your heels up and down ten times.

Wear support hose. Thick support hose can help control the development of varicose veins. You can get them at most department stores, or you can get a prescription from your doctor for stockings that provide extra support. Support stockings work by keeping your veins from bulging and by exerting pressure on your legs from the bottom up; when the pressure is greater on your calves than it is on your thighs, blood is, in effect, squeezed upward. This helps your body pump the blood back to the heart. The stockings are an effective aid, but some people complain because they can be uncomfortably hot and because they come in a limited choice of colors.

Wear spandex leggings. These work the same way as non-prescription support pantyhose.

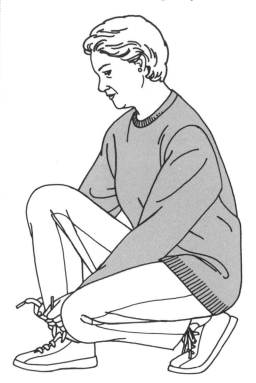

Wear lace-ups. If your feet swell habitually, consider wearing tennis shoes or other shoes with laces or ties that can be loosened to relieve the pressure on your feet.

Put your feet up. Raising your legs makes it easier for your body to move blood back to the heart. If you raise them so they are higher than your heart, you'll have gravity working for you rather than against you. Lie flat on the floor or the couch and prop your legs up with pillows or cushions. Do this up to ten

minutes every hour, if possible. If you have chronic swelling in your lower legs, it may help to put a few pillows under your feet while you sleep.

Exercise your feet. Working the muscles in your feet and ankles will get things moving from the bottom up; the action of the muscles down there will help to force blood up and out of your legs. There are a number of exercises you can do almost anywhere and almost anytime. Flex your feet up and down as you would when you pump a piano pedal or gas pedal; rotate your feet, first clockwise and then counter-clockwise; bend your knees and slide your heels forward and back.

Become a master of disguise. Don't stop wearing shorts or skirts because you're embarrassed about your varicose veins. Instead, try covering them up with makeup specially made for legs. It comes in a variety of colors to match your skin tone, and it won't rub off on clothing or stockings. Some brands are waterproof and include a sun block, so they're perfect for the beach.

Watch for warning signs. Blood clots can form in varicose veins; this event is rare, but it is dangerous. Thrombophlebitis occurs when a clot causes inflammation in the vein. A clot that begins to move within a vein can travel up to the heart or lungs and block the flow of blood, causing heart failure or a pulmonary blockage, or embolism.

If a clot does form in your leg, you may experience tenderness or pain in a small area, or you may have swelling or tenderness in much or all of the leg. If any of these symptoms occur, see your doctor.

You can help avoid the formation of clots by keeping active, maintaining a healthy weight, and by getting up and stretching your legs now and then when you are sitting for a long period of time.

AT THE DOCTOR'S

Most cases of varicose veins can be successfully treated at home. However, in very severe cases, they may require a surgical procedure called vein stripping, in which the afflicted veins are tied off and removed; other healthy veins in the area will take over the job of pushing blood toward the heart. A chemical can also be injected into the veins, closing them off and forcing the blood to find other channels to the heart.

Sources: **Alan M. Dietzek, M.D.,** Vascular Surgeon, North Shore University Hospital, Manhasset, New York; Assistant Professor of Surgery, Cornell Medical College, New York, New York. **Hugh Gelabert, M.D.,** Assistant Professor of Surgery, Section of Vascular Surgery, University of California at Los Angeles School of Medicine, Los Angeles, California. **Luis Navarro, M.D.,** Author, *No More Varicose Veins*; Founder and Director, Vein Treatment Center, New York, New York. **Richard Ottaviano,** President, Covermark Cosmetics, Moonachie, New Jersey. **Frank J. Veith, M.D.,** Professor of Surgery, Chief, Vascular Surgical Services, Montefiore Medical Center-Albert Einstein College of Medicine, New York, New York.

10 WAYS TO MINIMIZE OR PREVENT VARICOSE VEINS

- Find out whether varicose veins run in your family.
- Start an exercise program.
- Lose excess body weight.
- Don't spend too much time standing or sitting.
- Wear support stockings or spandex leggings.
- Cover the veins with leg makeup.
- Elevate your feet.
- Do foot exercises.
- Wear shoes that lace up.
- Keep an eye out for signs that a blood clot has formed.

•WARTS

How to Erase

Them

THEY'RE UGLY. THEY'RE CONTAGIOUS. They feel tender and itchy. And if you've got some, you definitely want to get rid of them. They're warts, unsightly infectious growths in the outer layers of the skin, caused by a virus called the human papilloma virus (HPV).

Many of us have had one or more of these raised, rough-textured, gray-ish growths. They can vary in size from that of a pinhead to a large mass. Usually, they're found on the hands and fingers, although they can appear anywhere on the skin. A smaller, smoother, flat variety of wart sometimes shows up on the hands or face. When warts appear on the bottoms of the feet (plantar warts), they can become large, grow inward rather than out, and cause problems with walking. Sometimes warts appear on the genital and anal areas.

CAUSES

Doctors know that warts are caused by the human papilloma virus, but they don't know why warts appear, disappear, and then seemingly spontaneously reappear without warning. Usually, the HPV enters through a break in the skin— a cut, crack, or scratch. Then the virus sits quietly, incubating for up to six months before it erupts into the raised lesion we know as a wart.

The human papilloma virus is a "contact virus." That is, it's passed from direct skin-to-skin contact with an infected person. If you have a wart, you can spread the virus to other parts of your body by touch-ing, scratching, shaving, or biting your nails. Warts are often spread on the scalp by brushing or combing the hair. Moist areas of the body such as the soles of the feet provide perfect breeding grounds for the virus's growth. You can get warts no matter what your age. People do seem to develop an immunity to the virus as they age, however, which is why you'll often see more children than adults with warts.

Common skin warts are the most prevalent type. In children, you'll often see the flat type of skin wart. These warts usually appear smooth, flat, and yellowish-brown in color.

Plantar warts are warts that appear on the soles of the feet. These warts can grow to two inches in diameter. They can be quite debilitating because they grow inward. With each step you take, the tissue swelling pushes inward and creates a sensation that resembles walking with a pebble in your shoe.

Warts that appear in the genital or anal area are extremely contagious. Once rare, genital warts are becom-ing increasingly common. Usually they're spread through sexual con-tact with an infected individual. It's possible for a mother infected with genital warts to pass the virus on to her fetus during pregnancy or birth. Women who have genital warts and are pregnant should inform their obstetrician about their condition, get regular prenatal care, and discuss possible alternate birthing options.

AT-HOME TREATMENT

Try the following strategies to wipe out your warts. If you're dia-betic, never use home remedies on warts. See your physician instead. Genital warts have been shown to increase the risk of cervical cancer in women. If you have genital warts, have them evaluated and treated by a physician.

Be sure of your diagnosis. Before you begin any treatment, be sure you have warts and not some other skin problem. You can usually identify warts (except the flat variety) by the red "seeds" on the surface of the wart. These aren't really seeds at all, but tiny blood vessels supplying the wart. In contrast, moles are usually smooth, regularly shaped bumps, darker than normal skin color. If you find patches of rough, raised skin with skin lines running through them, you most likely have a callus or a corn.

Some lesions may be skin cancer (malignant melanoma). Usually, skin cancers have irregular borders and colors. If you have a question about a skin eruption, don't delay in seeing a dermatologist for proper diagnosis.

Hands off. If you don't want to spread your warts to others or to other parts of your body, don't touch them. If the surface of a wart is broken, either intentionally or accidentally, it could lead to infection. Let children know that picking, touching, or chewing warts can cause them to spread. Wash your hands (and your children's) often and thoroughly with soap and hot water to avoid spreading the virus.

Tape it up. An inexpensive method of wart removal that leaves no scar involves wrapping the wart in adhesive tape. It's especially effective on finger warts. Wrap the wart completely with four layers of adhesive tape. The first piece should go over the

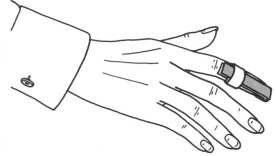

top of the finger; the second, around the finger. Repeat these two steps with two more pieces of tape. The tape should be snug, but not too tight. Leave it on for six and a half days. Then remove the tape for one-half a day. Repeat the procedure until the wart disappears. You may have to do this for three or four weeks. This technique also works on plantar warts, but you have to be sure the strips of tape are long enough to securely fasten the adhesive to the wart.

Bring on the castor oil. Put some castor oil on a cotton swab and apply it directly to the wart. The acid in the castor oil irritates the wart (and presumably the virus). This technique works especially well on small, flat warts on the face and back of the hands.

Try vitamin C. Make a paste by crushing vitamin C tablets and adding a little water. Apply the paste directly to the wart (don't get it on the surrounding skin). Cover the wart with gauze and tape. The acid in the vitamin C may be enough to irritate the wart away.

Get hot. Soaking your plantar warts in very hot water softens the warts and may even kill the virus. Be careful that the water

10 WAYS TO TREAT YOUR WARTS

- Be sure you have warts.
- Don't scratch, pick, or touch your warts.
- Wrap your warts in adhesive tape.
- Try castor oil.
- Apply vitamin C paste.
- Soak your warts in hot water.
- Keep your feet dry.
- Cover cuts.
- Use over-the-counter products with caution.
- Use the power of your mind.

is not so hot that you burn your skin.

Stay dry. Viruses, especially those that produce plantar warts, flourish in damp environments. To prevent the growth of these viruses, keep your feet as dry as possible at all times. Change your socks often, whenever your feet become sweaty. Use a medicated foot powder. And switch shoes every day to allow your shoes to dry out properly between wearings.

Cover up. The human papilloma virus enters the skin through cuts, scrapes, cracks, and scratches. Keep the virus out from under your skin by keeping your injuries covered with sterile bandages.

Use OTC medications with caution. Many topical wart removal products available over the counter work fairly well. In fact, the Food and Drug Administration has just approved the use of products containing 26 percent salicylic acid that work even better than before

(in the past, products couldn't contain more than 16 percent). Be careful to apply these preparations only to your wart and not to the surrounding skin. If you're using a liquid medication, smear a ring of petroleum jelly around the wart before applying the product. This should protect the non-affected skin around the wart. If you're using medicated wart pads or patches, carefully cut them exactly to the size of the wart and no larger. Whenever possible, leave over-the-counter products on overnight, uncovered.

Use your mind. Studies using hypnosis and visualization to remove warts have had some amazing results. One researcher at Massachusetts General Hospital in Boston used hypnosis to treat 17 patients with warts. He told them they would feel a tingling sensation in the warts on one side of the body, and only those warts would disappear. Nine of the 17 patients lost more than 75 percent of all their warts; four of them lost all the warts.

Use your imagination to visualize the warts becoming smaller. Feel them tingle slightly as they shrink. Try using a visualization like this several times a day over a few weeks and see if it improves your warts.

PREVENTION

The best advice is to prevent warts before you become infected.

Keep those feet covered. Millions of virus particles can leak from

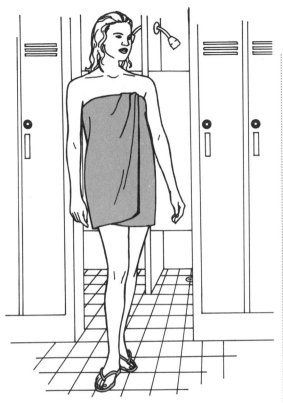

warts. That means if you're walking around barefoot in public areas like locker rooms, pools, showers in fitness centers, or on carpets in hotel rooms, you're putting yourself at risk for contracting plantar warts. The best advice is to wear shoes, sandals, or slippers. In wet areas, use rubber thongs.

Avoid contact. Since the human papilloma virus is a contact virus, the way to keep from getting infected is to avoid direct, skin-to-skin contact with anyone who has warts. If you do come into contact with someone's wart, wash your hands immediately with soap and hot water.

Know your partner. In these days of sexually transmitted diseases like genital warts and AIDS, "casual" sex can be life threaten-ing. Know your partner and his or her sexual history before you have sex.

Look for lesions. It may not sound romantic, but take the time to look over your sexual partner's genitals before you have sexual contact. Look for any lesions, redness, or other abnormalities.

Use condoms. No matter how well you know your partner, insist on using condoms every time you have sex.

Stay healthy. Your immune system is what fights viruses like HPV. Do everything you can to keep your immune system strong. Eat a well-balanced diet, exercise regularly, don't smoke, get enough rest, and manage your stress.

---

6 STRATEGIES FOR PREVENTING WARTS

- Avoid contact with infected individuals.
- Know your sex partner.
- Examine your partner's genitals.
- Use condoms.
- Don't go barefoot.
- Adopt a healthy lifestyle.

Sources: **Joseph P. Bark, M.D.,** Chairman of Dermatology, St. Joseph Hospital, Lexington, Kentucky; Author, *Retin-A and Other Youth Miracles* and *Skin Secrets.* **Andrew Lazar, M.D.,** Assistant Professor of Clinical Dermatology, Northwestern University School of Medicine, Chicago, Illinois. **Jerome Z. Litt, M.D.,** Author, *Your Skin: From Acne to Zits*; Assistant Clinical Professor of Dermatology, Case Western Reserve University School of Medicine, Cleveland, Ohio. **Anne Simons, M.D.,** Coauthor, *Before You Call the Doctor*; Family Practitioner, San Francisco Department of Public Health; Family Practitioner and Assistant Clinical Professor, Family and Community Medicine, University of California San Francisco Medical Center, San Francisco, California.

•WEIGHT GAIN

How to Slim

Down Safely

and

Permanently

ASK ANY AMERICAN WOMAN YOU know if she's happy with her body. Chances are, she'll say no. Although only an estimated one-fourth to one-third of all Americans are overweight, the majority of women believe that they have a weight problem.

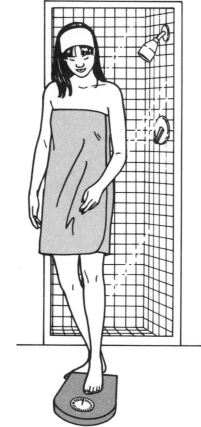

Here are the hard facts: At any given moment, 33 to 40 percent of American women are actively dieting. These women are big spenders, too. In fact, the money they spend comprises the largest part of the $30 billion a year spent in this country on various weight-loss products and programs. (Just think what that huge sum of money could do for the homeless and the hungry!)

Sadly, much of the money spent on diet products and programs is coming out of the pockets of repeat customers. In other words, these products aren't working. While they may help you lose weight in the short term, as much as two-thirds of that weight is generally regained within a year and almost all of it within five years.

Dieting becomes a way of life for some people, particularly women, who lose weight and gain it back over and over again in a syndrome of "yo-yo" dieting. A 1991 study published in *The New England Journal of Medicine* indicates that you may be shortening your life span if you engage in such practices. And most research has shown that such weight cycling probably makes it easier to regain the weight by altering your metabolism (the rate at which your body burns calories). The general pattern is this: You lose eight pounds of fat and two pounds of muscle the first time you diet. Then you gain back ten pounds—all of it fat. The net result is that you've increased your amount of fat by two pounds. You've also lost muscle mass, and muscle actually helps burn more calories.

The old school of dieting ran on the equation that 3,500 calories equaled one pound of weight. Cut the calories or burn more of them than you consumed, and you would drop pounds. Nice theory, but it didn't hold water. The problem is that weight loss is more complicated than a simple equation, according to researchers who participated in a conference sponsored by the National Institutes of Health in the spring of 1992. Those experts also concluded that being overweight wasn't just a question of restraint. Instead, they decided that it was "a complex disorder of energy metabolism."

If you really want to keep the weight off for the rest of your life, you have to change your definition of the word "diet." In fact, the word refers to what you eat on a day-to-day basis, not what you don't eat for a limited time.

Obesity researchers have discredited the calorie-control theory of weight loss. One expert interviewed for this chapter summed it up nicely: "Someday," he said, "I hope we'll look back on semistarvation diets the way we currently view such archaic practices as bleeding and purging. A weight problem is not like having pneumonia where you can take a course of antibiotics and cure it. You have to keep working on your weight."

AT-HOME TREATMENT

Keeping in mind the reality of the success rates of most diets, the question becomes not simply how can you lose weight, but how can you lose fat wisely and increase your chances of keeping it off. First off, you have to decide if you truly need to lose weight.

Unfortunately, most women don't care what the various charts say about our height-weight ratios. We're striving for a certain look, a body image that may be impossible for some of us to attain. To make a responsible decision about whether you need to lose weight, you'll have to consider your shape, height, weight, and history of obesity-linked diseases, as well as the history of those factors in your family. For a guideline on what your weight should be, you can check the Metropolitan Life Insurance Company Height and Weight Tables, which were revised in 1983. To determine your risk for weight-related health problems, consider the following:

- Are you at risk for high blood pressure, type II diabetes, or heart disease? Your physician can help you with those answers by examining your medical and family history, along with performing certain diagnostic tests.

- Where's your fat located? If it's concentrated around your belly, you need to lose. If it's around your hips and thighs but your belly's flat, you can relax a bit. That's because abdominal fat is linked with a higher risk for medical conditions—especially heart disease—than is fat on the hips and thighs. Divide your waist measurement by your hip measurement to get your waist/hip ratio: 0.70 to 0.75 is considered healthy for women.

- Calculate your body mass index (BMI). Divide your weight in pounds by 2.2 to get kilograms, and your height in inches by 39.37 to get meters. Your BMI equals your weight in kilograms divided by your height in meters squared. (In other words, multiply your height by itself, then divide your weight by that number.) Normal BMI is considered to be between 19 and 27.

If, after deliberating, you have decided that you truly need to lose weight, then consider when your weight problems began: Have you gained weight recently as the result of a traumatic event such as a marital separation or a job loss? Or has this been a gradual pattern since your teens?

16 STEPS TO A SLIMMER YOU

- Set a realistic target weight.
- Don't lose weight too quickly.
- Don't pick a high-stress time in your life to try to lose weight.
- Start with small goals; build to bigger ones.
- Keep high-fat, unhealthy foods out of your house.
- Learn to judge appropriate portion sizes.
- Don't count calories.
- Eliminate alcohol from your diet.
- Eat regularly; don't skip meals.
- Don't restrict your calorie intake to very low levels.
- Don't quit after one setback.
- Follow the U.S. Department of Agriculture's dietary guidelines.
- Cut down your fat intake.
- Start a program of mild aerobic exercise and strength training.
- Join a support group.
- Be wary of programs and products promising magical routes to weight loss.

You should also analyze your eating and activity patterns. For example, if you're starving and bingeing, you first have to learn how to eat normally—when you are hungry (not sad, depressed, lonely, tired, or bored) and only until you are comfortably full.

Experts now believe that constant dieting and erratic eating habits can reduce your metabolic rate, forcing your body into a starvation mode that hoards fat. So, if you have been practicing unhealthy habits for a number of years, your body may have to go through some healing before you try another weight-loss plan. Otherwise, no matter how much you cut down on food, you may continue to gain weight.

To get a handle on what you are eating, you can try keeping a food diary for two weeks. Write down everything you eat, when you eat it, and how you're feeling at the time— bored, angry, or hungry, for example. A food diary can be very illuminating. It may show you that you eat automatically, without thinking. Your diary can also be helpful if you decide to visit a registered dietitian for assistance.

Finally, remember that it is possible to be too thin. Very few women can match the body measurements of magazine fashion models. The rest of us risk endangering our health when we try too hard to reach those dimensions. What's most important is to be fit and healthy at whatever weight and size.

The tips that follow can help you design your own program of weight loss. However, one word of caution: These suggestions are only appropriate for adults who are in good health and who are not pregnant or nursing a baby. Even if you are overweight, pregnancy is not an appropriate time to cut back on your food intake. According to experts, even if you weigh 400 pounds, you still need to gain at least 20 pounds during pregnancy. Inadequate weight gain can pose a significant risk to the fetus. That means you must eat regularly and never skip a meal. Skipping meals can cause the body to break down its fat reserves, which creates certain by-products known as ketones that may harm the fetus. If you have any significant health problems, you should consult your physician before beginning any diet or exercise program.

Be realistic. Genetics is one factor in the complex weight equation. Large studies of adopted children have shown that the weight of children is determined more by genetics than by the eating habits of the adoptive homes. (Keep in mind, though, that eating habits are still an important factor in determining your weight.) If you're thinking about losing some weight, take a look at other family members. Do you see a general trend toward a certain body type? If you have a hereditary tendency toward a heavier profile, you may find that you have to work harder to lose weight. Don't become discouraged; you can trim down. The keys are to realize that you are fighting against genetics and to set a realistic weight-loss goal for yourself. Decide on a target weight that is healthy for you, given your hereditary tendencies. Always remember that the most important thing is to be strong and fit, not to match some imagined standard of thinness.

Make a patience pact with yourself. Don't plan to lose too much weight too soon. Rapid weight loss may cause the body to go into a starvation response, holding onto its fat reserves for impending famine and slowing your metabolism. This can lead to a rapid weight gain down the road. In general, try to lose no more than half a pound per week.

Be kind to yourself. Pick a good time to take on new lifestyle changes. You don't want to choose a period of high stress. In other words, the week before your wedding is not the best time to start. Since success tends to breed success, pick a time when you are most likely to succeed.

Take baby steps. If you try to take on too much at once, you may be setting yourself up for failure. Don't try to change all your bad habits overnight. Make changes gradually. For example, instead of vowing to eat only low-fat foods from now on, try starting with a few low-fat meals a week. Then add a whole low-fat day, and so on. The same goes for exercise. Start with a five- or ten-minute walk every day, then build up slowly to longer and more strenuous exercise periods.

Create a healthy environment to reduce temptation. This is a piece of simple but effective advice. When you don't have potato chips or chocolate in the house, avoiding them is much easier. Instead of keeping those high-fat snacks handy, have raw vegetables or your favorite fruit around. Same goes for what gets cooked for meals. If you're the family food shopper, you can control this area yourself. If someone else does the grocery shopping, hand them a list. Overweight tends to run in families, partly because of shared eating habits.

Throw out your calorie counter. Not all the experts agree about this one, but most suggest that changing the way you eat is more effective than simply limiting your caloric intake.

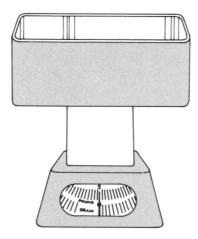

Get a handle on portion sizes. Weighing and measuring your food for a few days will train your eye to recognize portion sizes.

Just say "no" to the evening martini. Cutting alcohol out of your diet is one lifestyle change that is apt to make your Levi's fit better. Alcoholic beverages are empty calories, meaning that they carry absolutely no nutritional benefits. Also, some studies show that alcohol may promote distribution of fat around the waist. On average, Americans get ten percent of their calories from alcohol. So for some, simply cutting out the cocktails would mean a substantial drop in calories. In fact, some people may be able to lose weight just by giving up beer.

Never skip a meal. Eat breakfast, lunch, and dinner. Missing meals can lead to binges later. Your body will try to make up for the lack of food intake as it goes into starvation mode. An added benefit of regular meals is that if you get one-third or one-fourth of your calories at each meal, you won't want to snack as much in between.

Don't undereat. Very low-calorie diets can lead to bingeing and a slowdown in metabolism that can eventually result in rapid regaining of weight. Also, believe it or not, your metabolism is at its highest while it's digesting a meal. That doesn't mean you should eat constantly; just eat sensible, regular, nutritious meals.

Take one day at a time. Don't throw your whole plan out the window just because you succumbed to the chocolate mousse at your favorite restaurant. Instead of chastising yourself for your failings, learn to concentrate on your successes.

Feed your body what it needs. What your body needs is nutrients. According to the U.S. Department of Agriculture's dietary guidelines, you need two to three servings a day of meat, fish, poultry, or meat substitutes like eggs, legumes, or nuts; two to three servings of dairy products (preferably low-fat); two to four servings of fruit; three to five servings of vegetables; and six to eleven servings of breads, cereals, pastas, and other grains. If you are sedentary, you should consume the number of servings at the lower end of the range. If you are active, find a middle path. If you are very active (meaning that you engage regularly in rigorous sports, such as backpacking, cross-country skiing, long-distance cycling, and so on), consume the number of servings at the higher end of the range. Even at the low end of the range, you definitely won't go hungry while you eat healthy.

Get the skinny on fat. A dieter should always be on the lookout for fat. Cutting high-fat foods from your diet not only trims the figure but can also lower your risk of heart disease and some cancers.

Fat is nature's way of storing energy; nine calories of energy are crowded into each gram of fat, whereas a gram of protein or carbohydrate has only four. Also, the body tends to store fat calories as (you guessed it) body fat, while carbohydrates and protein are more likely to be used for energy.

How much fat does a proper diet include? The average American is consuming about 37 percent of her calories from fat these days, down from 40 percent a few years ago. The American Heart Association recommends that no more than 30 percent of your calories come from fat. However, if you're serious about losing weight (or lowering your cholesterol), you may have to go much lower than that—down to ten to 20 percent of your daily calories. However, you should never go below 20 grams of fat per day. This amount is necessary for good health.

Follow these pointers to cut the fat out of your diet:

- Switch to reduced-fat or fat-free salad dressing.
- Buy nonstick pans and use a tiny amount of oil or nonstick spray.
- Eat less meat and cheese; both can be high in fat.
- Buy lean cuts of meat and trim the fat before cooking. Remove the skin from poultry.
- Don't fry. Instead, roast, bake, broil, or simmer meat, poultry, and fish.
- Choose low-fat dairy products, such as skim milk.
- Fill up your plate with vegetables, fruits, beans, and grains, and don't drown them in butter or high-fat sauces.
- Learn about spices; use them to flavor your foods.
- Avoid nondairy creamers and toppings, which often contain high amounts of saturated fats from palm or coconut oils.

Move it. Exercise seems to be a key factor in losing weight. And it may not necessarily be a simple equation in which this or that activity burns off so many calories. (You've probably heard that it takes miles of walking to burn off one cookie.) But what exercise may do, according to some researchers, is speed up your metabolism, for as long as 18 hours after your work out. Your body continues to burn off the calories even after you've stopped exercising. Also, exercise tends to build muscle mass, and muscle burns more calories.

How exercise will affect your life depends on how active you already are. The less active

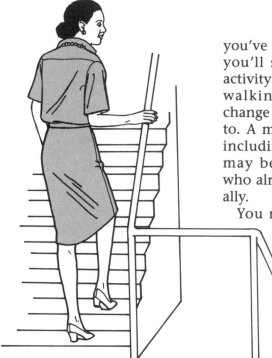

you've been, the more benefit you'll see in increasing your activity level. A routine of brisk walking could dramatically change the life of a couch potato. A more aggressive regimen, including running or cycling, may be needed by someone who already exercises occasionally.

You may find it helpful to work on changing your eating patterns before you add physical activity to your life. Get comfortable with those changes, and then move on to the physical aspect of your program. You can get advice from your local YMCA, or you can hire a personal trainer.

If you have been sedentary, try starting with these tricks to get your body moving:
• Take the stairs instead of the elevator.
• Park your car farther away from the office.
• Walk there instead of riding or driving.
• Take several short walks if you can't fit one 30-minute workout into your schedule or if it seems too strenuous.

If you think more strenuous exercise is in order:
• Cross-train. It takes about 48 hours for your muscles to replace the tissue that is broken down by an intense workout. You can take the day off, or you can choose to work on another muscle group while the first one recovers. For example, use a rowing machine on Monday and run on Tuesday.
• Alternate difficult and easy workouts. This practice is also helpful for avoiding injury. (Sixty-five percent of the people who take up running or aerobics quit within six weeks because of injury.) Try working out hard one day and gently the next: Run, then walk, for example. Alternating activities and intensity can make sticking with it easier.
• Say "I'll be baaack," to the gym. You don't have to develop biceps like Arnold Schwarznegger's to reap the benefits of strength training. As mentioned above, lean body mass, or muscle, requires more calories than fatty tissue does. Resistance training creates muscle mass, which raises your metabolism.

Get some support. Many overeaters have an unhealthy relationship with food. After all, food is our original source of comfort in life. We derived security and pleasure—not just sustenance—when we suckled at our mothers' breast or on a bottle. Now that you're an adult, you can find other, healthier, more appropriate ways to nurture yourself. To help you achieve that goal, consider finding support in the form of a group such as Overeaters Anonymous (look for a local listing in your newspaper or phone book). You may also find groups at a nearby hospital or church. A support group can also help you reinforce your new, healthier habits.

Don't be taken in by the promise of a free lunch. There is plenty of money in the weight-loss game, and every quack and fraud seems to promise more than they can possibly deliver. In fact, the Federal Trade Commission has investigated the advertising and marketing claims of many diet products and programs over the last two years. Here are a few claims that you should watch out for:

• Words like "melt away," "no effort," "painless," "no exercise."

• Plans that promise excessive weight loss, such as a pound a day.

• Programs that depend on artificial food or pills.

• Claims that a food, such as grapefruit, possesses magical properties to get rid of excess weight.

• Diets or gadgets that claim to cause weight loss from just one part of the body, such as the buttocks or the chin.

• Multilevel marketing plans that involve purchasing products from or selling them to people you know.

AT THE DOCTOR'S

Once you decide that you're ready to change your lifestyle to reach a desirable weight, you'll have to design a plan you can live with that will help you achieve your goals. The basic tenets of such a plan are: making nutritionally sound food choices, eating an adequate amount of food each day, and starting a program of mild aerobic exercise.

You may find the advice of your family physician, a registered dietitian, or an exercise physiologist helpful. However, in consulting professionals, you'd be wise to avoid "one-stop shopping." In other words, make sure that the dietitian sticks to nutritional counseling and the exercise physiologist to exercise. Some university medical centers and hospitals are adopting a multidisciplinary team approach to handle weight loss; a registered dietitian, a physician, an exercise physiologist, and a behavioral psychologist join forces to work on all aspects of the weight problem.

Sources: C. Wayne Callaway, M.D., Member, 1989-1990 Dietary Guidelines Advisory Committee to the U.S. Department of Agriculture/Department of Health and Human Resources; Associate Clinical Professor of Medicine, George Washington University in Washington, D.C. **Barbara Deskins, Ph.D., R.D.,** Associate Professor of Clinical Dietetics and Nutrition, University of Pittsburgh, Pittsburgh, Pennsylvania. **Johanna Dwyer, D.Sc., R.D.,** Director, Frances Stern Nutrition Center, New England Medical Center Hospitals; Professor, Tufts University Medical School, Boston, Massachusetts. **Gabe Mirkin, M.D.,** Author, *The Mirkin Report*, a monthly newsletter on health, fitness, and nutrition; Associate Professor, Georgetown University Medical School, Washington, D.C. **John H. Renner, M.D.,** President, Consumer Health Information Research Institute; Member, Board of Directors, National Council Against Health Fraud, Kansas City, Missouri.

●WRINKLES

How to Prevent

Them from

Developing

AH, THE FOUNTAIN OF YOUTH. IF ONLY we could find it: Our bodies would be restored to their youthful firmness. Our gray hairs would magically disappear. And the wrinkles on our faces would be smoothed away as the skin was pulled taut over our newly baby-soft, plump faces.

Unfortunately, until we find that fountain of youth, we will have to settle for less-than-miraculous remedies for the facial lines that all too often accompany our bodies' aging processes. But just think: Even if you don't manage to completely prevent wrinkles from appearing, you can always wear them proudly as badges of a life well lived.

You may have heard numerous suggestions for preventing or removing wrinkles. Unfortunately, many are no more than wishful thinking. The truth is:

- Drinking at least eight glasses of water a day won't prevent wrinkles. All that water is supposed to plump up your skin, so wrinkles won't show as much. This is completely untrue. The kidneys closely regulate water intake. Keeping up your fluid intake has other health benefits, but it won't do a thing for your wrinkles.

- Getting a massage won't smooth away your wrinkles. Massaging the skin is no more effective at getting rid of wrinkles than massaging the scalp is at causing hair to grow. Of course, if facial massage relaxes you, maybe it will cause you to frown less and develop fewer worry lines.

- You can't scrub away wrinkles. The idea of using an abrasive cleanser or a scrubbing pad as an orbital sander to get rid of wrinkles is

a mistake. In fact, dermatologists say that they have seen terrible skin problems develop from attempting this strategy. Wrinkles are caused by damage below the skin surface, not on the top. However, procedures such as chemical skin peels and dermabrasion, where the top layers of skin are sanded away, can minimize wrinkles' appearance. These procedures should only be done by a licensed professional.

CAUSES

Before considering any treatments for wrinkles, it is important to understand how skin ages and why we end up with wrinkles. Most people think that aging of the skin is the main cause of wrinkles, but there are other, more important factors. The big gun as far as wrinkle-producers go is the sun. The bottom line is that getting a "healthy-looking" tan is not so healthy for your skin.

Aging does play a role in wrinkle production. As we grow older, our skin begins to wear out. The skin and skull gradually become thinner and the underlying fat disappears. However, this type of wrinkling doesn't begin to happen until very late in life, at least not until the seventh or eighth decade.

Another factor that comes into play over the years is gravity. This insidious force slowly pulls everything toward the center of the earth, as if trying to reclaim it. The corners of the lips are the first thing to come down. The eyelids fall next. Then, the jowl forms, the upper lip begins to disappear into the mouth, the tip of the nose begins to point down, and the ears get longer.

Lastly, sleep lines can add to your facial etchings, as can the expressions you've worn throughout the years. Those lines occur simply from muscles pulling on the skin when you laugh, cry, wink, blink, kiss, and so on.

PREVENTION

You can't avoid aging, obviously, but you don't have to end up with a prunelike complexion. If you follow some common-sense measures, you can prevent some wrinkling and continue to put your best face forward.

The following tips can help you minimize the effect of the wrinkle-makers.

Avoid sun damage. The first and most important measure you can take is to wear sunscreen on your face every day, with no excuses or exceptions. By doing this and by avoiding direct sunlight between the hours of 10:00 A.M. to 2:00 P.M., you'll protect yourself from wrinkles and skin cancer. Despite how glorious the warm sun may feel, the ultraviolet radiation is nothing short of disastrous for your skin. The sun's radiation destroys two substances in the lower layer of the skin: collagen (a fibrous protein) and elastin. The elastin fibers are literally fragmented into little particles, making the skin less elastic and promoting wrinkles.

Not everyone is equally susceptible to the sun's harmful radiation. Fair-skinned individuals have more to worry about than do darker-skinned individuals, because they have less protective pigment.

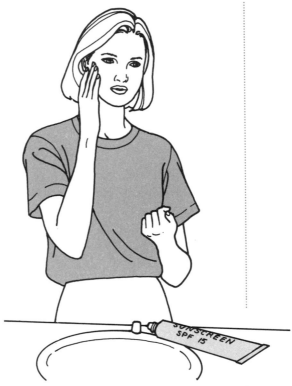

Regardless of what type of skin you have, however, the sun can still damage it. Make applying sunscreen part of your morning routine (or use make-up that contains sunscreen). Every day that you delay only hurts your skin. According to dermatologists, patients who have taken extra care to avoid the sun or conscientiously protected their skin with sunscreen are relatively age-proof. There is other encouraging news for people who have not been so careful in the past. A study of older people with sun-damaged skin who moved to a nursing home and stayed out of the sun revealed that their wrinkles and blotchiness actually lessened. So, if you start protecting your skin now, some of the damage may be reversed.

Don't snuggle up to your pillow. Over the course of many years, wrinkles can develop from something as simple as sleeping with your face pressed into the pillow. This process is similar to putting a folded napkin away in a drawer. When you take it out, you'll find creases in it. These creases can also appear on your face if you consistently sleep on one side. Try to break the habit of sleeping on your side or your stomach, and learn to sleep on your back. This may help you wake with a smoother face.

6 WAYS TO FIGHT WRINKLES

- Wear sunscreen on your face every day.
- Avoid the sun between 10:00 A.M. and 2:00 P.M.
- Sleep on your back.
- Quit smoking.
- Modify your facial expressions.
- Use a moisturizer.

Put out that cigarette. A study conducted at the University of Utah Health Sciences Center in Salt Lake City showed that premature wrinkling increased with amount of cigarette consumption and number of years as a smoker. Heavy smokers are almost five times more likely to have excessive wrinkling than are nonsmokers. Smoking may damage the collagen in the lower layer of the skin, but it can also more directly cause crow's-feet and vertical lines around the mouth—by making you squint from smoke irritation and purse your lips to take a puff.

Stop frowning. Constantly knotted brows, frowning mouths, or squinted eyes can eventually form wrinkles. Most of the time, we're not even aware of our habitual expressions, but by watching yourself in the mirror, you may notice some of your own facial tendencies. If the lines you see are not to your liking, you may be able to modify some of them.

Keep it moist. Using a moisturizer won't have a long-lasting effect, but it can remove some wrinkles temporarily by plumping up your skin. Moisturizers seal in the moisture on the surface of the skin. Apply moisturizer to damp skin and then pat your skin dry. You may want to look for a moisturizer that gives you the extra benefit of being a sunscreen, too.

AT THE DOCTOR'S

No at-home treatment will erase wrinkles once they've developed (although you can go a long way toward preventing them and minimizing their severity). However, depending on your line of work, your vanity, and your pocketbook, you can take advantage of a dermatologist's or a plastic surgeon's magic bag of tricks. Insurance companies usually do not cover any of the following treatments.

Retin-A. High doses of Retin-A, a drug that is used to treat certain types of acne, has also been shown to be very effective in minimizing wrinkles. The drug, which is smoothed onto the skin nightly, stimulates more rapid regeneration of skin cells. The treatment may be continued for years. It may not be used during pregnancy or while breastfeeding. One caveat of Retin-A treatment is that it causes heightened sensitivity to the sun and may hasten the development of skin cancer if treated skin is exposed to excessive amounts of ultraviolet rays. The manufacturer suggests wearing sunscreen every day while using the product.

Dermabrasion. This is a procedure in which the top layer of skin (called the epidermis) and part of the second layer (the dermis) are sanded off using of a tool made especially for this purpose. Depending on the type of dressing used, skin may take between six and 14 days to heal. Besides minimizing the appearance of wrinkles, dermabrasion can also make scars less noticeable. The downside of this treatment is that it can be expensive, is usually not covered under medical insurance policies, and carries a small risk of complications. It should only be performed by a licensed dermatologist (and be choosy about selecting one).

Chemical peels. This involves an application of acid to the face. The acid removes the top layers of skin and exposes the smoother skin underneath. The effect is similar to dermabrasion. Again, this procedure carries a risk of complications, and so should be performed only by a licensed dermatologist.

Incidentally, there are a number of products sold over the counter that contain fruit acids and claim to minimize the appearance of facial lines by "exfoliating" the top layers of skin. These products do not produce the same effects as a professional chemical peel, but are far less dangerous.

Face lift. Fashionable in celebrity circles, this surgical procedure pulls the skin taut across the face. Like any form of surgery, it carries a risk of complications.

Sources: **Melvin Elson, M.D.,** Medical Director, The Dermatology Center, Inc., Nashville Tennessee; Coauthor, *The Good Look Book*; Director, Cosmeceutical Research Institute, Inc., New York, New York. **Donald Kadunce, M.D.,** University of Utah Health Sciences Center, Salt Lake City, Utah. **David J. Leffell, M.D.,** Assistant Professor of Dermatology, Chief of Mohs Surgery, Yale University School of Medicine, New Haven, Connecticut. **Gary Rogers**, M.D., Associate Professor of Dermatology and Surgery, Boston University School of Medicine, Boston, Massachusetts.

•YEAST INFECTION

Get Rid of the

Itch

IT STARTED OUT AS A SLIGHT BURNING and itching sensation in your vaginal area. Now you've got a thick vaginal discharge that smells like bread yeast and looks like cottage cheese, your genital area is red and inflamed, your lower abdominal area feels painful, and the itching is about to drive you crazy. You've got a yeast infection, one of the more common—and miserable—aspects of being a woman.

Most women are bothered at some time or another by a vaginal infection. They can be caused by any number of organisms. One of the most common causes is the fungus *Candida albicans*. This organism, which is normally found on the skin, in the membranes of the mouth, in the intestines, and in the healthy vagina, can overgrow and cause what's commonly called a yeast infection because of the thick discharge that smells like baking bread. (Yeast infections are also called candidiasis, candidosis, moniliasis, or candida vaginitis.) The waste products produced by the rapid overgrowth of *Candida* (and other organisms) cause the itching, burning, pain, and discharge.

Sometimes *Candida* organisms can infect the mouth, where it is called thrush. Newborns who pass through a birth canal infected with *Candida* often contract thrush. When yeast organisms infect the skin, they cause an inflamed rash (diaper rash is often caused by *Candida*). These microorganisms can also infect the nails, esophagus (food tube), and digestive tract. In people whose immune systems are severely impaired, yeast organisms can infect the blood and cause serious infections of the organs.

CAUSES

A yeast infection, especially if it is recurrent, is a signal that your body is out of balance. Normally, the slightly acidic pH in your vagina keeps *Candida albicans* and other organisms from overgrowing. However, plenty of things can alter the vaginal pH and let the growth of these organisms go wild.

Women are especially vulnerable to yeast infections under these conditions:

- Pregnancy. When you're pregnant, the hormonal changes alter the vaginal pH and increase carbohydrate (glycogen) production, which provides food for infectious organisms like *Candida*.

- Menstrual period. The fluctuating hormones associated with menstruation can also alter the vaginal pH and make a woman more vulnerable to yeast infections.

- Antibiotics. Many women find when they take antibiotics like tetracycline or ampicillin to clear up a health problem, they end up with a vaginal yeast infection. That's because *Candida* lives in balance with other organisms in the vagina, particularly lactobacilli. Antibiotics kill the beneficial lactobacilli and alter this delicate balance. In addition, some antibiotics such as tetracycline actually stimulate the growth of yeast organisms.

- Diabetes/high-sugar diet. When you have diabetes or when you regularly eat excessive amounts of sugar, you alter your blood sugar levels. High blood sugar can, in turn, change the vaginal pH enough to allow yeast organisms to grow unchecked. Some women drink a great deal of high-sugar fruit juices, believing they will prevent bladder infections. However, these drinks may promote yeast infections.

- Stress. Doctors aren't willing to say that stress causes vaginal yeast infections. However, many women say that when they're excessively stressed, they tend to experience more yeast infections.
- Birth control pills. Researchers haven't found a clear cause-and-effect relationship between birth control pills and yeast infections. They do know that oral contraceptives increase the body's production of glycogen, a perfect food for yeast organisms.

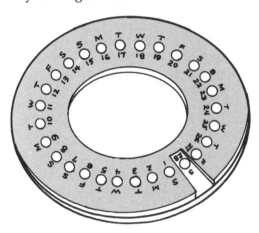

- Tight clothing. Wearing tight clothing like leotards that restrict the flow of air to the vaginal area and make the area hot and moist provides the perfect conditions for yeast growth.
- Immune-compromising conditions. If you have a health condition that compromises your immune system like lupus or AIDS, or if you're receiving chemotherapy, you're at greater risk for yeast infections. This is also true if you're taking any medications that suppress your immune system or if you're addicted to certain drugs.

IS IT YEAST?

It's important to be sure that *Candida* organisms are the culprit before you begin treating your vaginal infection at home. Yeast organisms cause itching, caked discharge that smells like baking bread, reddening of the labia and sometimes upper thighs, and lower abdominal discomfort. However, other organisms like *Trichomonas* ("trick"), a one-celled protozoan, can cause vaginitis-type symptoms. If your discharge is foul-smelling, yellowish, and frothy, suspect *Trichomonas*. Your vaginal symptoms might also be caused by a bacterial infection (bacterial vaginosis) from *Gardnerella* or other organisms. Bacterial infections generally cause little irritation and a heavy discharge that has a "fishy" odor, especially after intercourse.

An even more serious cause of vaginitis-like symptoms are sexually transmitted diseases like gonorrhea or chlamydia. *Trichomonas*, bacterial vaginosis, and sexually transmitted diseases cannot be self-treated. They require professional medical attention. If you have any vaginitis symptoms, be sure to have your symptoms evaluated by a physician to ensure proper diagnosis and proper treatment.

Some women suffer from yeastlike symptoms, but the problem isn't an infectious agent at all. The irritation and other symptoms are caused by chemical irritation (noninfectious vaginitis) rather than by the overproduction of an organism. The culprit in noninfectious vaginitis might be excessive douching, feminine hygiene sprays, bubble baths, talcum powder, or scented or colored toilet paper.

At-Home Treatment

When you can't avoid a yeast infection, home remedies can help. Remedies for treating vaginal infections focus on restoring the vaginal pH, repopulating the vagina with beneficial organisms, and/or reducing the population of overgrown organisms. If you visit the doctor for a diagnosis, don't douche at all before you go (it can interfere with diagnosis). Also, don't use feminine hygiene sprays or powders.

Many women who suffer from recurrent yeast infections have had their symptoms diagnosed by a physician and know all too well the signs and symptoms of a yeast flare-up. If you are sure that your vaginal symptoms are caused by yeast organisms, try these strategies:

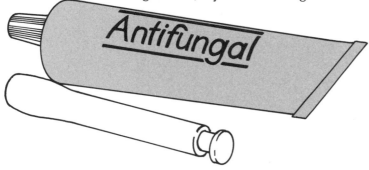

Head to the pharmacy for an antifungal. Effective antifungal vaginal creams, miconazole (Monistat) and clotrimazole (Gyne-Lotrimin), once available only by prescription, are now available over the counter at pharmacies. Use the suppositories nightly for three days or insert the cream once a day for seven days. Use the full course of medication required. Often your symptoms will subside almost immediately, but don't stop using the medication. If your symptoms recur or persist, try using the medication for a longer period of time than indicated on the package instructions. Also, try applying the antifungal cream to the outside of your vagina (vulva) and to your partner's genitals twice a day for ten days.

Women who have recurrent vaginal infections can use antifungal creams a few days after and/or before menstrual periods to prevent problems. Use antifungal products while you're taking antibiotics to prevent infection.

Bring on the vinegar. Routine douching isn't good for vaginal health, but douching with a mild vinegar or yogurt solution at the first sign of infection can help restore the natural pH and repopulate the beneficial bacteria. To make a vinegar douche, use one to three tablespoons of white vinegar to one quart of warm water. For a yogurt douche, use live culture, plain *Lactobacillus acidophilus* yogurt, and make a dilute mixture with warm water.

An effective douche should take about ten minutes. For the best douche results, follow these steps:

1) Clean the container, tube, and irrigation nozzle well with a good antiseptic solution. Fill the container with the douche solution.

2) Lie in the tub with your legs parted, a folded towel under your buttocks. (You cannot perform an effective douche sitting on the toilet.)

3) Suspend the douche container 12 to 18 inches above your hips.

4) Insert the nozzle two to four inches into the vagina with a gentle rotating motion until it encounters resistance.

5) Allow the solution to flow into the vagina very slowly. Use your fingers to close the vaginal lips to control the flow and allow a little pressure to build up inside so that the solution reaches all the internal surfaces.

Go for the boric. Boric acid, available over the counter in pharmacies, is one of the safest, least expensive, and most effective remedies for a yeast infection. When you feel yeast symptoms, insert one boric acid capsule for seven days into the vagina. If you can't find boric capsules ready-made, you can make your own by purchasing size "O" gelatin capsules (available in pharmacies or health food stores) and filling them with boric acid. If you're pregnant, don't try boric acid. Talk with your physician about other treatment options.

Go for yogurt tabs. Some women find yeast relief using Lactinex (*Lactobacillus*) tablets (available in health food stores). Insert them vaginally once or twice a day and douche with vinegar twice a day for two days for symptom relief.

Wash 'em away. It's not the yeast organisms but the by-products they secrete that cause irritation. Often you can get symptom relief by simply washing with water or a douche. (This does not cure the infection.)

---

9 WAYS TO TREAT YOUR YEAST INFECTION

- **Douche with vinegar or yogurt solutions.**
- **Try boric acid suppositories.**
- **Use antifungal creams or suppositories.**
- **Consider using Lactinex tablets as suppositories.**
- **Wash away yeast secretions.**
- **Have both you and your lover(s) treated.**
- **Wash up before lovemaking.**
- **Practice good oral hygiene.**
- **Call the doctor.**

Get treatment for partners. Too often, when a woman contracts a yeast infection, only she gets treated. But her partner could be reinfecting her with yeast organisms. Men may exhibit no symptoms, but often harbor yeast organisms, especially in the foreskin of uncircumcised penises. Some medical authorities suggest also using antifungal creams around your anal area and between the anus and vagina to prevent spread to the vagina.

If you engage in frequent oral sex and suffer from yeast infections, both partners should use an antifungal mouthwash.

Make it clean. When you have a yeast infection, it's particularly important to practice good hygiene. Be sure that your lover washes conscientiously before you make love.

Use a condom. You may not feel like engaging in sex while you have a vaginal infection. However, if you do have intercourse while infected, be sure to use a condom.

Don't share towels, baths. Sometimes yeast organisms can be passed through shared baths or towels. While you're infected, bathe alone, don't share towels, and wash your hands frequently with soap and water. Also, wash your clothing in hot water, or hot water with an added cup of vinegar or bleach, to kill yeast organisms.

Watch for symptoms. Usually you can effectively self-treat mild cases of yeast infection. However, call the doctor if you may have been exposed to a sexually transmitted disease or if you have any of the following symptoms:
- Abdominal pain or tenderness.
- Bloody discharge that is recurrent or that occurs between periods.
- Discharge that gets worse or persists for two weeks or more despite treatment.
- Recurrent yeast infection symptoms. Diabetes or a prediabetic condition might be contributing to your problem.
- Thin and foamy, grey, or yellowish-green discharge.
- Chills or fever.
- Back pain.
- Puslike discharge.

PREVENTION

If you've ever had a yeast infection, you're surely in no hurry to have one again. Use these strategies to reduce your risk of getting a yeast infection:

Avoid tight clothing. Don't encourage yeast growth by wearing tight clothing and building up heat and moisture. Opt for looser garments, cotton underwear, and cotton-lined panty hose that allow your genital area to breathe.

Keep your genital area dry. Dry your genital area thoroughly after bathing or showering. Gently towel your genital area or use a blow dryer on a low setting.

Cut the vaginal deodorants. Advertisers would have women believe that they need to deodorize their genital areas with feminine hygiene sprays, harsh soaps, and other perfumed products. These contain alcohol and hundreds of other chemicals that can dry out and irritate sensitive vaginal tissues and throw off the vagina's natural balance. Opt instead for mild, unscented soaps or non-soap cleansers without fragrances.

Watch your sugar intake. Many women's health authorities say that a diet high in sugar and artificial sweeteners may contribute to yeast infections. Too much of these foods can alter vaginal pH and increase the body's production of glycogen, which provides food for organisms.

Eat live-culture yogurt. Some studies have shown that eating yogurt that contains live cultures of *Lactobacillus acidophilus* can help prevent yeast infections. The problem is that most commercial yogurts don't contain live cultures. Try buying yogurt in a health food store,

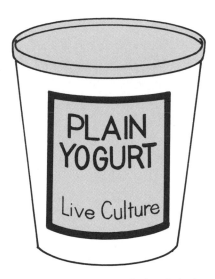

and be sure to read the label to ensure that it contains the right cultures.

Consider alternative birth control. If you take birth control pills and suffer from recurrent yeast infections, you might want to talk with your doctor about other forms of birth control. Oral contraceptives change the body's estrogen/ progesterone balance and increase the vaginal glycogen. IUDs decrease vaginal secretions, making the vagina more hospitable to yeast overgrowth. Some doctors speculate that vaginal sponges also alter the vaginal environment and make it more susceptible to yeast. If you suffer from recurrent yeast infections, you might consider a barrier form of contraception like condoms, a diaphragm, or a cervical cap.

Anticipate yeast. If you are susceptible to yeast and know that you are entering a high-risk situation, such as taking antibiotics, start home treatments for yeast right away. Don't wait for an outbreak.

Manage your stress. Excessive stress can depress the immune system and make you more vulnerable to infections like yeast. Take a class and learn an effective stress management technique like meditation, biofeedback, visualization, or progressive relaxation.

Try menstrual pads instead of tampons. Anything that interferes with the normal flow of menstrual blood can alter vaginal pH. Studies haven't definitely linked tampon use with an increase in yeast overgrowth, but some women find they have fewer yeast infections when they use menstrual pads instead of tampons.

Nix routine douching. Women have been told they should routinely douche with a variety of feminine hygiene products to "clean" the vagina. The vagina doesn't need help in cleansing itself. It does so naturally. All routine douching does is alter the vagina's pH and encourage yeast infections. It can also increase the risk of pelvic inflammatory disease (PID), a potentially deadly infection of the uterus, ovaries, or fallopian tubes. PID often causes scarring of the fallopian tubes, which can result in fertility problems. If PID is allowed to spread systemically, it can cause death. Symptoms of pelvic inflammatory disease include fever, chills, lower abdominal pain or tenderness, back pain, spotting, pain during or after intercourse, and puslike discharge. Usually,

10 WAYS TO PREVENT YEAST INFECTIONS

- Avoid tight-fitting clothing.
- Keep your genital area dry.
- Don't use harsh products.
- Cut down on sugar.
- Eat yogurt that contains live *Lactobacillus acidophilus* cultures.
- Consider using barrier-type contraceptives.
- Anticipate possible yeast infections.
- Effectively manage your stress.
- Try menstrual pads instead of tampons.
- Don't routinely douche.

women show some, but not all of these symptoms. If you experience any of these symptoms, see your doctor immediately.

Some researchers also believe that routine douching may increase your risk of cervical cancer. One study showed that women who douched more than once a week were nearly five times as likely to get cervical cancer as women who douched less often or not at all. Doctors speculate that the normal vaginal bacteria somehow protect the vaginal area and that routine douching may invite organisms that trigger cancer.

Sources: **Amanda Clark, M.D.**, Assistant Professor of Obstetrics and Gynecology, Oregon Health Sciences University, Portland, Oregon. **Sadja Greenwood, M.D.**, Assistant Clinical Professor, Department of Obstetrics, Gynecology, and Reproductive Services, University of California at San Francisco, San Francisco, California. **Anne Simons, M.D.**, Coauthor, *Before You Call the Doctor*; Family Practitioner, San Francisco Department of Public Health; Family Practitioner and Assistant Clinical Professor, Family and Community Medicine, University of California San Francisco Medical Center, San Francisco, California. **Felicia Stewart, M.D.**, Coauthor, *My Body, My Health* and *Understanding Your Body*; Gynecologist, Sacramento, California. **Susan Woodruff, B.S.N.**, Childbirth and Parenting Education Coordinator, Tuality Community Hospital, Hillsboro, Oregon.

•Health Information Resources

AIDS Hotline

American Social Health Association
P.O. Box 13827
Research Triangle Park, NC 27709
800-342-2437
800-243-7889 hearing impaired
800-344-7432 Spanish

Call for information about transmission and prevention of AIDS, pamphlets and fact sheets, and referrals to testing sites and counseling.

American College of Obstetricians and Gynecologists

Attn: Resource Center
409 12th Street, S.W.
Washington, D.C. 20024-2188
Send business-size self-addressed stamped envelope for order form listing pamphlets concerned with women's health.

American Institute for Preventive Medicine

30445 Northwestern Highway, Suite 350
Farmington Hills, MI 48334
313-539-1800
Call for self-care and wise-consumer booklets and for women's workbook, *Healthy Life for Women.* Catalog of publications available.

American Heart Association

7272 Greenville Avenue
Dallas, TX 75231-4596
800-AHA-USA1 (800-242-8721)

Call for connection to your local affiliate of the American Heart Association; to inquire about dozens of pamphlets on heart disease, diet, exercise, smoking (some of which are specific to women); and for information on educational programs in the community and at the work site.

American Diabetes Association

1660 Duke Street
Alexandria, VA 22314
703-549-1500

Information available in printed form and by telephone, including physician referrals. Newsletter and monthly magazine printed for members. Also contact your local American Diabetes Association office (listed in the white pages of your telephone directory).

American Cancer Society

1599 Clifton Road N.E.
Atlanta, GA 30329
800-227-2345

Call for referrals to local American Cancer Society offices and for information on obtaining some of the hundreds of pamphlets available on cancer and other health topics, including nutrition, mammography, breast cancer, and smoking.

Arthritis Foundation Information Line

P.O. Box 19000
Atlanta, GA 30326
800-283-7800

Call for brochures as well as information about local chapters available by phone (contact local chapter for physician referrals). Write for access to additional resources.

Asthma and Allergy Foundation

1125 15th Street, N.W., Suite 502
Washington, D.C. 20005
800-7ASTHMA (800-727-8462)

Call for a general information packet and list of publications.

Endometriosis Association

8585 North 76th Place
Milwaukee, WI 53223
800-992-3636

Call for free introductory material and a catalog listing additional information including books, video tapes, and a newsletter.

National Headache Foundation

5252 North Western Avenue
Chicago, IL 60625
800-843-2256

Send self-addressed stamped envelope with 52 cents postage for physician member list. Information on headaches—including hormonally triggered migraines—is available, along with a quarterly newsletter for members.

National Herpes Hotline

American Social Health Association
P.O. Box 13827
Resource Triangle Park, NC 27709
(919) 361-8488

Call for information, counseling, and referral to one of 88 local agencies. A wide range of publications is available, including a quarterly journal on herpes.

National Osteoporosis Foundation

2100 M Street, N.W., Suite 602-B
Washington, D.C. 20037
800-223-9994

Call for free copy of 22-page booklet, *Stand Up to Osteoporosis,* and a questionnaire about risk factors. Write for other information.

PMS Access

P.O. Box 9326
Madison, WI 53715
800-222-4PMS

Call for packet on premenstrual syndrome that includes information on diet and exercise. Additional information available on infertility, menopause, and endometriosis as well as a bimonthly newsletter. Pharmacists available to answer specific questions.

Sexually Transmitted Diseases Hotline

American Social Health Association
P.O. Box 13827
Research Triangle Park, NC 27709
800-227-8922

Call for printed material (some in Spanish, some specific to women), a catalog, and referrals to clinics nationwide.

●INDEX

Cold sores, 57, 68, 83-84, 324
  prevention, 84
  recurrences, 83
Cold treatment, 21, 29, 50, 61,
  109, 217, 244, 264, 265, 271,
  291, 327, 331, 352
Colitis, mucous, 236
Colitis, ulcerative, 121, 122,
  336
Colloidal oatmeal bath
  treatment, 110, 217
Computed tomographic (CT)
  scan, 188
Condom dermatitis, 108, 111
Condoms, 322, 328, 367, 383.
  See also contraception.
Conjunctivitis, 148
Constipation, 85-89, 291, 300,
  338
  and bowel habits, 85
  treatment, 85-89
Contraception, 254, 255, 262,
  275, 328
Contraceptives
  and acne, 7
  and bladder infection, 40
  and depression, 103, 105
  and fluid retention, 170
  oral, 190, 211, 317, 381, 385
Corn pads, 92
Corns, 90-93, 117, 173, 175, 365
  hard, 90
  salicylic acid as treatment, 93
  soft, 90
Corticosteroids, nasal, 13, 17
Cortisone, 217, 307
Cranberry juice, 39
Crohn's disease, 121
Croup, 164
Cryosurgery, 324
CTS. *See* carpal tunnel
  syndrome.
Curvature of the spine, 28
Cystitis. *See* bladder infection.

D
Dairy products, 281, 373
  and cholesterol, 203, 204, 207
  and diarrhea, 125, 126
  and flatulence, 161
  and lactose intolerance, 247-
  249, 337
Dandruff, 94-96, 276, 304
Dawn-simulator therapy, 311-
  312
Dead Sea salts, 309
Decongestants
  for colds, 80
  and constipation, 86
  for ear discomfort, 135, 136,
  140
  for eye redness, 149
  for postnasal drip, 286
  for sinus infection, 188
  and sore throat, 334
Dehydration
  causing uterine contractions,
  262
  and colds, 78
  and diabetes, 118
  and diarrhea, 123, 154, 268
  and fever, 154
  and incontinence, 222
  from morning sickness, 289
  and muscle cramps, 267
  and postnasal drip, 286
  from vomiting, 268
Delhi belly. *See* traveler's
  diarrhea.
Denture discomfort, 97-99, 119,
  180
Deodorants, 45-46
Depilatories, 143-144
Depression, 100-106, 300, 343
  biochemical, 102
  bipolar disorder, 102
  and CFS, 70
  and hormones, 102, 255, 257
  and insomnia, 230
  manic, 102

Depression *(continued)*
  and post-pregnancy, 102
  postpartum, 102, 103
  premenstrual, 300
  reactive, 101
  SAD, 101-102, 106, 310-312
  and sexual difficulties, 320
Dermabrasion, 376, 379
Dermatitis, 107-113
  allergic contact, 107, 111
  atopic, 108, 112
  condom, 108, 111
  irritant contact, 107, 111-112
  localized neurodermatitis, 109
  nummular, 109
  seborrheic, 109
  stasis, 109
  treatment, 109-110
Deviated septum, 284
Diabetes, 114-120, 262
  and bad breath, 34
  and bladder discomfort, 38
  and CTS, 60
  and decongestants, 80
  and diabetic retinopathy, 119
  diarrhea as symptom, 121
  and flu, 167
  foot care in, 117
  and foot problems, 90, 93, 228
  gestational, 115, 120
  and gingivitis, 177
  high risk groups, 120
  and obesity, 115, 120
  and oral hygiene, 119
  and pregnancy, 119
  treatment, 115-120
  Type I, 114, 115
  Type II, 114, 115, 120
  and yeast infection, 380, 384
Diaper rash, 380
Diarrhea, 121-126, 300, 338,
  359
  and dehydration, 121
  in the elderly, 121
  and food poisoning, 121